Becoming a reflective practitioner

Becoming a reflective practitioner

Third edition

Christopher Johns

With contributions by Simon Lee, Susan Brooks, Sally Burnie, Jill Jarvis, Ruth Morgan and others

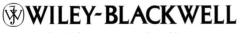

WILEY-BLACKWELL

A John Wiley & Sons, Ltd., Publication

This edition first published 2009
© 2009 by Christopher Johns

Blackwell Publishing was acquired by John Wiley & Sons in February 2007. Blackwell's publishing programme has been merged with Wiley's global Scientific, Technical, and Medical business to form Wiley-Blackwell.

Registered office
John Wiley & Sons Ltd, The Atrium, Southern Gate, Chichester, West Sussex, PO19 8SQ, United Kingdom

Editorial offices
9600 Garsington Road, Oxford, OX4 2DQ, United Kingdom
2121 State Avenue, Ames, Iowa 50014-8300, USA

For details of our global editorial offices, for customer services and for information about how to apply for permission to reuse the copyright material in this book please see our website at www.wiley.com/wiley-blackwell.

The right of the author to be identified as the author of this work has been asserted in accordance with the Copyright, Designs and Patents Act 1988.

Library of Congress Cataloging-in-Publication Data

Johns, Christopher.
Becoming a reflective practitioner/Christopher Johns; with contributions by Simon Lee . . . [et al.]. –
3rd ed.
    p. ; cm.
    Includes bibliographical references and index.
    ISBN 978-1-4051-8567-7 (pbk. : alk. paper) 1. Nursing – Philosophy. 2. Holistic
nursing. I. Title.
    [DNLM: 1. Philosophy, Nursing. 2. Models, Nursing. 3. Thinking. WY 86 J65b 2009]
    RT84.5.J636 2009
    610.73–dc22
                                                                                2008053128

A catalogue record for this book is available from the British Library.

Set in 10 on 12 pt Sabon by SNP Best-set Typesetter Ltd., Hong Kong
Printed in Singapore

1 2009

Excerpts of text have been reproduced from Blackwolf and Gina Jones, *Listen to the Drum* (1995) and *Earth Dance Drum* (1996), in chapters 1, 3, 6, 9 and 16 of this book, with kind permission of Blackwolf and Gina Jones and Hazelden Publishing.

Contents

Foreword

And just what are we to make of becoming a reflective practitioner? Are we to learn? Are we to change? Are we to work toward transformation of self and other?

This work by Christopher Johns brings us face to face with the human elements and human dilemmas, the deep level of humanity that clinicians encounter daily, moment by moment, the blessings and challenges of living, suffering, changing, evolving, dying, leading us to nothing less than a rebirthing of self and work. And how are we to live this practice of reflection? How are we to be? To become? To evolve? To alter? To repattern? To rethink?

We do so by stepping into practice moments; we do so by honouring our own inner humanness; we do so by stopping, being present, listening to stories, life narratives, filled with inner meanings, myths, metaphors and by reflecting on one's own presence of being and becoming in the moment. It is through the reflective moment that we both seek and gain insights, dynamics of wisdom and depth of meanings revealed whole to us but only when we stop, pause and are present to such profound human mystery and wisdom that is already contained on the margin, in the shadows, in the distant haze of our own existence.

It is here, when we are still and witness to our own openness, that we connect with self and other in shared moments of human being and becoming. A multifaceted jewel, the diamond net of refracted light contained within each human moment of human encounter . . . a clue, a coloured hue, contributing to a human canvas, a human studio of caring moments, each one a possibility for hope, for movement through pain, suffering, loss, challenge, while being present to the joy; the aesthetic, the paradox, the dilemma, the eternal, uncovered from the journey toward wholeness. In the nurse's presence, in listening to and becoming part of another's story, life drama, myth for meaning and hope, we are able to promote health or become true instruments of timeless healing that transcend self, other and system alike.

Reflective stories in this text offer models of insight; they reveal the hidden subtext of paradox, inner drama, unaddressed questions, unknowns, that lead to ethical grids and maps on the reflective journey – a reflective journey, into context, discovery, relationships, non-objectivist, non-formulaic notions and moods that guide not by convention and rationalistic principles but rather by intentional consciousness, by awakening. Awakening to presence, relationships, being and becoming part of the connections, patterns and processes that mirror human-to-human caring and healing. This reflective subtext of nursing invites us into and through informed, reflective, appropriate skilled action of human connectivity, creativity and intuition. Through internal and external existential dialogue and story and guidance we journey into the spiritual, the aesthetic, the ethical, the arts, that touch and celebrate the non-quantifiable, that once again reunite the profession and the practitioner alike, with the compassion and passion of nursing's life and work.

It is here through the Johns Reflective Practice Model and its evolving process for self-reflection and guidance that we discover, once again, that the 'personal becomes the professional'. It is here that we learn to grow in caring by becoming instruments of healing, first by learning about our own inner healing and health processes and needs that flow from self to other. These lessons transcend yet inform each caring moment, consciously or unconsciously. It is through reflective practice that nurses and nursing learn about nursing as never known before. It is here, in honouring the whole, in gleaning and seeking meaning from parts and particles of light in the institutional and often individual darkness, that we find new hope for transforming nursing and nurses alike.

Finally, it is through reflective practice, as continually explored and explicated by Johns and colleagues, that we are offered a method, a mode, a mood, a model of being and becoming that allows us to face and live through, if not be blessed by, our own woundedness. This model is a guide that informs and invites us, in uniquely individual ways, to engage in authentic caring and become part of a process of healing and wholeness that is required for a new era in human history and futuristic nursing.

In the past, nurses and nursing have tried to escape the inner learning and healing that is required for the practice journey; we have done this by succumbing to medical science, medical-nursing tasks, industrial-system demands. It has turned out that these routes to nursing have been a detour from our human caring practices and commitment to processes of wholeness and healing that have motivated, inspired and informed individuals and communities across time.

It is through the breakdowns of conventional practices, combined with breakthroughs of reflective practice, which can now be integrated with the most up-to-date knowledge and skills, philosophies and theories, that we enter a new world of professional care practices that embrace, encompass and more fully actualise the paradigm of hope spread before and behind nursing in its history and traditions. It is only by stopping, pausing and reconsidering our encounters and relationships with self and other that we mature as a distinct caring, healing and health profession.

However, it is the reflective practice processes and approaches that may be the most threatening, yet at the same time offer the greatest hope for growth, maturity and personal and professional maturity. If nursing turns its back on reflection, it is turning its back on its woundedness and core humanity, which is the ground of being and becoming. In not pausing to consider reflection, we remain technical assistants, trying to defend ourselves from our own wounds and suffering, forever stranded on the shoreline as humanity and health care itself sets out to pursue new horizons of possibilities contained within the depths of our shared humanity and the oceanic changes possible for human evolution and growth.

Will we choose reflection and human transformation as a path to the future or succumb to robotic mutation? Which route will we take? Reflect upon it and choose but do so with passion and purpose. As we individually and collectively ponder the future, this text offers a holistic lesson that will serve us well into the next millennium.

Jean Watson

Preface

Welcome to the third edition of this book. The major aim of the book remains the same as previous editions: to pose and respond to the question 'What does it mean to be a reflective practitioner?'.

In the second edition I asserted that being a reflective practitioner is a way of being in practice rather than something I do – for example, something I write in a journal on an educational course or something I do in clinical supervision – that reflection is something lived. This is of fundamental significance. Reflective practice is fundamental to professional practice, because I assume that all professionals are concerned with knowing and realising desirable and effective practice, yet work in conditions where for one reason or another such realisation is often difficult.

Whilst the third edition has been entirely revised, some narrative from the second edition remains. However, I give significantly greater emphasis to the process of reflective writing rather than the realisation of desirable practice.

The book is organised as 19 chapters divided into three parts.

Part 1

In Chapter 1, I set out some ideas of reflection. My perceptions of reflective practice have been informed by various influences from cognitive approaches, characterised by the construction of models and the application of technique, to more esoteric 'wisdom' approaches. The cognitive approaches reflect Western roots in rationality whereas the more esoteric approaches reflect Eastern traditions rooted in mysticism and spirituality. It is perhaps not surprising that Western influences have dominated my thinking simply because it has been my own way of thinking and the expectations of students and reviewers alike. Yet, as I study and understand the more esoteric influences, notably Native American lore and Buddhism, I find myself dwelling in the mystery of experience and increasingly uncomfortable with the dominance of the rational approach to reflective practice. My esoteric turn has been influenced by two events. The first was reading Blackwolf and Jones' book *Earth dance drum* (1996) culminating in their participation at the 5th International Reflective Practice conference in Cambridge in 1999. The second event was embracing Buddhism as a more satisfactory and enlightening way to live my life and give greater purpose to my practice as a palliative care nurse and complementary therapist. A key message to esoteric approaches to life is harmony and balance. As such, the purpose of this chapter is to begin to move reflective thinking into a greater balance.

In Chapter 2 I set out a reflective model for clinical practice based on the Burford NDU model: caring in practice that I developed at Burford Hospital between 1989 and 1991. At the core of a reflective model is a *valid* vision for practice that gives meaning and direction to practice and poses the question 'If we hold these values, how can we realise them as a lived reality?'. I assume that reflective practice flourishes in reflective environments. In response I set about creating reflective systems and organisational culture to support reflective practice in action.

In Chapter 3 I set out the process of learning through reflection as movement through six dialogical movements. This is a significant appreciation of reflective theory. The first dialogical movement is dialogue with self to write a rich description of experience. The second dialogical movement is to stand back from the descriptive text and move into reflective mode with the intention of gaining insights, using a model for structured reflection.

In Chapter 4 I explore the third and fourth dialogical movements to check out, deepen and affirm tentative insights through dialogue with literature and with peers and guides within guided reflection. In doing so, I explore the nature of guidance.

In Chapter 5 I explore the fifth and sixth dialogical movements. The fifth movement is weaving the coherent and reflexive narrative: reflection is presented as narrative that adequately portrays the journey of self-inquiry and transformation towards the practitioner realising desirable practice. I explore imagery, art and poetry in shaping the narrative, and consider the nature of coherence for narrative writing, drawing on the work of Ben Okri and the increasing influence of autoethnography.

In Chapters 6 and 7 I set out the being available template as a way to know and monitor the development of desirable practice based on holistic values. This work has been considerably condensed from the second edition, reflecting the shift in emphasis toward the process of reflection. However, this work remains essential, revealing the way reflection enables the practitioner to develop clinical practice around the therapeutic relationship with the patient and family. At the core of knowing the person is 'empathic inquiry', the ability to connect with the experience of the person. Compassion is healing energy yet needs to be nurtured and focused. I explore the 'aesthetic response', the ability to make effective clinical judgements, and on this basis to respond with appropriate, effective and ethical action, and reflect on its impact. I reflect on the significance of knowing and managing self within relationship. This is the flipside of compassion and empathy – to tune into and flow with the person in ways that ensure that our own 'stuff' does not get in the way.

In Chapter 7, I explore the significance of creating and sustaining an environment in which it is possible for the practitioner to be available and which places the nurse–patient relationship into its organisational context. I also explain my understanding of those factors that may constrain the practitioner's ability to be available: issues of tradition, authority and embodiment. This chapter also deals with issues such as managing change, assertiveness, managing conflict, stress and support.

In Chapter 8 I explore the therapeutic value of patient reflection through enabling and listening to their stories.

Part 2

I offer four narratives written by students whilst on academic post-registration degree programmes. These are all examples of realising desirable practice although they do not explicitly refer to the being available template to achieve this.

These narratives are examples of reflective writing through the dialogical movements, illuminating different styles yet with a common purpose.

In Chapter 9 Jill Jarvis reflects on her palliative care with one patient through touch and paying attention to the care environment. In Chapter 10 Simon Lee reflects on the personal impact of being with a patient and family as the patient approaches death. In Chapter 11, Jim takes a post-punk perspective on challenging power issues in his practice in advocating for his patient within a psychiatric setting. In Chapter 12, Clare, similarly working in a psychiatric setting, reflects on her relationships with patients. These narratives are evocative and powerful.

Part 3

Part 3 offers chapters concerned with creating the reflective environment both within clinical practice and within education. In Chapter 13, I explore reflective communication, both verbal and written. The core value of communication is that it must be both practical and meaningful. The nursing process is critiqued and exposed as an absurd model for the reflective practitioner. Instead I assert the movement towards narrative forms.

In Chapter 14 I explore a reflective approach to ensuring quality and responding to the clinical governance agenda through the reflective techniques of clinical audit and standards of care in order to get valid feedback that our visions of practice are indeed realised as a lived reality. I use the first of two narratives written by Lazell to illuminate the significance of quality. I assert that quality must be the responsibility of each practitioner intrinsic to everyday practice rather than something abstract and imposed. As before, I use Lazell's narrative to emphasise the quality of her reflective writing as much as the topic of quality.

Chapter 15 is an exposition of transformational clinical leadership through examples of students on the Masters of Clinical Leadership programme at the University of Bedfordshire. Transformational leadership is reflective leadership dedicated to establishing the learning organisation, yet can transformational leadership shift the prevailing transactional culture of healthcare or is this just another example of rhetoric? I use narratives by Susan Brooks and Sally Burnie as context.

In Chapter 16 I develop the ideas of the learning organisation and clinical supervision as reflective milieu, extending ideas introduced in the previous two chapters using my own example of working with Trudy, a district nurse, in clinical supervision with me over six sessions.

In Chapter 17, using a second narrative by Lazell, I explore reflection as chaos theory. Lazell's narratives are examples of Masters level reflective writing.

In Chapter 18 I pull together narrative strands into considering the nature of the reflective curriculum. This is creative work I am currently pursuing, more a work in progress being developed through various projects worldwide. I argue that reflection must be the core of the curriculum throughout the programmed duration in dialogue with clinical practice and informed by specialist knowledge modules as appropriate.

In Chapter 19 I take a performance turn, to consider the development of performance to present narrative, shifting from the representation of self through narrative. This has led me to work with drama and dance teachers in my doctoral work with practitioners using guided reflection/narrative as a process of self-inquiry and transformation. This work is again creative and experimental and will be the focus of a revised edition of *Guided reflection: advancing practice*. I give two examples of performance: the first is Ruth Morgan's performance of 'Musical Chairs' and the second is 'RAW'.

I have endeavoured to write the book in a reflective style, in contrast with a more traditional text, through the extensive use of stories taken from my reflective journal or those shared with me in guided reflection or clinical supervision. As readers acquainted with the second edition will notice, some of the narratives remain although my reflections on them have been developed. In addition, the reader will find many new narratives as examples of reflective writing and guided reflection. The beauty of story is the way it can illuminate the contextual meaning of complex theory in ways the reader can sense in relation to their own experiences. Story draws out the subtlety and nuances of caring from its apparent mundaneness and its significance within healthcare. As the reader will note, the stories are emotional, reflecting the intimacy, anguish and beauty of the human caring encounter. In this respect, story is a way of honouring caring work.

Writing in a more traditional style would be a contradiction to what I view as the essential nature of reflective practice. It would only reinforce the idea that reflective practice is a technology with specific techniques to apply. Perhaps as novices, we need techniques to access the artistry of reflective practice yet I urge the reader to keep this point in perspective because, as you develop expertise, the techniques can become a burden, constraining rather than liberating the self.

The reflective practitioner has an open and curious mind in order to be receptive to what the text has to say. As a consequence I have not always drawn out the significance of the stories. Where I have, these are only my view. I do not intend to impose these. Indeed, as a 'reflective reader', you will relate to the stories in terms of your own experiences and make your own interpretations. This is the value of 'reflective texts'; it is possible to relate to the stories because they are deeply subjective and contextual.

Over time, as I engage with Buddhism, I find myself naturally assimilating ideas from Buddhism into my everyday practice. In appreciating the Buddhist influence, I am not suggesting that the reflective practitioner need be a Buddhist, but simply that some of these ideas may offer the practitioner a guide to journey through their experiences to ease their suffering as manifest within their everyday experiences. In doing so, they become ever more able to realise desirable practice, i.e. to ease the suffering of others. So, as a Buddhist, I work daily on nurturing my compassionate self through meditative and reflective practice.

Note: for convenience, throughout the book I refer to nurses/therapists as 'she' and 'her'.

Christopher Johns

Acknowledgements

Thanks to Moira Vass, who requested that I publish her account of living with motor neurone disease in Chapter 8 that offers valuable insight into the therapeutic benefits of journalling.

Thanks to Simon Lee, Susan Brooks, Sally Burnie, Jill Jarvis and Ruth Morgan for contributing their stories. Thanks to Clare, Jim and Lazell (pseudonyms) for also giving permission to share their stories.

My thanks to Beth Knight and Rachel Coombs at Wiley-Blackwell.

Special thanks to Blackwolf and Gina Jones and Hazelden Publishing for the extensive quotes from *Earth dance drum* (1996) and *Listen to the drum* (1995). Their work continues to teach and inspire me. Thanks also to Ben Okri for his wisdom, and Phoenix Publishing. Thanks to Vintage Books for permission to use Jeannette Winterson's words from *The powerbook* and to Penguin for the use of AA Milne's words from *Winnie-the-Pooh*. Thanks also to Quartet Books for permission to use Ann Dickson's 'rights of women' and Sigridur Halldorsdottir for allowing me to use her 'modes of being'.

Indeed, thank you for all the authors' words throughout the book that have inspired and taught me.

Part 1
Basic structures

Chapter 1
Exploring reflection

Reflection is learning through our everyday experiences towards realising one's vision of desirable practice as a lived reality. It is a critical and reflexive process of self-inquiry and transformation of being and becoming the practitioner you desire to be. As such, reflection is always purposeful, moving towards a more reflective, effective and satisfactory life. Reflection is a special quality of being. It is necessary to learn its right posture to tap into its mystery to gain most benefit from its learning potential. The idea of developing the right posture is compelling. Shunryu Suzuki (1999:28), writing from a Zen Buddhist perspective on meditation, says:

> So try always to keep the right posture, not only when you practice zazen, but in all your activities. Take the right posture when you are driving your car, and when you are reading. If you read in a slumped position, you cannot stay awake long. Try. You will discover how important it is to keep the right posture. This is the true teaching. The teaching which is written on paper is not the true teaching. Written teaching is a kind of food for your brain. Of course, it is necessary to take some food for your brain, but it is more important to be by yourself by practicing the right way of life.

The true teaching of reflection, like *zazen* (meditation), is through doing it and reflecting on doing it with guides who, like *zazen* masters, point you in the right direction. You cannot easily learn reflection from books but yet you can take brain food to inform the journey. Books give you ideas about reflection, just as they give you ideas about being a nurse or any other practice discipline.

Opening the *Compact Oxford English Dictionary* (2005:86) I read:

Reflect:
- throw back heat, light, sound without absorbing it
- (of a mirror or shiny surface) show an image of
- represent in a realistic or appropriate way
- bring about a good or bad impression of someone or something (on)
- think deeply or carefully about.

Interpreting this definition, reflection might be described as a mirror to see images or impressions of self in context of the particular situation in a careful and realistic way. The image of a mirror is helpful for viewing and keeping and adjusting the right posture moment by moment, bending to the shifting moment.

A reflective practitioner is someone who lives reflection as a way of being. And yet, in my experience, when people refer to reflection they are generally referring to reflection-on-experience. Indeed, most theories of reflection are based on this idea – looking back at an experience or some event that has taken place. The idea of an *experience* is difficult to grasp – where does one experience begin and another end? Is experience not the endless flow of life? Is anticipating a forthcoming event an experience in itself? I consider an experience as thinking, feeling or doing something. Each intake of breath is an experience. Each thought is an experience.

Reflection is awareness of self within the moment, having a clear mind so as to be open to possibility of that moment. It is the wisdom that helps us see things clearly. Only when we can see things clearly, for what they really are, are we able to make the best decisions mindful of the potential consequences, what Aristotle described as phronesis. We come to see and appreciate the barriers that limit possibility. Hence our reflections are stories of resistance and possibility; chipping away resistance and opening up possibility, confronting and shifting these barriers to become who we desire to be as nurses, doctors and therapists is a life-long learning quest.

Our biggest barriers are ourselves, notably those fears that limit our potential. Rosenberg (1998:145) says:

> We may have been seeing our fear, for instance, as a big boulder that stands in our way, but now we can see that it is more like a cloud.

Rosenberg's words help us to see that reflection is often shifting things subtly, quietly almost, rather than instantly or dramatically.

The significance of reflective practices for professional life

Schön's (1983, 1987) critique of an epistemology of professional practice is vital to appreciate. He opens Chapter 1 of his book *Educating the reflective practitioner* with these words:

> In the varied topography of professional practice, there is the high, hard ground overlooking the swamp. On the high ground, manageable problems lend themselves to solution through the application of research-based theory and technique. In the swampy lowland, messy, confusing problems defy technical solution. The irony of this situation is that the problems of the high ground tend to be relatively unimportant to individuals or society at large, however great their technical interest may be, while in the swamp lie the problems of greatest human concern.
>
> The practitioner must choose. Shall he remain on the high ground where he can solve relatively unimportant problems according to prevailing standards or rigor, or shall he descend into the swamp of important problems and non-rigorous inquiry? (1987:1)

Schön's notion of the hard high ground and the swampy lowlands reflects two types of knowing. The metaphor of *swampy lowlands* draws attention to the type of knowing that practitioners need in order to respond to the problems of everyday practice that defy technical solution, where the practitioner faces issues of distress and conflict within the unique human–human encounter on a daily basis. This resonates strongly with a profession like nursing where each clinical moment is a unique human–human encounter grounded in suffering. There are no easy answers to the life problems that face patients and nurses who strive to care. When we think we know the solutions to complex situations, we endeavour to apply such knowledge, yet when we seek to impose control of events through applying such knowledge, we somehow miss the point. No two things are the same, everything is unique within the human–human encounter. Practice is a mystery drama unfolding. We may have had similar experiences but not this one. We draw parallels but it is not the same. We have to be mindful, to read the particular signs or we may get it wrong. These signs are often subtle, requiring perception, imagination and intuition. Subtle differences between this experience and previous experiences demand subtle shifts of response that cannot be known outside the unfolding moment. Hence the reflective practitioner is mindful of subtle shifts and responds appropriately. No mean feat. There are no prescriptive solutions.

However, I must take issue with the implication that the practitioner must choose which land to inhabit. Both are essential for the effective practitioner to comfortably dwell within because of the nature of everyday practice. The practitioner must dwell in the swampy lowlands and yet be comfortable with visiting the high hard ground in order to appropriately assimilate relevant theory and research into practice.

Schön turned on its head the established epistemological hierarchy of professional practice, suggesting that swampy lowland knowing is more significant than technical rationality because it is the knowledge practitioners need to practise. Such knowing is subjective and contextual, yet is often denigrated as a lesser form of knowing, even dismissed as 'anecdote' by those who inhabit the hard high ground of technical rationality. People got locked into a paradigmatic view of knowledge and become intolerant of other claims because such claims fail the technical rationality rules for what counts as truth.

Researchers have endeavoured to understand why research is not used by practitioners in practice (Armitage 1990, Hunt 1981). These authors suggest that blame lies with the practitioners because of their failure to access and apply research. However, as Schön (1987) argues, little research has been done to address the real problems of everyday practice and research always needs to be interpreted by the practitioner for its significance to inform the specific situation. The decontextualised nature of most research, with its claims for generalisability, makes this problematic. Any claim for generalisability must be treated with extreme caution to inform unique human–human encounters. Such encounters are essentially unpredictable. The insensitive application of technical rationality is likely to lead to stereotyping – fitting the patient to the theory rather than using the theory to inform the situation. Schön exposes the illusion that research can simply be applied.

Technical rationality (or evidence-based practice) has been claimed as necessary for nursing's disciplinary knowledge base because it can be observed and verified (Kikuchi 1992). Historically, professions such as nursing have accepted the superiority of technical rationality over tacit or intuitive knowing (Schön 1983, 1987). Visinstainer (1986) notes that:

> Even when nurses govern their own practice, they succumb to the belief that the 'soft stuff' such as feelings and beliefs and support, are not quite as substantive as the hard data from laboratory reports and sophisticated monitoring. (p37)

The consequence of this position in nursing has been the repression of other forms of knowing that has perpetuated the oppression of nurses and of their clinical nursing knowledge (Street 1992). Since the Briggs Report (DHSS 1972) emphasised that nursing should be a research-based profession, nursing has endeavoured to respond to this challenge. However, the general understanding of what 'research-based' means has followed an empirical pathway reflecting a dominant agenda to explain and predict phenomena. This agenda has been pursued by nurse academics seeking recognition that

Box 1.1   The pathway from novice to expert

Novice	→	Expert
Linear thinking and acting	**→**	**Intuitive**
View parts in isolation from whole	→	**Holistic or gestalt vision**
Reliance on external authorities	→	Reliance on internal authority
See self as separate from situation	→	See self as integral to the situation
Application of knowledge	→	Wisdom

nursing is a valid science within university settings. Whilst such knowledge has an important role in informing practice, it certainly cannot predict and control, at least not without reducing patients and nurses to the status of objects to be manipulated like pawns in a chess game.

Dreyfus and Dreyfus (1986) note that for the expert practitioner, clinical judgement is largely intuitive, learnt through holistic pattern appreciation and past experiences. For this reason, models and theories of reflection have limited value. They may offer the novice reflective practitioner a way to access the breadth and depth of reflection, yet it is folly to think that they can 'know' reflection in this way. These models threaten to impose an understanding of reflection that skims the surface of its potential depth and subtlety. At some point the practitioner must break free from the shackles of models in order to swim within the vast ocean of life.

Benner (1984) and Benner *et al* (1996) draw heavily on Dreyfus and Dreyfus's model of skill acquisition (1986), in determining the pathway from novice to expert (Box 1.1).

In contrast to novices, experts intuit and respond appropriately to a situation as a whole without any obvious linear or reductionist thinking. The novice simply does not have this tacit knowledge accumulated from past experience. Reflection as a learning process enables practitioners to bring to consciousness, scrutinise and develop their intuitive processes and, *ipso facto*, to develop their tacit knowing. As Holly (1989) notes:

> It [keeping a reflective journal] makes possible new ways of theorizing, reflecting on and coming to know one's self. Capturing certain words while the action is fresh, the author is often provoked to question why… writing taps tacit knowledge; it brings into awareness that which we sense but could not explain. (pp71-5)

This is subliminal learning, revealed in light of reflection. Learning through reflection also takes place on a more deliberative level. Indeed, through reflection, practitioners become more mindful and increasingly sensitive to their intuitive responses.

Cioffi (1997) draws on the work of Tversky and Kahneman (1974) to suggest that judgements made in uncertain conditions are most commonly heuristic in nature. Such processes are servants to intuition. The heuristics intend to improve the probability of getting intuition right by linking the current situation to past experience, being able to see the salient points within any situation, and having a baseline position to judge against. Without doubt, the majority of decisions practitioners make are intuitive. King and Appleton (1997) and Cioffi (1997) endorse the significance of intuition within decision making and action following their reviews of the literature and rhetoric on intuition; they note that reflection accesses, values and develops intuitive processes. The measured intuitive response is wisdom.

As significant as this exposition on expertise is, it only scratches the surface of practice. The real value of reflective practice is its emancipatory potential as reflected in

Jack Mezirow's (1981) idea of *perspective transformation* and Paulo Freire's (1972:15) idea of *conscientization* that refers to 'learning to perceive social, political and economic contradictions [with being fully human] and to take action against the oppressive elements of reality'.

> To surmount the situation of oppression, men must first critically recognise its causes, so that through transforming action they can create a new situation – one which makes possible the pursuit of a fuller humanity. (Freire 1972:24)

This notion resonates with nursing's quest in society – what does nursing exist to do? What does it mean to be a nurse? These questions are challenges that go to the heart of reflective practice. The answers to these questions are the background for reflective practice. I will simply say that nursing's quest must be to enable patients to become more fully human. In doing so, nurses must confront and shift their own oppression as a subordinate workforce that diminishes their own humanness and which limits their potential to enable others to become fully human. Without freedom to practise, talk of expertise is fool's gold. Expertise *is* freedom.

Knowing reflection

Picking up Suzuki's idea of *brain food*, there is much brain food to inform reflective practice. When I teach reflection, I might draw the students' attention to theories of reflection as espoused by Boud *et al* (1985), Boyd and Fales (1983), Gibbs (1988), Mezirow (1981) and Schön (1987) with a view to using these theories within their own reflective practice. These theorists all espouse a rational approach to reflection. Definitions of reflection are characterised as learning through experience toward gaining new insights or changed perceptions of self and practice. Indeed, my own work has contributed to this body of knowledge (Johns 2004a).

Boyd and Fales (1983:101) describe reflection as:

> the process of creating and clarifying the meaning of experience [present and past] in terms of self [self in relation to self and self in relation to the world]. The outcome of the process is changed conceptual perspective. The experience that is explored and examined to create meaning focuses around or embodies a concern of central importance to the self.

They identify six stages for reflection:

- a sense of inner discomfort
- identification or clarification of concern
- openness to new information from external and internal sources
- resolution
- establishing continuity of self with past, present and future
- deciding whether to act on the outcome of the reflective process.

Boyd and Fales' last stage – deciding whether to act on the outcome of the reflective process – suggests that acting on perceptions and insights gained through reflection is deliberative. Perhaps on one level it is but on another, deeper intuitive level, changed perceptions of self must inevitably lead to changed action.

Mezirow (1981) viewed reflection as emancipatory action, strongly influenced by a critical social science perspective. Mezirow's work suggests the depth of reflection through a number of processes spanning from consciousness – the way we might think about something, to critical consciousness where we pay attention and scrutinise our thinking processes. This is a very significant idea, because it acknowledges that the way we think about something may itself be problematic. Mezirow describes the outcome of reflection as *perspective transformation*.

Powell (1989), in a small study with eight nurses on a post registered diploma course, utilised Mezirow's six levels of reflectivity to demonstrate that all students, with one exception, did not reflect at the level of critical consciousness. The one person who demonstrated some critical consciousness thinking was very experienced. The study doesn't outline the extent or quality of the guidance given. Although it is impossible to generalise from this study, it does suggest that critical consciousness thinking is not within the scope of people's normal thinking. Of course, this will differ with individuals, in that some people may be more naturally reflective than others.

Boud *et al* (1985) posit reflection as moving through three key stages:

- returning to experience
- attending to feelings
  - utilising positive feelings
  - removing obstructing feelings
- re-evaluating experience
  - re-examining experience in the light of the learner's intent
  - associating new knowledge with that which is already possessed
  - integrating this new knowledge into the learner's conceptual framework
  - appropriation of this knowledge into the learner's repertoire of behaviour.

Such theories enable practitioners to frame their reflective approach, often as a linear progression through a number of stages with the aim of developing insights into self and practice that can be applied to future experiences. My purpose is to draw the reader's attention to different approaches rather than to critique these approaches for their relevant merits. The reader will only find their way through the intentional experience of being reflective and reflecting on that experience.

The rational approach reflects a generally Western technological approach to learning that can be contrasted with more esoteric approaches reflected in ancient wisdom traditions (Johns 2005). As I study and understand the more esoteric influences, notably Native American lore and Buddhism, I delve more deeply into the nature of reflection, seeking to balance the dominant rational approach through appreciating its holistic or whole-brain thinking. These ideas are threaded through the book's text.

Whole-brain stuff

The right side of the brain is the centre for certain qualities of mind: creativity, imagination, perception, intuition, synthesis, wonder and spirit. It counterbalances the more dominant left side of the brain that is concerned with qualities of mind associated with analysis, reason, rationality and logic (Table 1.1).

Daniel Pink (2005) notes that 'the left hemisphere analyses the details; the right hemisphere synthesises the big picture' (22).

Table 1.1 Qualities of mind

Left brain	Right brain
Reason	Creativity
Logic	Imagination
Rationality	Perception
Analysis	Curiosity and wonder
	Intuition
	Spirit
	Synthesis

Virginia Woolf (1945) noted that the great mind is the androgynous mind where the faculties of left and right brain are integrated as a whole. Through rich story description and art, the practitioner *paints* a big canvas of the experience. As I explore in Chapter 3, this descriptive phase is the first dialogical movement, the data for reflection. The descriptive phase is opening and nurturing the right brain that has been severely neglected by left brain domination. Play has become a lost art (Pink 2005). The imagination has become trimmed (Paramananda 2001). Only then is the left brain invited to join the game to analyse the experience with the intention to seek meaning. In the weaving of the narrative, the right and left sides of the brain synthesise in common endeavour. I must emphasise the idea of reflection as spirit; that reflection is essentially life giving, paying attention to one's being, acknowledging that health care is at its core a spiritual practice. It is vital to appreciate this amidst the sterility of reason when the human factor is often lost amongst the facts. Wisdom traditions such as Buddhism and Native American are grounded in spirit.

A typology of reflective practices

Reflective practice can span from *doing* reflection towards reflection as a *way of being* within everyday practice (Fig. 1.1).

Schön (1983, 1987) distinguished reflection-*on-action* from reflection-*in-action* as a way of thinking about a situation whilst engaged within it, in order to reframe and solve some breakdown in the smooth running of experience, influenced by Heidegger's idea of breakdown. Heidegger (1962, cited in Plager 1994: 72-3) describes three interrelated modes of involvement or engagement with practical activity we have in day-to-day life:

- ready to hand – in this mode of engagement, equipment and practical activity function smoothly and transparently. The person is involved in an absorbed manner so that the activity is for the most part unnoticed
- unready to hand – in this mode, some sort of breakdown occurs in the smooth functioning of activity, becoming conspicuous to the user
- present to hand – in this mode, practical everyday activity ceases, and the person stands back and reflects on the situation.

Reflection-on-experience	Reflecting on a situation or experience after the event with the intention of gaining insights that may inform my future practice in positive ways.	*Doing reflection*
Reflection-in-action	Pausing within a particular situation or experience in order to make sense of and reframe the situation in order to proceed towards desired outcomes.	
The internal supervisor	Dialoguing with self whilst in conversation with another in order to make sense.	
Reflection-within-the-moment	Being aware of the way I am thinking, feeling, and responding within the unfolding moment whilst holding the intent to realise my vision. It involves dialoguing with self to ensure I am interpreting and responding congruently to whatever is unfolding and having mental acuity to change my ideas rather than being fixed to certain ideas.	
Mindfulness[1]	Seeing things for what they really are without distortion, whilst holding the intention of realising desirable practice.	*Reflection as a way of being*

[1] My appreciation of mindfulness has shifted from the second edition.

Figure 1.1 A typology of reflective practices.

The practitioner usually adjusts to minor interruptions within the smooth flow of experience without overtly thinking about it, because the body has embodied knowing. Sometimes, the practitioner is faced with situations that do not go smoothly. The practitioner must then pause and stand back to consider how best to proceed, to shift posture. Schön termed this *reflection-in-action*, a type of problem solving whereby the problem (or breakdown) is reframed in order to proceed. This requires a shift in thinking and contemplating new ways of responding.

It is easy to misunderstand reflection-in-action as merely thinking about something whilst doing it.

Schön (1987) drew on examples from music and architecture – situations of engagement with inanimate forms. His example of counselling is taken from the classroom, not from clinical practice. The classroom is a much easier place in which to freeze and reframe situations, in contrast with clinical practice which is involved within the unfolding human encounter.

The internal supervisor

Casement (1985), a psychoanalyst, offers a more satisfactory concept of reflection-in-action as the ability to dialogue with self whilst dialoguing with a client. He calls this dialogue with self the *internal supervisor*.

Practitioners pay attention to the way they are interpreting what the client is saying and weighing up how best to respond. Speaking as a psychoanalyst, this degree of attention and awareness is essential to successful psychoanalytical practice and yet, considering how nurses and doctors are with patients, the impact of self on the other is an important therapeutic moment and demands an awareness of self in relationship with the other.

Reflection-within-the-moment

The idea of paying attention to self within the unfolding moment defines *reflection-within-the–moment*; the exquisite paying attention to the way self is thinking, feeling and responding within the particular moment, whilst holding the intention to realise one's vision. Such self-awareness moves reflection away from techniques to apply to a way of being in practice. It is opening a mental space and developing mental acuity.

Reflection-within-the-moment is developed through constant reflecting-on-experience: the more reflective on experience I am, the more reflective I become within practice, especially around those issues on which I have reflected and gained insights. Although I cannot prove this point in conventional research terms, all practitioners I have guided demonstrate this ability. Try this for yourself. It is profound.

Without doubt, reflection-on-experience sensitises the practitioner to self within practice. Reflection-within-the-moment is an exquisite ability, perhaps the hallmark of expertise. It characterises the *reflective practitioner*.

Being mindful

Being mindful is *seeing things for what they really are without distortion, whilst holding the intention of realising desirable practice.* Understanding the nature of mindfulness is not easy simply because it is beyond conceptual appreciation. Hence words grasp at its essence. Goldstein (2002:89) notes:

> Mindfulness is the quality of mind that notices what is present without judgment, without interference. It is like a mirror that clearly reflects what comes before it.

The idea of being without judgement, without interference, is very significant, as if being mindful is a precursor for making good judgements based on clear understanding; a precursor for wisdom.

Goldstein writes from a Buddhist perspective. I too draw on the deep wellsprings of Buddhist psychology to explore the nature of mindfulness or *smrti*, which implies being aware moment to moment:

- of things and the world around us
- of self – body, feelings and thoughts
- of self in relationship with others
- of ultimate reality.

Ultimate reality can be viewed on two levels: the mundane level is concerned with holding and intending to realise a right vision of practice, however this might be expressed; the transcendental level is concerned with spiritual growth. Realising the mundane is inevitably a movement towards the transcendental. Being mindful, I know what I am doing and why I am doing it, and that what I am doing right now fits with my intention.

> Awareness sees everything as unique. Awareness brings an understanding that even the most common sight is never to be repeated and that to see something as it really is, we must be free from the habitual tendency to label and categorize. Only then can we truly recognize things for what they are. (Paramananda 2001:138-9)

Being mindful, I am vigilant against unskilful actions and negative mental events that are constantly trying to distract the mind, for example anger, arrogance, resentment, envy, greed and so on (Sangharakshita 1998). In Buddhism, this quality of mind is called *apramada* or non-heedlessness, the guard at the gate of the senses ever watchful for those negative emotions that would distract me.

Setting out my stall

I describe reflection as being mindful of self, either within or after experience, like a mirror in which the practitioner can view and focus self within the context of a particular experience, in order to confront, understand and move toward resolving contradiction between one's vision and actual practice. Through the conflict of contradiction, the commitment to realise one's vision, and understanding why things are as they are, the practitioner can gain new insight into self and be empowered to respond more congruently in future situations within a reflexive spiral towards developing practical wisdom and realising one's vision as praxis. The practitioner may require guidance to overcome resistance or to be empowered to act on understanding.

By reflexive, I mean 'looking back' to see the self emerging towards realising desirable practice through a series of experiences. Practical wisdom is the moral knowing I use in making clinical judgements mindful of their likely consequences. I use praxis to mean informed, intentional, moral action. In earlier descriptions of reflection I had realising one's vision as a lived reality. I use praxis in a similar way – that lived reality is always manifest in certain kinds of action in tune with one's intention (i.e. desired practice).

Bimadisiwin

An altogether more poetic description of reflection is offered by Bimadisiwin.

> Bimadisiwin is a conscious decision to become. It is time to think about what you want to be. The dance cannot be danced until you envision the dance, rehearse its movements and understand your part. It is demanding for every step needs an effort in becoming one with the vision. It takes discipline, hard work and time. Decide to be an active participant in your life journey. It is rewarding. Embrace the joy your vision brings you, it is yours to hold forever. It is freeing, for it frees the spirit. It releases you to become as you believe you must. (Blackwolf and Jones 1996:47)

Blackwolf is of the Obijway nation and offers a timeless wisdom. Such words stimulate the imagination. The idea of caring as a dance captures its performance; the fluid and knowing movement of my hands across someone's feet is poetry in motion. Yet to be a skilful dancer requires effort, discipline, commitment, patience, compassion and wisdom.

> Believe in the vision of you.
> Practice the vision.
> Become the vision. (Blackwolf and Jones 1996:p47)

Let these words stir the mind and heart. Blackwolf and Jones' book *Earth dance drum* has influenced the way I view and develop reflection. At every turn of the page there is some new message to inspire:

Reflect periodically throughout the day. See clearly who you are, what you are experiencing. Like brother eagle, preen your emotional feathers throughout the day. They are the feathers that help you fly to greater heights. (p15)

Prerequisites of reflection

Fay (1987) identifies certain qualities of mind that are necessary to reflection: openness, curiosity, wilfulness or commitment, and intelligence. I can add energy, passion, discipline and playfulness to this list. These qualities of mind are significant to counter the more negative qualities of mind associated with defensiveness, habit, resistance, laziness, stress, and no doubt many other adjectives.

Commitment

I meet many practitioners whose commitment to their practice has become numb or blunted through working in non-challenging, non-supportive and generally stressful environments where the realisation of caring values is constantly threatened by inadequate resources and unsympathetic attitudes. Perhaps satisfaction is making it through to the end of the shift with minimal hassle rather than fulfilling caring ideals. Often, when things get overly familiar, we take them for granted and get into a habitual groove.
    John O'Donohue (1997:122-3) notes:

> People have difficulty awakening to their inner world, especially when their lives become familiar to them. They find it hard to discover something new, interesting or adventurous in their numbed lives.

Practitioners who are numb will not enjoy reflection. Indeed, they will turn their heads away from the reflective mirror because the images are not positive. These practitioners do not want to face themselves and their responsibility to care. Yet, if they can face the mirror, perhaps with guidance, reflection offers the practitioner a way to rekindle commitment and reconnect to caring ideals. Things wither and die if not cared for. When those things are people then the significance of commitment becomes only too apparent. Commitment harmonises or balances conflict of contradiction – it is the energy that helps us to face up to unacceptable situations. As Carl Rogers (1969) notes, the small child is ambivalent about learning to walk; he stumbles and falls, he hurts himself. It is a painful process. Yet the satisfaction of developing his potential far outweighs the bumps and bruises. As I know only too well, through years of guiding practitioners to learn through experiences, nurses reflect on painful situations. Practice is not always a pretty sight. Yet with commitment, even in the darkest moments, the glimmer of caring shines through. The realisation of caring within such moments is profoundly satisfying and sustaining, it nourishes commitment and reaffirms our beliefs. No words express this sentiment better than those of Van Manen (1990:58):

> Retrieving or recalling the essence of caring is not a simple matter of simple etymological analysis or explication of the usage of the word. Rather, it is the construction of a way of life to live the language of our lives more deeply, to become more truly who we are when we refer to ourselves [as nurses].

Curiosity

Curiosity is fundamental to the creative life and yet many practitioners are locked into habitual patterns of practice. Worse, they resist looking at new ways as if these represent an inherent threat to their security. As John O'Donohue (1997:163-4) notes:

> Many people remain trapped at the one window, looking out every day at the same scene in the same way. Real growth is experienced when you draw back from that one window, turn and walk around the inner tower of the soul and see all the different windows that await your gaze. Through these different windows, you can see new vistas of possibility, presence and creativity. Complacency, habit and blindness often prevent you from feeling your life. So much depends on the frame of vision – the window through which we look.

The image of practitioners opening shutters to view themselves is a powerful visualisation of mindfulness.

Paying attention to my practice, I am open to what is unfolding. Being open, I am not defensive, but curious and open to new possibilities. Every situation becomes an opportunity for learning. Curiosity is being mindful. Why do I feel that way? Why do I think that way? Why do I respond that way? Why are the walls green? Does music help patients relax? Why is Jim unhappy – would a SSRI antidepressant work better than a tricylic? Etcetera. Everything enters into the gaze of the curious practitioner on the quest to realise desirable and effective practice. From this angle it is perhaps easy to see the scope of reflection. Gadamer (1975:266) notes how:

> the opening up and keeping open of possibilities is only possible because we find ourselves deeply interested in that which makes the question possible in the first place. To truly question something is to interrogate something from the threat of our existence, from the centre of our being.

Contradiction

Reflection is often triggered by negative feelings such as anger, guilt, sadness, frustration, resentment or even hatred (Boyd and Fales 1983). Negative feelings create anxiety within the person and bring the situation that caused these feelings into the conscious mind. The practitioner may *naturally* reflect either consciously or subconsciously to try and defend against this anxiety. The practitioner may distort, rationalise, project or even deny the situation that caused the feelings. They may take action to relieve the tension anxiety causes by attacking the source of the negative feeling or taking it out on someone else. They may more quietly talk it through with someone willing to listen or, more vigorously, take some exercise. We all have our own tactics for such moments. We may even write in a journal!

Negative feelings reflect contradiction between our values and our practice. Contradiction is *creative tension* – the tension that exists between our visions of practice and our understanding of our current reality (Senge 1990). For people concerned with doing what is best, this tension can feel uncomfortable or like a gnawing ache. Whilst it may be natural to pay attention to negative feelings because they disturb us, practitioners can also reflect on positive feelings such as satisfaction, joy and love. In my experience, this is less likely because such feelings are not viewed as problematic. Experiences that arouse no strong feelings are simply taken for granted, that is until the practitioner becomes *mindful*, in which case all experience becomes available for reflection.

Energy work

So, reflection encourages the expression, acceptance and understanding of feelings. Negative feelings can be worked through and their energy converted into positive energy for taking future action based on an understanding of the situation and appropriate ways of responding. As Lydia Hall (1964:151) succinctly puts it:

> Anxiety over an extended period is stressful to all the organ functions. It prepares people to fight or flight. In our culture, however, it is brutal to fight and cowardly to flee, so we stew in our own juices and cook up malfunction. This energy can be put to use in exploration of feeling through participation in the struggle to face and solve problems underlying the state of anxiety.

This conversion of negative energy into positive energy for taking action can be understood within Prigogine and Stengers' (1984) theory of dissipate structures as appropriated by Margaret Newman within her theory of Health as Expanded Consciousness (1994).

In my sketch in Figure 1.2, inspired by Newman (1994:38), the single curly lines represent effective self-organisation continuing until they hit a crisis, represented by a mass of curly lines. In crisis, normal patterns of self-organisation fail, resulting in anxiety (negative energy). Being open systems, people can exchange this energy with the environment and create positive energy for taking action based on a reorganisation of self as necessary to resolve the crisis and emerge at a higher level of consciousness; that is, until the next crisis.

Recognition of crisis may seem obvious but it is usually reflected in a subtle sense of breakdown and is not easy to discern within my normal patterns of thinking. Therefore, a guide may be a vital transformative catalyst. The word 'crisis' might be replaced with 'chaos'. Wheatley (1999:119) notes that:

> It is chaos' great destructive energy that dissolves the past and gives us the gift of a new future. It releases us from the imprisoning patterns of the past by offering us its wild ride into newness. Only chaos creates the abyss in which we can recreate ourselves.

Reflection is the vehicle for this ride. Hold on!

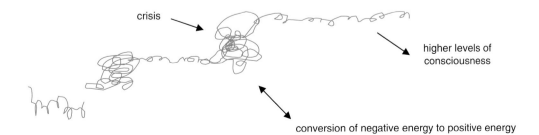

Figure 1.2 Converting negative energy to positive energy.

Understanding

Understanding is the basis for making good judgements and taking action congruent with realising desirable practice. It is only when practitioners understand themselves and the conditions of their practice that they can begin to realistically plan how they might respond differently. Yet, we do not live in a rational world. There are barriers that limit the practitioner's ability to respond differently to practice situations even when they know there is a better way of responding in tune with desirable practice. These barriers blind and bind people to see and respond to the world as they do.

I want to emphasise that reflection is always action oriented towards realising vision as a lived reality. In other words, reflection is not a neutral thing but a political and cultural movement towards creating a better, more caring and humane world. As such, the ideals of a critical social science are enshrined – firstly, that reflection is firstly a process of enlightenment or understanding as to why things are as they are (self in context); secondly, a process of empowerment to take action as necessary based on understanding; and thirdly, a process of emancipation whereby action actually transforms situations for a vision to be realised (in the understanding that visions actually shift in the process of realisation).

However, just because the practitioner can understand why things are as they are may not mean they can easily change things. Fay (1987) highlighted the limitations of rationality to bring about change due to three key aspects of culture: tradition, force and embodiment, that offers a typology of resistance.

- Tradition – a pre-reflective state reflected in the customs, norms and prejudices that people hold about the way things should be, and their habitual practices.
- Force – the way normal relationships are constructed and maintained through the use of power/force.
- Embodiment – the way people normally think, feel and respond to the world in a normative and largely pre-reflective way.

These barriers are powerful resistors to change that the practitioner must overcome to realise desirable practice. If people were rational they would change their practice on the basis of evidence that supports the best way of doing something. But even then two people may rationally disagree! Until practitioners become aware of these factors that constrain them, they are unlikely to be able to change them. However, because things are normative these barriers are often not perceived.

Reflection is then *critical* reflection, in the sense of a critical social science. The language of a critical social science may be intimidating with its rhetoric of oppression and misery yet it can be argued that nursing, as a largely female occupation, has been subjugated by patriarchal attitudes that render it politically passive and thus unable to fulfil its caring destiny. If so, then realising a holistic vision requires an analysis and eventual overthrow of oppressive political and cultural systems. The link between oppression and patriarchy is obvious, considering nursing as women's work, and the suppression of women's voices in 'knowing their place' within the patriarchal order of things. Images of 'behind the screens' where women conceal their work, themselves and their significance (Lawler 1991) and images of emotional labour being no more than women's natural work, therefore unskilled and unvalued within the heroic stance of medicine (James 1989), are powerful signs of this oppression.

Maxine Greene (1988:58) notes:

> Concealment does not simply mean hiding; it means dissembling, presenting something as other than it is. To 'unconceal' is to create clearings, spaces in the midst of things where decisions can be made. It is to break through the masked and the falsified, to reach toward what is also half-hidden or concealed. When a woman, when any human being, tries to tell the truth and act on it, there is no predicting what will happen. The 'not yet' is always to a degree concealed. When one chooses to act on one's freedom, there are no guarantees.

I feel my excitement tingle as I read and write these words. Reflection opens up a clearing where desirable practice and the barriers that constrain its realisation can be unconcealed and where action can be planned to overcome the barriers, whatever their source. No easy task, for these barriers are embodied, they structure practice and patterns of relating. Fear is a powerful deterrent for being different. Reflection enables practitioners to speak and know their truth, ripping away illusions.

The commitment to the truth is vital in Greene's words. Yet how comfortable are people in their illusions of truth? Is it better to conform than rock the boat? Is it better to sacrifice the ideal for a quiet life and patronage of more powerful others? Is it better to keep your head down than have it shot off above the parapet for daring to reveal the truth?

Empowerment

Reflection is empowering, enabling the practitioner to act on insights towards realising desirable practice. Kieffer (1984) noted that the process of empowerment involved:

> Reconstructing and re-orientating deeply engrained personal systems of social relations. Moreover, they confront these tasks in an environment which historically has enforced their political oppression and which continues its active and implicit attempts at subversion and constructive change. (p27)

Kieffer's words may not rest comfortably with many readers. Yet the truth of the situation is stark; if practitioners truly wish to realise their caring ideals then they have no choice but to become political in working towards establishing the conditions of practice where that is possible.

Being in place

Linked to the previous point, the reflective journey can be viewed as a movement from *knowing your place* – a place determined and controlled by more powerful others – to *being in place* – the place where I need to be to realise my vision as a lived reality (Mayeroff 1971).

Try this exercise.

- In each circle in Figure 1.3, write a description of 'knowing your place' and 'being in place'.
- Identify what factors constrain you from being in place.
- Now identify positive action you can take to be in place.

- Reflect each day on the difference positive action makes.
- Repeat the exercise at least weekly and mark along the line your progress toward being in place.

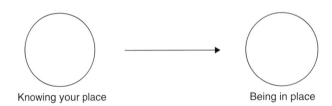

Knowing your place   Being in place

Figure 1.3 The reflective journey.

I shall assume that not *being in place* is a deeply disturbing idea that creates a strong sense of internal conflict. As such, I can pretend I am in a 'good enough place' as some sort of compromise to survive a hostile world. However, the movement to being in place is not easy. As suggested above, deeply embodied forces rally to uncomfortably remind me to know my place.

But that is OK. At least I am aware of this. It is my reality. It is a beginning. Perhaps all I can do is chip away at the edges, but if so, I can imagine being a sculptor chipping away slowly but purposefully at the granite slab toward creating a beautiful thing. For without doubt, my image of desirable practice is a beautiful thing. It is worth making the effort, isn't it?

Developing voice

As such, empowerment is developing an assertive and political voice that is heard and listened to within the corridors of power. And yet so many nurses' voices are silent or suppressed for fear of sanction. Such practitioners are not so much lost for words but have no words to say. Perhaps you can remember being silenced, not so much by others but by yourself. Practitioners often say 'I wish I had said something but …'

Is it fear of repercussion or humiliation? Either way, it is a reflection of knowing that your place is to be silent. Think of a recent experience when you would have liked to say something – write it down and ask yourself why you were silent. What would you have liked to say? How did you feel? What do you imagine the response of others would be?

Perhaps you did say something – what were the consequences?

Julia Cumberlege (DHSS 1986) observed at meetings concerned with discussion of her report on community nursing that doctors sat in the front rows and asked all the questions, whilst nurses sat in the back rows and kept silent. She commented how nurses needed to find a voice so they could be heard, otherwise they would have no future in planning healthcare services.

This comment reflects how nurses have traditionally been socialised into a subordinate and powerless workforce through educational processes and dominant patterns of relationships with more powerful groups (Buckenham and McGrath 1983). I remember as a student nurse sitting passively in the classroom being filled with facts, what Belenky *et al* (1986) describe as received knowing; the way practitioners listen and speak with the voices of others that they have embodied. They conceive themselves as capable of receiving, even reproducing knowledge from the all-knowing external authorities but not capable of creating knowledge of their own. I had no sense of being enabled to develop

critical thinking skills, and even if I had, the all-knowing authorities within clinical practice would have soon put me in my place. Despite the rhetoric of developing the practitioner as a critical thinker, the weight of tradition and authority continues to suppress
her emergence.

So when I ask a nurse 'Why do you do it like that?', she is likely to reproduce knowledge from an external authority that has been unquestioned. When I ask her how else
she might do it, she may struggle to think laterally because she has never been enabled
to think. Perhaps this scenario is shifting with university education.

So, reflection at its root level opens a door to find and express voice. Belenky *et al*
(1986) describe this as the subjective voice, finding the inner voice, listening to, valuing
and accepting one's own voice as a source of knowing. This may mean rejecting the
authoritative voice that has dominated the way the practitioner views, thinks about and
responds to the world.

The subjective voice is tentative, vulnerable in its uncertainty, and hence may need to
be nurtured in a community of like-minded people. It may be confusing because it is
competing with received voices. As such, it is easy to discount one's own subjective voice
as being unsubstantiated, even ridiculed by more 'knowing' others. Listening to self, the
self may see an uncanny stranger on display, a self that has been censored (Cixous 1996).
Belenky *et al* (1986:85) note:

> During the period of subjective knowing, women lay down procedures for systematically
> learning and analysing experience. But what seems distinctive in these women is that their
> strategies for knowing grow out of their very embeddedness in human relationships and the
> alertness of everyday life. Subjectivist women value what they see and hear around them and
> begin to feel a need to understand the people with whom they live and who impinge on their
> lives. Though they be emotionally isolated from others at this point in their histories, they
> begin to actively analyse their past and current interactions with others. (p85)

Reflection encourages the practitioner to pay attention to self within the context of human
relationships and encourages this alertness in everyday life. The idea that practitioners are
isolated is intriguing – many nurses talk of chatting with others, but to what purpose? Does
such chat reinforce prejudices and discontent or does it enable the growth of knowing? The
role of guided reflection within the curriculum opens this space but it needs to be a continuing space through the programme to have any real developmental impact.

Although the subjective voice is unsubstantiated, it does open the door to dialogue
with sources of knowing to become informed. Belenky *et al* (1986) describe this as the
procedural voice.

The procedural voice

The procedural voice has two complementary ways of knowing: connected and separate
knowing. Both are vital to effective practice. Connected knowing is informed by understanding the experiences of others through empathy. In contrast, the separate voice is
dispassionate in its ability to critique and reason. It is the rational voice that seeks to
understand things in terms of logic and procedures. It is the antithesis of received knowledge – no longer is knowledge accepted on face value but it is now challenged for its
validity and appropriateness to inform the particular situation. Perhaps the reader can
sense Schön's metaphoric swampy lowland as the world of the connected voice, and the
high hard ground as the world of the separate voice.

The connected voice is the yin voice, feminine, perceived, intuited whereas the separate voice might be viewed as the yang voice, rational, logical, reasoned. Both voices are significant in healthcare and when woven together result in what Belenky *et al* (1986) term the constructed voice.

The constructed voice

This voice is informed, passionate and assertive. Virginia Woolf (1945) considered that the great mind is androgynous, finding the balance between the feminine and masculine, the yin and yang, the right and left brain. She writes, 'It is when this fusion takes place that the mind is fully fertilised and uses all its faculties' (p97).

However, even practitioners who have a constructed voice may be silenced. As Belenky *et al* note:

> Even among women who feel they have found voice, problems with voice abound. Some women told us, in anger and frustration, how frequently they felt unheard and unheeded – both at home and work. In our society which values male authority, constructivist women are no more immune to the experience of feeling silenced than any other group of women. (p146)

The unbalanced mind leans too heavily towards the masculine, favouring reason over intuition, justice over care, outcomes over process, science over art. Perhaps the feminine has to be privileged to find balance? I wonder – do normal patterns of practice privilege masculine values and demean feminine values? Is management essentially masculine or patriarchal?

It is often said that to succeed in a man's world, women must become more masculine than men. Look about your practice – is there a grain of truth in this idea?

Writing as agentic action

Another way to view empowerment is in terms of realising and sustaining agency, shifting from a victimic to an agentic mode of being (Polkingthorne 1996). Agentic people are clear on what they want to accomplish, understand how intended actions will contribute to their accomplishments, and are confident that they can complete the intended actions and attain their goals. In contrast, the practitioner may perceive herself as a victim, feeling powerless to take action towards realising a vision of practice.

To view self as a victim is to experience a loss of personhood and to project the blame for this loss onto others rather than take responsibility for self. Victimic people depict their lives as out of their control, shaped by events beyond their influence. Others' actions and chance determine life outcomes, and the accomplishment or failure to achieve life goals depends on factors they are unable to change. Bruner (1994) notes that people construct a victimic self by:

> reference to memories of how they responded to the agency of somebody else who had the power to impose his or her will upon them, directly or indirectly by controlling the circumstances in which they are compelled to live. (p41)

Bruner's words highlight that the construction of life plots is always in relation to others. The plots are oriented more towards avoiding negative possibilities than to actualising positive possibilities. In contrast, Cochran and Laub (1994) considered that the change from a victimic to an agentic identity consisted of two correlative movements: the progressive construction of a new agentic life story, and the destruction of and detachment from the victimic life story. The victimic plot does not simply fade away; it must be actively confronted, which can generally be seen moving through four phases.

Phase 1

This first phase is dominated by the person's sense of entrapment or incompleteness, being controlled, helplessness – described as 'trapped in a world in which most of what makes life worthwhile is gone, and threatened by the possibility that this bleak existence might extend indefinitely' (Cochran and Laub 1994:90).

Phase 2

People become involved in activities that will assist in (re)gaining an agentic life. Escape from phase 1 begins with the formation of a goal that is worthwhile and attainable (vision). The person takes ownership of her practice, and can see that her efforts make a difference and affect outcomes. The person monitors her progress and establishes standards for success in achieving progressively more difficult goals. Experiences of success in achieving these goals are crucial to validate the person's capacity to make a difference and fuel her optimism for a better future and produce a sense of freedom and control.

Phase 3

People engage in activities more closely related to their goals in more self-directed ways – what Cochran and Laub (1994) describe as actually playing the game, whereas phase 2 was practising the game. The person becomes aware that the remaining major barriers to a fuller and more agentic life reside as much in her own beliefs and attitudes as in factors outside herself.

Phase 4

People experience a liberating sense of completing their goals. Cochran and Laub (1994) note: 'Now one lives with a sense of life being on course, full, open to possibilities, unrestricted' (p94). The person has achieved a sense of wholeness that is no longer threatened by former recollections. She has become the author of her own life and taken control of her existence.

Reflection and writing would enhance the core ingredients of personal agency: self-determination; self-legislation; meaningfulness; purposefulness; confidence; active striving; planning; and responsibility (Cochran and Laub 1994). The person's work is to create a plot out of a succession of actions, as if to direct the actor in the midst of action. Locating ourselves within an intelligible story is essential to our sense that life is meaningful. Being an actor at all means trying to make certain things happen, to bring about desirable endings, to search for possibilities that lead in hopeful directions. As actors, we require our actions not only to be intelligible but to get us somewhere. We act because we intend to get something done, to begin something which we hope will lead us along a desirable route; we act with what Kermode (1966:813) calls the 'sense of an ending':

> Because we act with the sense of an ending, we try to direct our actions and the actions of other relevant actors in ways that will bring the ending about.

Evaluating reflection

Reflective practice has been criticised for its lack of definition, modes of implementation and its unproven benefit (Mackintosh 1998:556). Mackintosh singles out the Burford reflective model for criticism. She states:

> The benefits of reflection are largely unaddressed by the literature [*that is, beyond unsubstantiated claims*], and instead the underlying assumption appears to be that reflection will improve nursing care or the nursing profession in some intangible way. This is demonstrated by Bailey (1995), who although describing the introduction of reflection into a critical area and claiming that an improvement in problem-solving skills occurred, gives no evidence that the quality of care was improved in any way. These failings can also be found in much of the literature describing the Burford reflection in nursing model [Johns 1998a, b, c] which attempts to integrate reflective practice into a clinically grounded nursing model through use of a series of 'cues'. Much of the published evidence regarding the model's impact on clinical practice appears to be based on personal anecdote, and again, evidence in support of its impact on patient care is of a mainly qualitative and descriptive mature. (my italics)

Of course, reflective accounts are subjective and singular. The accounts within *The Burford NDU model: caring in practice* (Johns 1994) were not cited in the above references. Yet in this book there are four collaborating accounts from Burford practitioners and accounts from four other nursing units besides Burford – accounts that testify to the impact of the Burford model on clinical practice. In other words, Mackintosh reviews the literature with her own partial eye, seeing or interpreting what she wants to read to support her prejudice against reflective accounts and qualitative methodologies. As Wilber (1998) highlights, different paradigms have their own rules for injunction as to what counts as the truth, and who better to know her own truth than the practitioner? To dispute that truth would mean that every survey, interview and pyschometric test is flawed, tainted with the 'suspicion of authenticity', and perhaps more so because the truth is obscured behind an objective illusion.

As I explore in Chapter 3, the role of the guide is to help the practitioner see herself more objectively and to challenge the basis for perceptions and assumptions.

The limitations of reflection as a mode of learning have been highlighted by, amongst others, Platzer *et al* (2000). They noted that students may be resistant to revealing self, a point also highlighted by Cotton (2001), that reflection becomes a type of surveillance, assessment and control. Yet education has always been a socialisation process. Where teachers use reflection from a teacher-centred perspective, then it may be resisted. Platzer *et al* further note that embodied ways of learning and organisational culture impose tremendous barriers to reflecting on and learning from experience. Without doubt, there are barriers, but the barriers are a focus for learning and shifting, both within self and within the organisational culture. Real education is not necessarily easy. Students may prefer to be fed what they need to know but is that an adequate preparation for developing critical thinkers? The Model for Structured Reflection (MSR) has been tested and found to be beneficial in enabling students to develop self-awareness and caring potential (Novelestsky-Rosenthal and Solomon 2001).

Burton (2000) has noted:

> It will be argued that reflective theory and practice has not yet been adequately tested and there is a pressing need for evidence to demonstrate irrefutably the effectiveness of reflection on nursing practice, particularly with respect to patient outcomes. (p1009)

Burton challenges why the UKCC and ENB insist that nurses at all levels of experience should reflect, when the evidence to support its benefits is unsubstantial. Perhaps she should ask why do people think in the first place and read research findings? Yet Burton's words, again like Mackintosh, reveal the way people who inhabit a behavioural paradigm view reflection. They impose their own rules of injunction without appreciating the nature of reflection.

Reflection is *not* primarily a technology to produce better patient outcomes and yet it follows that if reflection does enable practitioners to realise desirable practice, desirable practice is always concerned with best meeting patient needs and that this realisation is best illuminated through reflexive narratives. For example, doctoral work by Jarrett (2008) clearly demonstrates her appreciation and realisation of spasticity nursing over a 4-year period. My work with leaders within the masters of leadership programme, designed as a collaborative research project, enabled me to analyse 24 dissertation narratives to gain insight into being and becoming a leader within NHS organisations. Examples of reflexive narratives have been published in my other books (Johns 2002, 2005, 2006) that demonstrate the impact of guided reflection on knowing and realising desirable practice. Reflection is essentially about personal growth and that impact on personal growth can only be known through the stories these people tell. As narratives can exquisitely illuminate, the impact on patient care shines through yet not in any reductionist sense (for examples, see the research narratives published in Johns 2002).

Conclusion

In this chapter I have explored the nature of reflection grounded in a critical social science as a process of self-inquiry and transformation towards realising desirable practice as a lived reality. I suggest that this is the hallmark of professional responsibility to ensure that self is best fit to deliver effective practice. In Chapter 2, I explore how clinical practice can be structured through a reflective model, on the premise that reflective practitioners thrive in conditions that value and support reflective practice.

Chapter 2

A reflective framework for clinical practice

Peter and Sam[1]

Mid February.

Another cold morning driving to the hospice along dark slippery lanes.

I'm late, but a whisper tells me be patient, do not rush into the darkness where danger lurks for the careless.

Someone asks if I can do anything for the odour in Peter's room.

I do not know him. I am told he is close to death. Just 52 years old.

I am often asked as an aromatherapist to combat unpleasant odour – what is euphemistically referred to as *perfuming*.

Christine (a staff nurse) pulls me aside: 'Could you also offer Sam, Peter's wife, something? She's very distressed.'

Peter's room opens onto a corridor shared by several single rooms. Walking down the corridor, I observe the woman who sits outside Peter's room. People are gathered around her.

She looks up and gazes at me as I slowly approach. I know it is Sam even though we have not met before.

I gently inquire 'Sam?'.

She nods. Her distress is palpable, rippling through her even as she endeavours to contain it.

'I'm Chris, the complementary therapist ... have you been here all night?'

Again she nods.

'You must be tired?'

'Yes ... I am but it's OK. ... [silence]. ... I need to be here.'

'I know.'

I know because I can read the signs. I have heard this story many times before. It is legend.

We move into Peter's room and gaze at him. He looks peaceful, his breathing slightly noisy.

---

[1]A version of this narrative was published in my book *Engaging reflection in practice* (2000:123-6) and also formed my editorial to *Complementary therapies in clinical practice*.

She holds one hand and I take the other. He is not responsive even though yesterday Sam says he had a jacuzzi bath.

Today is another story. An unfolding drama.

Holding his hand, I listen, feeling for his wavelength to connect with him and tell him through my touch that I care for him. Such *intent* is vital – it is a gateway for healing. No words spoken. We dwell in the silence that lies thick between us.

Words by John O'Donoghue – sometimes we listen to things but we never hear them. True listening brings us in touch even with that which is unsaid and unsayable. Sometimes the most important thresholds of mystery are places of silence. To be genuinely spiritual is to have great respect for the possibilities and presence of silence.

Meeting a family for the first time under these conditions is never easy. The air is thick with emotional tension. Uncertain about how best to respond, I buy myself time by continuing to hold Peter's hand and sit silently with him, listening to him, being mindful of what is happening about me and within me, bringing myself into the right space to give therapy.

And yet I feel pressure from both myself and from Sam to act quickly, to grasp at a solution to ease Peter's suffering in the face of the other's and my own anxiety. I am *mindful* of not falling into a *fix-it* mentality.

Being mindful is being *patient*, mindful of not rushing into the darkness, of being careless.

I remember my task was to combat the odour. The odour isn't pleasant. I imagine it oozing from the rotting cavities. To sit by your dying husband waiting for his death is not easy. To sit with the smell of his rotting body must exacerbate the suffering.

I do not mention the odour to Sam. I wonder if she has acclimatised herself to it. I suggest to Sam that therapeutic touch might help Peter.

'Anything that might help, please try.'

Seeing her so vulnerable, so desperate, I want to hold her and say it's OK.

She gives a thin smile as if she knows and seeks to reassure me.

She doesn't ask what therapeutic touch involves and I do not inform her. She is absorbed in his and her own suffering.

I place my hand above Peter's chest and abdomen and sense the heat and pressure of the cancer.

Sam, intrigued, asks 'What are you doing?'.

'I intend by moving my hands across Peter's body it will help reduce the heat and pressure from his body and ease his suffering.'

Saying *ease his suffering* seems to reassure Sam.

These are powerful words. The word *suffering* is so evocative, confrontational even, as if it dares to name the palpable tension.

I might have added – 'and ease your suffering as well'. I don't say this because I know it would be a distraction – that she would say she didn't want any attention for herself. I know that to treat Peter is to treat Sam, especially as she continues to hold his hand.

I centre myself, tuning into the healing spirit that flows about. And for 20 minutes or so we dwell in silence as I practise.

Afterwards Sam says 'Peter seems so much more peaceful and his breathing is easier.'

The room is very still and I sense that she, too, is now easier.

I had intended the therapeutic touch would also combat the odour, and indeed the odour has diminished. I have noted before the ability of therapeutic touch to reduce odour, as if the odour emanates from a restless spirit (Johns 2004b). In calming Peter, the odour diminishes. The significance is to treat the cause of the odour rather than the odour itself.

Sam says she has been at the hospice at his bedside since Peter's admission. She knows he is dying and waits anxiously.

Waiting – a constant theme through my narrative. As a therapist I journey alongside people so they are not alone but mindful not to be intrusive in the waiting. Reading the signs to position myself therapeutically.

Sam seems to welcome my company.

She says 'It's only a week since his diagnosis. For 8 months he was treated for stomach reflux whilst the cancer ate away his pancreas. He experienced great pain, had lost 5 stone in weight, then the jaundice appeared and now this. …'

Her words trail off as her tears move close to the surface.

Such history is not uncommon. Questions that require answers but not now. Contained anger alongside the despair of his dying fuelling the deep conflict she feels. But now she must give her attention to Peter. Sam suffers not just Peter's dying but the anguish of his misdiagnosis. Peter is a young man, his life ripped away.

I try and empathise with Sam but struggle to connect with the turmoil I sense inside her, inside the container. How do I begin to understand her thoughts and feelings?

The empathic demand.

I ask 'How are you feeling?'.

No words. Perhaps no words are needed to feel her despair as she sits by Peter. Perhaps my inquiry was futile, banal … I seek the right words to express this …

A momentary sense of helplessness.

Sam follows me outside his room and says 'I am bursting inside … it is our wedding anniversary today… '

She pauses … 'I couldn't sleep last night … I kept dreaming I was at home and reaching for him in the empty bed.'

She bursts open. Her tears cascade like a burn in full spring flow. She is tossed on a raging sea of grief. I feel as if I pick my way through the bobbing debris, the desolation that cancer leaves in its wake.

'Is there something I can offer you … to help you relax?'

I feel the unspoken demand to care for this life put into my hands.

Silence … and then as if she has been thinking deeply, she says 'That's kind of you … I've slept at times … I'm really tired, exhausted … struggling being with Peter … but no, I don't want any treatments … I want you to give attention to Peter.'

Her look is plaintive. Sam wants no distraction from her bedside quest. Like many spouses she feels that any attention for her would be taking attention away from Peter. However, I feel I have already treated her with the therapeutic touch.

I open my arms outwards. I do not know why. Perhaps an invitation? A posture of connection. As I write, I open my arms in a similar way and am reminded of angels' wings. Could I be an angel? Was the giving of therapeutic touch brushing Peter and Sam with angels' wings? I am drawn to this imagery because I firmly believe that my intent to ease suffering through therapy is a spiritual encounter.

Perhaps angels do accompany us? Certainly the Bodhisattva White Tara is about.

But I am also aware that the risk of spiritual inflation haunts me (Borglum 1997). I have written of this before – that the spiritual can become intoxicating.

I must never become complacent but always challenge my intention. It is vital to have the right posture (Suzuki 1999:84).

I remind myself – *be soft in your practice.*

'Shall I set up an aroma-stone to give the room a more pleasant odour?'

She accepts my offer but does not want a strong heady smell. I find myself deliberating – shall I use bergamot, neroli or lavender, or even a mixture? I do not give Sam the choice but choose bergamot. She likes its smell. Bergamot is well known to combat anxiety (Davis 1999). Worwood (1999:) notes: 'We may cry inside, our hearts aching, but bergamot will lighten the heart and dispel self-criticism and blame'.

Perfect words for the occasion? Sometimes I read these spiritual descriptors to those sitting at the bedside but not this time, even though I carry Worwood's book in my satchel. I sense the words would be inappropriate to say despite their appropriateness to the moment.

I know through experience that neroli infuses a room with a profound sense of stillness. Intriguingly, Worwood (1999:235) notes that 'neroli touches the realms of angels, and anyone who uses it is brushed with the light of angels' wings …'.

Umm … but neroli has a more heady smell, as does lavender. Often several aroma-stones are burning different essential oils, infusing the air with a heady cocktail that can cause headaches. No others are burning this morning but I must always be careful about using essential oils in public spaces.

Later I make a point of attending the shift report and give a short account of my work with Peter and Sam. I share my views on combating odour. I assert that it's too easy to assume the odour has a physical cause, that perhaps it is a manifestation of despair. Someone says the room definitely smells better. Successful perfuming.

Christine chips in: 'Did you give Sam a treatment?'.

'Not directly … only through giving Peter therapeutic touch … she held his hand … she didn't want any attention taken from him.' I tell them about Sam's wedding anniversary and her despair, emphasising my role of being with her and Peter.

No comment. The shift report moves on. I sense the way their partial listening has filtered out information that does not fit their agenda. They are not used to a complementary therapist imposing a view, reflected in the small space on the complementary therapy sheet allocated to 'comment' where I am expected to write (reflect?) on treatments. Other complementary therapists simply write 'relaxed' as if the therapist's role is simply that – to aid relaxation. I imagine the reaction if I wrote in the patient notes or invaded the multiprofessional meeting and talked about 'the spiritual', how the chaplain would feel elbowed; or if I wrote about despair, the psychologist would take offence; or about physical pain, the doctors would curtly rebuke me; or that if I gave advice on constipation or helped someone get to the toilet, I would be reprimanded by nurses for exceeding my role. The patient and holistic practitioner both fragmented within professional territorial. Holism an illusion people cling to for identity.

A ripple of despondency ripples over me. I sense the despondency hit the wall and ripple backwards yet no-one seems to notice. My *equanimity* on edge.

The illusion of the collaborative team exposed. I cannot pretend to shift it. I work in the margins.

Before leaving, I return to the room to say goodbye to Peter and Sam – to wish them well on their difficult journey. Sam remains by the bedside maintaining her death vigil. I can imagine the knots tightening in her neck and along her shoulders. Being a massage therapist shapes my gaze!

Like a stranger I appear and then disappear from their torn lives. It is an extraordinary privilege to dwell with people so intensely, so intimately, just for a short time. And for a brief moment I imagine Avalokitishvara, the Bodhisattva of compassion, wrapping us in his arms. Such a beautiful image and feeling.

I did not meet Peter or Sam again. He died 2 days later.

Such is my practice, entering the hospice and finding myself in the midst of such drama. Having written the story, I can reflect deeper, challenging myself, pulling out significant issues from the story text, developing insights to inform my future practice. I wonder – could I have been more available to Peter and Sam in the brief moment we dwelt together; to have known and eased their suffering more? Such is my quest.

The Burford NDU model: caring in practice

The hospice where I worked with Peter and Sam utilised *The Burford NDU model: caring in practice* as a way of framing clinical practice. The Burford model is a reflective and holistic approach to clinical practice. I might say that to be holistic is also to be reflective in the sense that the reflective practitioner always sees things mindfully in relationship against a background of the whole. In 1990, when the Burford model was developed, nursing models were fashionable, reflecting an era of nursing seeking a theoretical identity and credibility as a profession as it strived to emerge from the shadows of medical domination.

Vision

The heart of clinical practice is a living and valid vision for practice (Senge 1990).

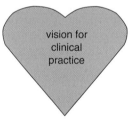

By 'living' I mean, it is something embodied and lived rather than just words on a piece of paper shut away in some file or drawer. A vision is fluid and dynamic, shifting to accommodate new meanings and ideas. A vision is the bedrock of practice, a springboard to guide all aspects of clinical practice and practice development. Where groups of practitioners work together it is self-evident that they need to share a common belief system that gives purpose and direction to practice and learning and ensures a consistent and congruent approach towards patients and families.

Senge (1990:206–8) so vividly states:

> When people truly share a vision they are connected, bound together by a common aspiration. Visions are exhilarating … they create the 'spark', the excitement that lifts an organisation out of the mundane.

In writing a vision, practitioners connect to their caring beliefs and values, beginning the process of empowerment that is central to realising the vision as a lived reality. Building a shared vision involves unearthing shared beliefs and values about the nature of practice that fosters genuine commitment rather than compliance (Senge 1990). Leaders learn the counter-productiveness of trying to dictate a vision, no matter how heartfelt. As such,

Box 2.1   Burford vision for clinical practice, 4th edition

We believe that caring is grounded in the core therapeutic of easing suffering and enabling the growth of the other through his/her health–illness experience, whether toward recovery or death. The practitioner is mindful of intent and is available to work with the person and the person's family in relationship, on the basis of empathic connection, compassion and mutual understanding, where the person's life pattern and health needs are appreciated and effectively responded to.

Caring is seamless across healthcare settings and responds to and promotes both the local community's and society's expectations of effective service. In this respect, we accept a responsibility to develop a culture of transformational leadership and the learning organisation that continually strives to anticipate and develop practice to ensure its efficacy and quality. By appropriate monitoring and sharing, we contribute to the development of the societal value of nursing and healthcare generally.

Our caring is enhanced when I work in relationship with our multiprofessional colleagues on the basis of mutual respect and care for each other within our respective roles. This means being free to share our feelings openly but appropriately, acknowledging that as persons, we are stressed and have differences of opinion at times. This is the basis of the therapeutic team that is essential to reciprocate and support our caring for patients.

constructing a vision must be a bottom-up approach to change that enables practitioners to grasp their own destiny rather than have it imposed on them. Then practitioners become active creators of their own practice and take responsibility for realising their beliefs in practice.

Vision sets up both resistance and possibility

In 1989, shortly after I arrived as General Manager and Head of the Nursing Development Unit, I challenged staff at Burford Community Hospital to reflect on the meaning of nursing within the hospital. I asked them to tell me about the hospital's philosophy. They struggled to articulate this. At that time, the hospital philosophy was 'imported', based on the philosophy of the Loeb Center in New York (Alfano 1971, Hall 1964). Hall's work was a vision of nursing as the primary therapy in its own right, alongside its role as complementary to medicine. In 1982, when Alan Pearson (1983) introduced this philosophy, it made sense in terms of his vision to establish nursing beds. Pearson had departed Burford some 3 years previous to my appointment. From the nurses' responses, it was apparent that the Loeb Center vision had faded. It was no longer *alive*. I realised that an 'imported' philosophy (vision) imposes a reality on practitioners which denies the expression of their own.

In response I facilitated the construction of a vision that reflected the individual practitioners' beliefs as a statement of collaborative intent that gave meaning and direction to our collective practice (Johns 2004a). The fourth edition (Box 2.1) has been amended from the original to reflect the development of my own understanding of holistic practice and the fact that a vision must always be dynamic, evolving to adequately represent the nature of changing clinical practice. I added 'a culture of transformational leadership' to the third edition (Johns 2004a).

Valid vision

To be *valid*, a vision for practice needs to address the three cornerstones (Johns 2004a).[2]

---

[2]This framework has been revised from the original work where I had identified four cornerstones (see Johns 2000).

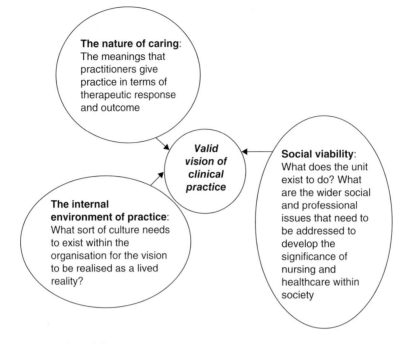

Figure 2.1 Cornerstones of a valid vision.

The nature of caring

So, what is holistic practice? The idea of holism seems to emerge from Smuts' view (1927) that the whole is greater than the sum of its parts. As such, people must be seen as a whole rather than the sum of their parts. Put another way, the parts must always be seen against a background of the whole person.

My personal vision, influenced by Buddhism, is to view caring as easing suffering and enabling the person to grow towards self-realisation, whatever that might mean for the person. Yet what is suffering? How can we respond to best ease it? What is growth? Such questions lie at the heart of caring practice and my reflective self-inquiry.

Suffering

Suffering is a disruption of the spirit. It manifests on the physical, emotional, psychological and spiritual planes. People suffer because they are afraid and feel alone. Hence, at the heart of easing suffering is connection – connection with self by listening to our own stories and connection with others who listen to our stories and say through skilful, wise and compassionate words and actions 'you are not alone'.

Nurturing growth

Mayeroff (1971:1) states:

To care for another person, in the most significant sense, is to help him grow and actualise himself.

There is no mystery or mysticism to this idea. It does not need to be wrapped up in a web of scientific jargon or elaborate artistic strokes. It is fundamental to life itself and as such must be expressed in its exquisite simplicity. To actualise self is to fulfil our human potential, whatever that might mean for the person (Maslow 1968). Newman (1994) illuminates how suffering creates the opportunity to stand back and take stock of self, especially when suffering becomes life threatening. Then our taken-for-granted mortality is shaken, forcing us to contemplate life as impermanent. Forced out of our complacency, we may question the very essence of our existence and the things that are really important to us. Illness confronts the sufferer with the taken-for-granted nature of health and much of life, prompting crisis – a breakdown where things no longer go smoothly, where things spiral out of control, creating anxiety. The breakdown is experienced as a period of disorganisation and uncertainty. Old patterns of organisation no longer work. The person feels threatened on a deep existential level and is thrown into crisis. To overcome the 'crisis', the person needs to learn new ways of organising self conducive with health.

As Remen (1996:156) suggests:

> In the struggle to survive our wounds, we may adapt a strategy for living which gets us through. Life threatening illness may cause us to re-examine the very premises on which we have based our lives, perhaps freeing ourselves to live more fully for the first time.

This can be very difficult as the person is locked into ways of living that are not so easily changed. The practitioner's role is to help the person 'see himself' and to guide the person to reorganise his life pattern so that the crisis is resolved.

A vision of caring is informed by caring philosophers or theorists who challenge practitioners to reflect on caring. For example, Jean Watson, in her transpersonal model of nursing (1988:49), states that the goal of nursing:

> is to help persons gain a higher degree of harmony within the mind, body, and soul which generates self-knowledge, self-reverence, self-healing, and self-care processes while allowing increasing diversity. This goal is pursued through the human–human encounter caring process and caring transactions that respond to the subjective inner world of the person in such a way that the nurse helps individuals find meaning in their existence, disharmony, suffering, and turmoil, and promotes self-control, choice, and self-determination with the health–illness decisions.

Savour Watson's words and sense the meaning. Can nursing be defined in this way? Would it suit all practice areas – health visiting, psychiatry, midwifery? Watson spirals nursing out of the shadow of the medical model into a world of existential suffering where the uniqueness and mystery of what it means to be human are fundamental to healing and fulfilment of human potential. Disease and illness are part of that pattern, although that part can so often create crisis for the person.

Watson's words are offered as a moment for reflection, as a challenge to widen the reader's vision of what caring might mean, not as a prescription of how the nurse should think about nursing. I know that such statements may seem far removed from the messy everyday world of practice. When I read this now so many years after it was first published, I find considerable resonance with the Burford vision.

Nurses have tended to view themselves in terms of what they do rather than in terms of what they believe or who they are. It is a functional as opposed to a philosophical/ontological understanding of self.

Nursing as functional gained prominence during the 1960s with the rise of technology and the medical model. Within the medical model, the ill person is reduced to the status of a patient with a set of symptoms that require investigation, diagnosis and subsequent treatment. Little significance is attributed to emotional, psychological, spiritual and social aspects of being ill or causes of illness. The nursing response is primarily to support the medical task. I am sure many readers will remember being told not to sit on the bed and talk to the patient – there is *work* to be done! The implication is that talking to patients is not work.

Within this culture nurses suspended their own (caring) beliefs as relatively unimportant to the medical task. Even today, caring has been increasingly subordinated to unqualified staff as nurses continue to embrace medical technology work despite the emergence of a holistic ideology.

As nurses have endeavoured to define nursing and construct nursing models, nursing as caring has become a subculture furtively taking place alongside the 'real work' of supporting the medical model. Whilst it is imperative to assume that all healthcare practitioners value caring, when the head is locked into the medical sphere and the medical sphere is most valued within organisations, then practitioners may lose sight of the caring ideal. I know many readers will have experienced this state of affairs when visiting family or friends, or experienced their own healthcare. It is important to bring this conflict to the surface because only then can nurses take action to resolve the contradiction to realise caring as a lived reality rather than as some nice ideal. Yet in a world where the health agenda is dominated by productivity and a culture of 'more for less', times are hard for caring. Practitioners may switch off their caring, simply because it is too painful to witness suffering and the failure to ease suffering. Indeed, as Halldórsdóttir (1991) suggests, suffering is caused by the lack of caring (see Tom and Joan story – Chapter 3).

From this exploration we can see that caring is the balance between *doing nursing*, reflecting theories and necessary skills, and *being a nurse*, reflecting ontological ideas about what it means to be a nurse in terms of selfhood and relationships. These are the outer foundations for a caring curriculum. These foundations support the inner foundations of practical wisdom, craft or praxis towards meeting patient need, and compassion. And then, flowing from the integration of these foundations we find caring unfolding mindfully. It is this balance that gives the practitioner a sense of identity as a nurse.

The *internal environment of practice* is reflected in the vision with its emphasis on the therapeutic team based on collaboration, mutual respect and care. It is concerned with the relationships between practitioners to support patient care. Ask yourself: does the pattern of relationship between colleagues reflect the holistic relationship with patients and families? To support holistic practice, relationships between colleagues must be invested in dialogue and consensus that acknowledge and value each person's view, which are mutually and genuinely supportive. Fine words but they need to be lived as a reality. It requires each practitioner to have an assertive voice, a voice that is connected to the patient's and their own experience – informed, ethical, passionate, respected and heard. As evidenced in the narratives throughout this book, a predominant focus for reflection is creating an environment to support clinical practice, notably dealing with conflict.

Social viability (Johnson 1974) is concerned with the role of the unit within society, i.e. what does the unit exist to do? It is responding to and influencing societal expectations, and wider professional issues such as research and teaching, challenging practitioners to look beyond the immediate context of the practice setting towards the wider social and professional communities. From this perspective, a vision can be a public statement that challenges society to 'see' nursing differently, as making a significant contribution to the lives of its members and more generally to the healthcare of the community. This is important considering that so many people in society view nursing as some subordinate role to medicine, and nurses as the ubiquitous 'doctor's handmaiden'. Make no mistake, the general practitioners who had admission rights to Burford Hospital would have been happy to patronise nursing. To re-orientate society to value nursing requires positive action, yet such positive action is also required to ensure that society's 'new perception' of nursing is constantly reinforced by nurses living out the holistic vision through their everyday dialogue and actions.

The context of Burford's practice was a community hospital. We felt strongly that the hospital was an extension of the community it served and provided inpatient services for those members of the local community who needed medical care but not admission to the local general hospital 20 miles away in Oxford. The hospital also took local people following major illness or surgery for rehabilitation, respite care and people with terminal illness.

In my experience, visions of practice do not profoundly influence practice. These visions are often written in vague rhetoric, often by a practice leader many years ago, pinned on office walls covered by layers of organisational memos or, worse, buried away in a policy file. The rhetoric is often grounded in caring clichés, such as 'we believe in holistic care', which have no meaning for practitioners and are clearly contradicted by even the most casual observation. It is one thing to say 'I believe in holism'; it is another thing to realise that as a lived reality. I shall assume that the failure to realise our vision is deeply felt and frustrating, eating away at our integrity. Reflection enables practitioners to use their frustration and resolve the contradictions so visions can be realised.

Jean Watson (1988:33) urges nurses to action. She writes:

> Caring values of nurses and nursing have been submerged. Nursing and society are, therefore, in a critical situation today in sustaining human care ideals and a caring ideology in practice. The human care role is threatened by increasing medical technology, bureaucratic-managerial institutional constraints in a nuclear age society. At the same time there has been a proliferation of curing and radical treatment cure techniques often without regard to costs.

Watson's words emphasise the significance of social viability. Practitioners may think that these *political* issues are above them but unless they accept a responsibility for caring on a societal plane as well as within their everyday practice, then there is little chance for nursing to become more valued or assert any political clout to realise its therapeutic potential. The caring ideal as love may be scorned when we as nurses are so damaged or wounded that we cannot care or love. Watson says that it is this love that provides the driving force to care. As I shall explore, it is this sense of love or compassion for the other that makes the practitioner more available to the other. Simply, without love for the other person, we cannot care because care is love. Without doubt, nurses, midwives, health visitors and all healthcare practitioners are aching to care. This ache is like a flower that has not bloomed, like a sun lost behind a cloud; if caring is unfulfilled then it turns to acid, to scarring and burnout. Without doubt, patients and families need to be loved by nurses. They ache for this love and when they do not receive it, they suffer.

From vision to reality

The descriptions of suffering, growth and caring are merely words. From a reflective perspective, they give direction. To know and ease suffering and enable growth is only known when experienced and reflected on, and only then does dialogue with the words of others become meaningful. As Rawnsley (1990:42) notes:

> Caring may be a desirable image for nursing, but is it meaningful? Is there congruence between the lived experience of nursing practice and the intellectual pursuit of caring as nursing's professional crest? When living the reality of their practice, nurses need ways through which they can connect the conceptual concerns of the discipline with the raw data of experience.

A structural view of a reflective framework for clinical practice

Rawnsley's words are apposite. To realise the Burford vision as a lived reality, I designed four reflective systems set against a background of the organisational culture. I present these as a mandala within a circle to represent wholeness (Fig. 2.2).

A system to ensure the vision is realised within each clinical moment

The basic question the practitioner must ask is: 'What information do I need to nurse this person?'.

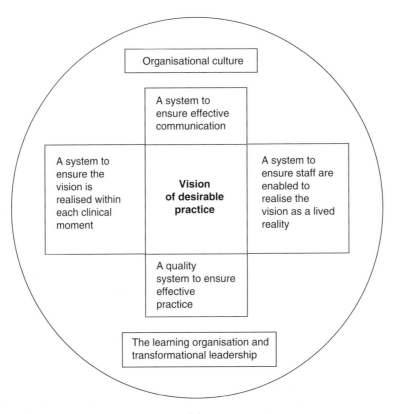

Figure 2.2 *The Burford NDU: caring in practice* mandala.

As Lydia Hall (1964) says, nurses can only nurse what the person reveals of themselves. As such, the nurse's skill is to create the conditions whereby the person can reveal self. This may be obvious in terms of the medical conditions but more subtle in terms of being a person and the impact of their medical condition on their life patterns and holistic well-being.

My audit of the Roper, Logan and Tierney activities of living model (1980) that the hospital was using indicated that the model was an inadequate representation of holistic practice. The model was inherently reductionist, breaking the person into bits of activity, with the consequent risk of losing sight of the whole. These models have rigid assessment criteria based on systems theory that 'encourage' the practitioner to fit the patient to the model, and to see the person as a set of parts in isolation from the whole. As such, they impose a reality that limits practitioners' imagination, creativity and reflection. A far cry from holism. Yet nurses in the UK, despite espousing holistic values, still persist in using such models despite their obvious contradiction.

My audit revealed that practitioners viewed assessment as a task they did on the patient's admission. The constant failure to adequately complete the boxes was apparent.

For example:

> Nutrition: 'likes a cup of tea in the morning'
> Sexuality: 'likes to wear lipstick'
> Dying: most often left blank.

These observations acknowledged the difficulty in seeing such 'activities' as part of everyday functional living. Sexuality reflects who people are. It is synonymous with the person's identity. Even responding to sexuality in terms of the 'sexual act' could not be addressed because of its social taboo. It is difficult to talk to a stranger about sex. It is even more difficult when one's sexuality may seem irrelevant to the healthcare experience. Then assessment can be insensitive and intrusive. Being assessed was also felt to be a ritual of depersonalisation – of transition from person to patient. The problem with assessment schedules is that they demand to be completed, especially when audit systems are linked to completion. Hence when an activity of living box is not completed, it indicates the practitioner had not assessed adequately. The effort was to complete the assessment sheet rather than to know the person.

Undoubtedly, the functional approach to nursing has encouraged practitioners to perceive models of nursing from a utility value, often extracting or modifying bits from the models, and thus breaking up their integrity. For example, *self-care* may have an attractive appeal because it suggests that a target for nursing care is to enable people to regain their independence and return to their level of functioning before the illness event. Yet on a philosophical level, self-care must mean self-determination, being able to take control of one's life in a positive frame of mind. If this is true, then the focus of self-care on functional issues would be misplaced because the functional would always need to be viewed within the meanings the illness or disease had for the person. The focus on functional self-care may lead practitioners to fail to see the person and their distress at a crisis point in their lives. Self-care at a functional level is a deficit model rather than a growth model, with its emphasis of returning the person to a normal level of activity. The patient becomes a series of deficits that need fixing rather than a person whose illness pattern is understood within the whole pattern of their life.

The Roper *et al* model is easily understood from a functional perspective because it seems to represent what nurses already do. Hence adopting the model requires minimal accommodation. Neither is it written in the obscure intellectual language that characterises so many American models of nursing. Pearson (1983:53), in justifying the use of the

Roper *et al* model at Burford, noted the way the model 'speaks to nurses in a language which is familiar and related to nursing in this country and hence its greatest advantage then is its ability to convey meaning to clinical nurses'.

Whilst a practitioner's identification with the model's language might be an advantage, it is also its weakness because, if it fits in with what nurses already do, then its impact on changing practice will be limited. Pearson seems to imply that models *should* convey meaning to nurses but this goes against the grain that the nurse must first find meaning for herself and then collectively with her colleagues. Only then are practitioners in a position to consider the value of external prescriptions of nursing to inform their practice. But if practitioners have developed their own vision for nursing, why would they want to use someone else's?

The outcome of the audit was to stop using the Roper *et al* model and to construct a reflective approach to appreciate the person's life pattern that emphasised the therapeutic relationship.

Such an approach must simultaneously:

- tune the practitioner adequately into the person within the holistic vision so that the vision is lived moment to moment
- tune the practitioner into self, so the practitioner is mindful of self moment to moment within the unfolding therapeutic relationship.

Core question

What information do I need to be able to nurse this person?

Cue questions

- Who is this person?
- What meaning does this illness have for the person?
- How is this person feeling?
- How has this event affected their usual life pattern and roles?
- How do I feel about this person?
- How can I help this person?
- What is important for this person to make their stay comfortable?
- What support does this person have in life?
- How does this person view the future for themselves and others?

Each cue is significant to pattern the holistic response to the person. The practitioner internalises the cues as a *natural* reflective lens to appreciate the unfolding clinical situation moment by moment. As such, pattern appreciation and pattern response are ongoing as a dynamic unfolding process.

The cues are *not* intended as a formulaic response to assess the patient, whereby each cue demands an answer; they cue the practitioner to pay attention to key processes within pattern appreciation. I emphasise the point because the practitioner who has embodied a reductionist systems approach may miss the reflective point and view the cues as another set of boxes to tick. As Sutherland (1994:68) noted:

> Although at first I did find myself going back to the Roper *et al*'s headings to make sure that I had not missed anything, omitting what was physically important, I did not need to do this for very long.

Sutherland further noted the impact of the reflective cues in changing her mindset:

> Because the emphasis is centred on feelings and the total picture of that person's situation rather than on their ongoing physical needs, it forced me to move away from a need to find things out, fill things in and get things done as soon as possible in an orderly fashion. It forced me to start listening to what patients themselves were saying was important to them and then to plan care with them from this basis ... it gradually became a welcome release for me. (p68)

There is something astonishing in Sutherland's words about the way she felt the Burford cues *forced* her to listen to the person, as if she hadn't really listened to the person before. I think it is true, as she suggests, that the 'old model' became the task; hence the effort was to complete it rather than really listen to what the patient or family were saying. As Sutherland suggests, the key is listening and connecting, and then working with the person toward meeting their health–illness needs.

The cues are explored in depth in Chapter 6 in response to *knowing the person* as a dimension of *being available*.

The apparent simplicity and profundity of the cues disarm people trapped within complex systems models. If we want to be reflective practitioners then clearly we need to frame practice through reflective approaches. Models are merely tools to enable something to be created. As such, they are chosen to be fit for purpose. Does a carpenter take a spoon to chisel wood?

A system to ensure effective communication

My audit revealed that the nursing process had no value either as a comprehensive record of care or in enabling the continuity of care. Indeed, the nursing process was considered a hindrance to effective practice because of its deterministic nature.

A more coherent approach than the nursing process to communicating meaningful information about the person's care and treatment was narrative. Simply put, narrative is a way of journeying with the person whereby significant issues of practice are clearly identified and recorded. Similarly, oral communication, for example shift reports, moved from giving information towards dialogue where significant issues of journeying with the person were explored. These aspects are explored in Chapter 12. Clinical practice *is* performance and narrative.

A quality system to ensure effective practice

How can we know whether our care is effective or not? Indeed, how might best practice be known? Here, we enter the world of clinical governance.

Reflective approaches to quality demand that quality is lived using double feedback systems that challenge not only care processes and outcomes but also the standard by which caring is judged. In other words, quality is always dynamic, evolving. It is never static. Things change constantly and so approaches to quality must be fluid in response. When quality is measured against external criteria that do not involve practitioners then quality becomes someone else's business and practitioners do not have to take responsibility for their own performance. As a responsible practitioner, I must take responsibility for ensuring my own effectiveness. This can be achieved by using:

- clinical supervision (see Chapter 15)
- clinical audit (see Chapter 13)
- standards of care (see Chapter 13).

Of course, other systems are necessary from an organisational perspective to enable government targets and benchmarking to be set. However, these tend to focus on arbitrary patient procedure and outcome measures rather than caring. If it is not acknowledged then caring is invisible, devalued, soft 'nursy' stuff that only emerges as an issue in response to patient complaint.

A system to ensure that staff are enabled to realise the vision as a lived reality

In 1990 I established a research project at Burford Hospital to explore the value of guided reflection to enable practitioners to become more effective (Johns 1998a). The project was the foundation work for developing my ideas about reflective practice. Initially I appointed an associate nurse on a 18-month contract on the understanding that she entered into a formal guided reflection relationship. We met approximately every 2–3 weeks for one hour in which she shared experiences of her practice and I guided her to learn through these experiences to enable her to make judgements about her clinical performance and effectiveness. What is interesting is that the standard of effectiveness was ascertained within the moment given the particular experience. Through reflection, the vision became increasingly meaningful as something lived rather than something abstract. Analysis of shared experiences led to the development of the being available template as a way of knowing holism, as explored in Chapters 6 and 7 and evidenced through the practitioner narratives presented in this book.

Organisational culture

What sort of organisational culture needs to exist to accommodate a reflective and holistic approach to clinical practice? I know that existing transactional or bureaucratic cultures cannot accommodate reflective practice simply because they are by their very nature static, reactive and unreflective. Such organisations are overly concerned with risk at the expense of creativity and professional responsibility.

What is required is a culture committed to creating and sustaining a learning environment and transformational leadership that invests in people.

Leadership

At Burford, at the time of developing the reflective model, I was mindful that my role as a clinical leader was to enable practitioners to accept responsibility through developing collaborative relationships about 'our' practice. A transformational leadership is vital to create and sustain the learning organisation. Reflective practice has a strong congruency with the notion of transformational leadership, in contrast with the transactional leadership that generally characterises healthcare organisations.

Burns (1978) defined transformational leadership as when 'one or more persons engage with others in such a way that leaders and followers raise one another to higher levels of motivation and morality [and achievement]'.

Chantal Cara (1999), in her study on nurses' perspective on how management can promote caring practice, notes that when leadership promotes working relationships congruent with caring values then practitioners can be more caring. When they don't, it leads to demoralisation and loss of caring. As Cara notes, 'This research reveals that both the environment and managers can create a significance influence on caring practice' (p27). I explore transformational leadership more deeply in Chapter 14.

The learning organisation

'The primary task of [a transformational] leadership is to establish and sustain the learning organisation' (Senge 1990:3). The learning organisation (LO) is:

> One where people continually expand their capacities to create the results they truly desire, where new and expansive patterns of thinking are nurtured, where collective aspiration is set free, and where people are continually learning how to learn together.

Senge identifies five inter-relating disciplines that constitute the LO: vision, mental models, systems thinking, team learning and personal mastery (Box 2.2) (see Chapter 15). As will

Box 2.2 The disciplines of the learning organisation

Vision	– is a collaborative consensual statement of shared beliefs and beliefs that gives meaning and purpose to clinical practice.
Personal mastery	– is the discipline of holding and resolving creative tension so that vision can be realised as a lived reality. It involves clarifying and deepening personal vision and seeing reality objectively. Senge (1990:141) notes: 'It [personal mastery] goes beyond competence and skills, though it is grounded in competence and skills. It goes beyond spiritual unfolding or opening, although it requires spiritual growth. It means approaching one's life as a creative work, living life from a creative as opposed to reactive viewpoint'.
Mental models	– are deeply ingrained assumptions or images that influence how the practitioner understands the world and how they take action. The discipline of working with mental models starts with turning the mirror inward; learning to unearth our internal images and assumptions of the world, to bring them to the surface and hold them rigorously to scrutiny, and subsequently shifting them in alignment with desirable practice.
Systems thinking	– is appreciating and critiquing the pattern of underlying systems that govern practice and shifting to align these systems with desirable practice when contradictory.
Team learning	– is collaborating with colleagues to realise a shared vision through dialogue – the capacity of members of a team to suspend their individual assumptions and engage in genuine thinking together, recognising and overcoming patterns of interaction that undermine learning. As Isaacs (1993) notes: 'Unfortunately, most forms of organizational conversation, particularly around tough, complex, or challenging issues lapse into debate (the root of which means 'to beat down'). In debate one side wins and another loses; both parties maintain their certainties, and both suppress deeper inquiry. (p24-5) There is nothing collaborative in the patterns of talk that Isaacs alludes to. Such talk reflects patterns of power relationships and rivalry, where people jostle for control typified by people lining up to get their point across and win the argument. Very little genuine listening takes place. People partially listen to what they want to hear, seeking feedback to reinforce their position rather than being open to new possibility through dialogue.

become apparent, personal mastery is the essence of reflective practice and the gateway for developing the learning organisation built on the foundation of shared vision towards shared success.

The Burford model's explicit assumptions

A reflective model or framework for clinical practice can be summarised as a set of explicit assumptions.

- Caring in practice is grounded in a valid vision for practice.
- The practitioner is mindful of easing suffering and nurturing growth as she goes about her practice moment to moment.
- The core therapeutic of nursing practice is the practitioner *being available* – a 'working with' relationship focused to enable the other to find meaning in their health–illness experience, to make best decisions and help take appropriate action to ease suffering and meet their life needs.
- Growth is a mutual process of realisation.
- Practitioners accept responsibility for working toward creating the learning organisation (Senge 1990) and transformational leadership.
- Caring in practice is a responsive and reflexive form in context with the environment in which it is practised.

Conclusion

In this chapter I have outlined a reflective model to structure clinical practice based on a valid collaborative vision that unites practitioners across disciplines in common purpose. Four systems are proposed to enable the vision to become a reality within a transformational leadership and learning organisational culture. In Chapter 3 I develop the idea of guided reflection and narrative construction through six dialogical movements.

Chapter 3
Becoming reflective

So far I have explored the nature of reflection and how clinical practice can be structured through a reflective model. In this chapter I establish the idea of reflection through six dialogical movements. I then explore the first two movements.

But first, a story I wrote following a nursing shift in a community hospital.

Tom and Joan[1]

I go with Marie, a healthcare assistant (HCA), to wash Mr Sturch. 'Hello Mr Sturch.' I introduce myself as Chris, a visiting nurse. 'Call me Tom', he says. I sense his need to be recognised and respected for who he is together with his need for familiarity.

At the shift report we had been informed how miserable Tom was being in hospital and being shut in a single room because of the risk of cross-infection due to his diarrhoea. We were waiting for results of a bowel culture. If Tom's stools were clear he could be moved back into the main ward.

As I was scheduled to work with Marie, I paid attention to knowing her. She is in her 50s and very committed to caring. She loves it and would love to be a nurse. She is experiencing some strain in her personal life with her mother very ill. She and her husband moved here some years ago. Now she travels every weekend, driving about 3 hours each way to care for her mother. I listen and help her talk through her feelings and options, even though we are little more than passing strangers. In doing so we begin to construct a therapeutic relationship.

Marie's approach to Tom is familiar and caring, but task focused. I immediately notice the characteristic pattern of parent–child communication. Tom is like a little boy, upset but trying hard to be good. Marie is mother, protective, kind, although her tolerance is limited to the extent that there is work to be done. I ask Tom how he feels this morning. He easily expresses his distress at being in hospital and shut up in this room. His tears are close to the surface. He is lonely in the side room and embarrassed that these poor girls have to clean him up. Marie kindly informs Tom that we are going to wash him. This is not negotiated with him. He needs considerable physical help as he has Parkinson's disease. His left hand in particular continues to tremor and his right side has been weakened by a previous stroke.

We begin to wash him as he lies on the bed. When he asks for the commode, I note the impact of his Ménière's disease characterised by his nausea on standing. The symptom is poorly controlled. Ensuring he feels safe, we leave him to use the commode. Afterwards, we help him complete his wash whilst sitting on the commode. I help him stand whilst

---

[1] A version of this narrative was first published in *Nursing Inquiry* (Johns 1998c).

Marie washes his bottom. On seeing Tom like that I am struck by Mary Madrid's (1990) account about the nurse imagining who the patient is in terms of his past. Tom tells me he had been a staff sergeant in the army during the Second World War, working in recruitment training. I can imagine him like that. How straight and proud he must have been and now, what a different way to parade. And yet I can say that to him with humour, acknowledging his past while being empathic with this moment. I realise the significance of this approach in respecting people. After the war, Tom had been an engineer in microwaves, work that reflected his intelligence. I resist a sense of pity at his current state. Instead I feel a wave of compassion towards him. I have learnt from previous experiences about acknowledging self-discomfort towards patients and families and confronting this through enabling the other to talk through their experience.

After his wash, Tom cleans his own teeth. He is normally shaven using an electric razor because the nurses feel clumsy with wet shaves even though Tom likes a wet shave. He appreciates the wet shave I give him. I am mindful how this 'little thing' (Macleod 1994) of shaving Tom makes a difference in caring. I know this informs Tom of my concern for him.By paying him attention, my concern is fed and grows. I experience a mutuality in his response. He begins to care for me.

Although we have only just met, I have been involved with him in intimate physical care – washing him, being here while he was on the toilet, wiping his bottom, shaving him – and emotional presence.Tom easily discloses other aspects of his life. He has been married for 59 years to 'wifie', his endearing term for his wife. Indeed, his diamond anniversary was in February. He becomes alive talking about his wife and their life together. She visits in the afternoons. He desperately wants to go home but is anxious about the future. He is so dependent physically and even though they had a support package, he fears he will be too much of a burden for 'wifie'. I wonder if he would be happier with television, some music or a paper? No, he just wants 'wifie' and to go home. I sense my need to 'fix it' for him, an almost overwhelming need to take his distress away from him. But of course, I am becoming anxious on his behalf, beginning to absorb his distress, which I recognise and repattern to be available to him.

Rubbing his smooth face, he thanks me. It feels good. His offers me a 'Murray mint – too good to hurry mint' (for those who remember the TV advert) – his gift in return for my attention, my respect and kindness. In seeking to connect with me, he needs to give something back. By accepting, I honour this need and he can honour himself. We begin to tune into a reciprocal relationship, where I can respond with an appropriate level of involvement with Tom. In this way I synchronise our rhythms of relating with each other at this moment. In tune with him, I am most available to him.

I am mindful of the ways in which I paid attention to him in response to his feelings and needs, which had made him so happy this morning when he had been so miserable. Nurses are focused on the tasks of the morning and don't necessarily see him from his perspective. They may see him as a person but that's not their frame for responding. Marie noticed the difference in him this morning and passed this off as 'male company being good for him'. I was able to say when his doctor visited that Tom's stool was now semi-formed and to assert Tom's desire to move back into the main ward. This request was granted. I could also challenge the adequacy of the medical treatment for Tom's Ménière's disease, to prompt a review of the medical response. The doctor welcomed my feedback. I felt good. I also had several 'Murray mints'.

At lunchtime I move over to the dinner trolley. Cook–chill. The domestics say the quality is quite good. They are serving dinners. I express my surprise at the absence of a nurse. 'That's all right, the nurses are often busy so we get on.'

One patient, Joan, has severe arthritis. She struggles to eat one-handed with an adapted fork, chasing the food around the plate. She has neither plateguard nor slipmat. The adapter fork is not effective as she holds the handle below the padded stem. I fix a plateguard. These things are so obvious – why can't others see them?

After lunch I sit with Joan considering whether I might offer her some therapeutic touch. My agenda – yet I am sensitive not to impose this on her. I am always mindful of Hall's (1964) challenge of nurses 'strutting their new skills'. These people are so passive, it would be so easy to impose a parental, 'we know best' stance, as a natural response to this passivity. We talk. I need to know this woman, who she is, to understand her experience of being here in hospital and her perceptions of the future. Joan is only 78 although she looks older, small and wrinkled but always with a smile on her suffering face. She is stoic and courageous, and would never make a fuss. Her twisted wrists give visual evidence to her advanced arthritis. She is in hospital for respite care. Her stay has been extended following a new mild stroke she experienced 5 days earlier. She is extremely anxious and distressed. We explore these emotions. She is afraid she won't go home because her husband can no longer manage to care for her. He is 80 and not in good health. She cries. Clearly it was deeply in her mind. Behind this brave and cheerful face she presents to the world she doesn't want to be a burden to anyone. She needs to be the co-operative, uncomplaining patient. Perhaps she has learnt this way of being through her chronic illness career.

I help her explore her home possibilities, that 'we' need to sit down with her and her husband and see what can be done. For example, her major fear is getting to the toilet but she has not considered the possibility of a commode. She has not walked for 5 days since the 'stroke'. I note she has not yet been referred to the physiotherapist. I offer to help her take a few steps. She is happy with this idea. She stands by herself. She struggles to grip the Zimmer frame, her normal walking aide, but refuses my help, murmuring through gritted her teeth 'I will do it'. She walks six steps before losing her right-hand grip.

Her notes are scanty. They tell me nothing about her and are associated with activities of living; Joan has difficulty washing, going to the toilet, with obvious goals of assistance.

I write in her care plan (Table 3.1):

In writing these notes I remind myself of the Burford cue questions (see Chapter 2): 'How does this person see the future for self and others?', 'What support does this person have in life?'. I write these two questions together with a brief summary of our work together within the 'progress' notes to help others see her as I have done.

Table 3.1 Joan's care plan

Problem	Goal	Intervention	Evaluation
4. Joan is anxious to recover her mobility. She managed to walked six steps this afternoon with Zimmer frame (her normal walking aide) before losing right-hand grip. (date)		Can we refer to the physiotherapist for assessment?	
5. Joan is very anxious about the future.		Can we sit down and talk with her and her husband about their future/fears? He is very deaf.	

I am reminded of Hall's words (1964): 'It is impossible to nurse any more of a person than that person allows us to see'. I thought 'how blind we have been'. Perhaps there is a taken for grantedness by staff because Joan is a respite patient despite her stroke. The staff seem well disposed to her, although I sense that they unwittingly contribute to her suffering by not seeing and responding to her and her husband in terms of their concerns. Her husband does not seem to be in the nurses' gaze at all. Perhaps his needs are met by providing respite care. Even in this ward dedicated to elderly people with chronic illness, the nurses essentially view practice through a medical/physical-oriented lens. The inappropriateness of this lens is stark and yet no-one can see it.

Considering the paucity of the notes, I realize that notes are not an effective way to communicate these concerns. I decide to reinforce my notes by talking it through with the nurse in charge. She is receptive to my feedback, although again I am wary about overstepping my welcome as some interfering academic. Better to avoid potential conflict. I think to myself 'how easy it is to marginalise self and become ineffective as a consequence' – another fine line to tread. Yet in doing so, do I compromise my integrity? I share with Joan what I have written and urge her to express her fears with the staff, that the staff will be receptive. But I doubt whether she will be able to do this. Later I see her husband and go to talk with them. He is small like Joan and very deaf. She is pleased to be with him and thankful for my intervention.

I never get to do my therapeutic touch but I feel good. I have experienced the mutuality of caring. I have quickly established a connected relationship with Joan and later with her husband. I feel certain that she, like Tom, connected with my concern.

Later, reflecting, I begin to doubt myself; did I enable the staff to see Tom and Joan in their humanness and plight well enough? I realise that practice culture is deeply embodied and not easily shifted.

Narrative

I was tired after the shift but thoughts and feelings about this experience were swimming in my head. I had to write about them and get them out of my head as authentically as I could. My journal is littered with expletives about how I felt, expletives edited out of the narrative and yet important to acknowledge.

Writing my journal is the first step towards constructing the narrative as a process of self-inquiry and transformation towards realising desirable practice – or being and becoming the practitioner I wanted to become.

It is the movement through six dialogical movements within the hermeneutic cycle (Fig. 3.1). The *hermeneutic circle* refers to the idea that one's understanding of the text as a whole is established by reference to the individual parts and one's understanding of each individual part by reference to the whole. Neither the whole text nor any individual part can be understood without reference to one another and hence, it is a circle (Wikipedia). In other words, the part receiving attention is always viewed against the background of the whole which constantly changes in response, ever deepening and unfolding the level of understanding.

Dialogue

Before exploring the six dialogical movements, I must first give attention to the idea of dialogue. Dialogue comes from the Greek word *dialogos*, which can be taken to mean

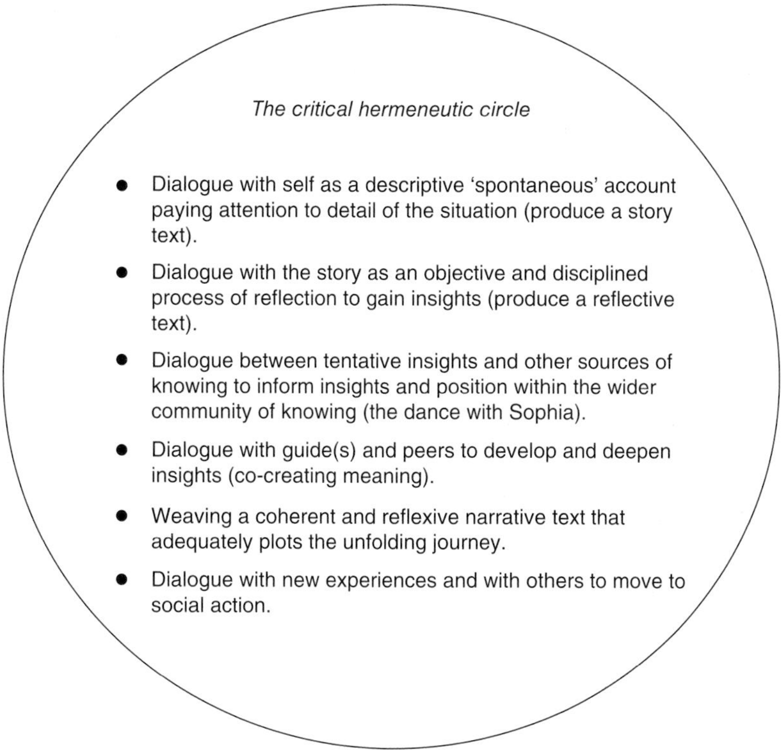

The critical hermeneutic circle

- Dialogue with self as a descriptive 'spontaneous' account paying attention to detail of the situation (produce a story text).

- Dialogue with the story as an objective and disciplined process of reflection to gain insights (produce a reflective text).

- Dialogue between tentative insights and other sources of knowing to inform insights and position within the wider community of knowing (the dance with Sophia).

- Dialogue with guide(s) and peers to develop and deepen insights (co-creating meaning).

- Weaving a coherent and reflexive narrative text that adequately plots the unfolding journey.

- Dialogue with new experiences and with others to move to social action.

Figure 3.1 Narrative as six dialogical movements.

'meaning flowing among and through us ... out of which may emerge some new understanding (Bohm 1996:6).

Isaacs (1993:25) describes dialogue as:

a discipline of collective thinking and inquiry, a process for transforming the quality of conversation and, in particular, the thinking that lies beneath it ... a movement towards creating a field of genuine meeting and inquiry where people can allow a *free flow of meaning* and vigorous exploration of the collective background of their thought, their personal predispositions, the nature of their shared attention, and the rigid features of their individual and collective assumptions ... as people learn to perceive, inquire into, and allow transformation of the nature and shape of these fields, and the patterns of individual thinking and acting that inform them, they may discover entirely new levels of insight and forge substantive and, at times, dramatic changes in behaviour. As this happens, whole new possibilities for co-ordinated action develop.

Based on Bohm's work, I identify six rules of dialogue:

1. commitment to work with others towards consensus for a better world
2. awareness and suspension of one's own assumptions and prejudices
3. proprioception of thinking
4. to be open to possibility and free from attachment to ideas
5. to listen with engagement and respect
6. to have a mutual appreciation of dialogue.

Dialogue can be with oneself, as if self is both object and subject, or with groups of people. It is always *moving towards* consensus for a better world. The emphasis on *moving towards* acknowledges a *letting go of attachment* to old ideas. The idea of a better world suggests that all action is moral social action towards this end. To dialogue, people must not only know and suspend their assumptions and opinions, but also be aware of the thinking that gave rise to these assumptions in the first place. Where do they arise from, how tenaciously do we cling to them? Why do we cling to them? This requires a *proprioception of thinking*, an awareness of where the mind is at the moment. Within the dialogical process there is a shift from problem solving towards acknowledging and resolving paradox that requires thinking about the way people think about things. If we use the same thinking that caused the problem to try and solve the problem, we fail. Hence we need to change the way we think to view the problem differently.

Bohm (1996:25) writes:

> We could say that practically all the problems of the human race are due to the fact that thought is not proprioceptive. Thought is constantly creating problems that way and then trying to solve them. But as it tries to solve them it makes it worse because it doesn't notice that it's creating them, and the more it thinks, the more problems it creates – because it's not proprioceptive of what it's doing.

Mezirow (1981) calls this critical consciousness – the ability to be conscious of our consciousness, alert to our mental models and how these influence the way we are thinking and feeling within the unfolding moment. In other words, *being mindful*. Only then can people transform their perspectives to see things differently.

The key to dialogue is to listen; only when people *really* listen can they hear what is being said or not being said. We probably all claim to listen but do we listen carefully? Or do we listen to what we want to hear or distort what we hear in order to fit into our own scheme, to confirm our own assumptions?

Dialogue opens the gateway to creativity. Tuffnell and Crickmay (2004:41) note that:

> Creating becomes a conversation when we enter into a dialogue with whatever we are doing. In this conversation we are drawn along in the moment by moment flow of sensation, interchange and choice, rather than following a predetermined intention or idea.

Dialogue is compelling and yet it is not a natural way of communicating. Consider the types of conversations you have in your practice – to what extent are they creative and flowing towards shared meaning and shared success?

The first dialogical movement: doodles in my journal

Boud *et al* (1985:27) inform us that:

> one of the most useful activities that can initiate a period of reflection is recollecting what has taken place and replaying the experience in the mind's eye, to observe the event as it had happened and to notice exactly what occurred and one's reaction to it in all its elements, it may be helpful to commit this description to paper, or to describe it to others. By whatever means this occurs the description should involve a close attention to detail and should refrain from making judgments.

I write reflections or stories of my practice in a journal. In writing my journal I naturally focus myself in relation to others. Indeed, I define myself in relation to others. In deconstructing these relationships, I get glimpses of myself through the reflection of the other. I get glimpses of the relationship between my thinking and my action, between the relationship of my practice with knowledge, between my values and the assumptions I find myself holding, and with broader organisational and professional mores that are themselves a reflection of deeper social and cultural patterns of relating. Journal writing is listening to my voice. Inevitably, it is intensely personal.

Susan Brooks (2004) reflects on being invited to keep a journal with the intent of constructing her leadership narrative.

Having never attempted to keep a reflective journal before – the journey ahead seemed a little daunting as evidenced by the first recorded entry that reflects the fear that I experienced at that time.

March 2002 – Today I start my journal. What shall I write? I'm really worried about this whole thing –will I get time to do it – will I want to do it – will I do it right? If I'm honest in it will it matter if others read it? Reflective practice, reflective practice – what is it really? I think I know but I don't think I've ever really done it properly. I feel so uncertain about everything at the moment and a bit scared and threatened. I don't feel I know anything about myself really and I suppose I just do what I do to fit in. I need to get over this and get on with it – pull yourself together Sue – you know you can do it.

This first journal entry, when I read it in retrospect, clearly reveals my initial uncomfortable reactions to the prospect of journal writing. I had doubts about my capacity to write, felt threatened by having to face myself on paper, questioned my ability to manage my internal censors that may inhibit complete honesty and held the naïve assumption that there is a correct way to keep a journal – all classic reactions to journalling (Street 1995).

These initial fears were quickly dispelled as the value of my journal soon became evident. After a while, it seemed to become a powerful emancipatory tool in giving my innermost thoughts voice. I was the only person with access to the journal and, possibly because of this, it became a very cathartic experience to write. As the process continued, I soon recognised that I did not need to confront all the chaos of my personal or professional life at any one time and became more discriminatory about the events that I considered worthy of deeper reflection and subsequent action (Street 1995). The journal became, in a sense, my autobiography containing both positive and less than positive experiences – a non-hagiographic record of my daily life. My journal had, after just a few months on the course, become a silent but very powerful and challenging teacher – perhaps more persuasive and influential than any human embodiment that I had met. The following entry signifies just how my attitude had changed since that first entry at the start of the course.

July 2002 – I read of a teacher today who got very excited about writing his journal. He wrote that he felt especially good about writing for himself instead of someone else. His written thoughts were entirely his own regardless of lack of style, format or academic expression. He had never written like this before and felt that he was really communicating with and understanding himself. That's just how I feel now and I wish I had started writing like this ages ago. To be unrestricted by structural rigour, academic expectations and the approval of others is so liberating!

From the practical aspect, a double-entry technique was used with the factual account (data collection) of the experience written on the left of the page and the reflective thought (the analysis) on the right (Moon 2002). Both the ordinary and extraordinary events of everyday practice were included to prevent selective inattention, particularly to the seemingly mundane, where habitual routinized practice is thought most likely to occur. I considered myself to be the primary research tool here. If the journal was to accurately and consistently record my own experiential world I needed to maintain a strong sense of commitment to the task and demonstrate the skills necessary to the reflective cycle – self-awareness, description, critical analysis, synthesis and evaluation (Atkins and Murphy 1993).

Keeping a journal enabled me to enter into a dialogue between my objective and subjective self and it transformed my feeling self into a spectator and analyst of my own personal professional drama (Street 1985). Street (1985) writes that journalling provides the reflector with a process for meta-theorising, that is, thinking about the processes of thinking. This significantly developed not only my skills of reflection but also my skills as a learner in general, moving me away from my previously held attitude that knowledge (and not necessarily enhanced learning skills) was the goal to be achieved.

Some people like to tell their stories whilst others prefer to write them. Indeed, many practitioners get stuck between telling their story and writing it. It is as if they hit a mental block. Perhaps the oral telling is more spontaneous whilst writing is more considered, more cognitive, more self-conscious. I sense the presence of an internal censor at work in writing that tries to fit the description into learned ways of writing that dismiss or denigrate feelings and imagination. Whatever, some people struggle to write. Perhaps telling stories is essentially a creative right brain act whilst writing is essentially a left brain activity and between the two sides of the brain, the connections are fuzzy and censored. If so, the practitioner may need guidance to release the imaginative and creative power into her writing.

Schön (1983) suggests a difficulty even in saying what we know, that much of our knowing is tacit and not easily explainable.

> When we go about the spontaneous intuitive performance of the actions of everyday life, we show ourselves to be knowledgeable in a certain way. Often we cannot say what it is we know. When we try to describe it we find ourselves at loss or we produce descriptions that are obviously inappropriate. Our knowing is ordinarily tacit, implicit in our action and in our feel for the stuff with which we are dealing. It seems right to say that our knowing is in our doing. (p49)

Spontaneous writing taps the tacit; it brings it to the surface like a bubbling underground brook. Holly (1989:71) notes that 'writing taps the unconscious; it can make the implicit explicit, and therefore open to analysis'. It is bringing feelings and thoughts to the surface where they can be looked at. Ferruci (1982:41) says:

> Writing … can be much more powerful than we may think at first … we should not be surprised that unconscious material surfaces so readily in our writing though that may surface all sorts of demons that we may prefer to keep quiet.

Ben Okri (1997:22) writes:

> The creative self has one side facing the dark waters, and the other side facing the bright and joyful firmament. Paradoxically, it flows into all things: and your spirit, in approaching it, should be able to flow into all things, all thoughts, all possible realities. Do not disdain the idle, strange, ordinary, nonsensical, or shocking thoughts the mind throws up. Hold them. Look at them. Play with them. See where they lead. Every perception or possibility has its own life-span: some have short lives, others keep growing, and may open to infusions of greater life.

The emphasis on the creative side is such a vital perspective on writing. It should be approached with a playful and creative spirit. IT is YOU! In writing, you are writing yourself, your body, nurturing your precious and unique self. In writing, you change yourself on a subliminal level. As Ferruci (1982:42) says, 'It is like cutting a new pathway in a jungle'.

In the quiet evening

Although I usually carry my reflective journal around with me in my briefcase, I most often write my reflections in the evening when I can dwell with my thoughts and consider the events of the past few days with less distraction than at work. Even the most ordinary events have great significance for the mindful practitioner. Everyday experiences are a source of rich learning. Reflective writing brings events into focus, enabling the journal to act as a midwife, giving birth to new understanding (Pinar 1981). Yet, interestingly, I rarely reflect on my educational work as a university lecturer, at least in a written format. Part of the reason for this is that I use my practice reflections as educational material and research activity. I like to teach the palliative care students 'around the camp-fire' – where I share my own stories of palliative care to trigger stories in others and to role model the art of reflective writing.

So ask yourself – how might you write?

Reflective activity

Think of the last time you were at work. Now think about one particular situation. It needn't be dramatic. It can simply be something mundane or ordinary, something you wouldn't normally give a second thought – something you did that on the surface was unproblematic.

Now write a description of this situation for 15 minutes. Try not to take your pen off the paper. Try not to stop and think too much about the why's of the situation. Just let the pen flow, paying attention to detail, drawing on all your senses.

31 October 2008 – I am leading a reflective practice workshop for speech and language therapists in Scotland. First, I read a narrative of my own practice with Trevor, a patient with a cerebral tumour with speech and communication difficulties – a story they can relate with in terms of their own experiences. I then ask them to write for about 18 minutes about a recent experience that seems significant in some way that happened earlier in the week. Many are still writing as I call 'time'. I ask how this experience was for them. Many are surprised they can write so much. Paying attention to detail opens up many aspects of the experience they had not sensed. Often one thing had led to another as they followed their flow of consciousness. Some naturally pay attention to feelings, some find themselves problem solving, some work through difficult feelings realising the cathartic value of writing. All find the experience of writing meaningful, enlightening even playful. Time had flown by. Only a few of the 25 therapists had journalled previously.

The second dialogical movement: surfing the reflective spiral

Having written a rich description, I now step back and enter into a dialogue with the text with the intention of finding meaning in the text and drawing insights. Insights are changed perceptions: that gaining insight is changing self, that I come to see and respond to the world differently. To dialogue, I must stand back enough from the text to see it objectively – moving into a subjective-objective relationship with it. I must pull myself free from any entanglement in order to see my reality clearly. Easier said than done because the text reflects who I am. It reflects my mental models – deeply ingrained assumptions, generalisations and values that influence how I understand the world.

Cleaning this lens, opening it to scrutiny and questioning its images enables me to approach experiences in a new way, allowing me to have a more thoughtful engagement with the experience (Van Manen 1990). A guide might be helpful, especially if you are new to reflection. As you become more experienced this ability to work within an objective-subjective stance becomes easier. We literally learn to see ourselves as we develop proprioception of thought.

Someone approaching reflection for the first time might ask certain questions.

- What is reflection?
- How do I do it?
- How do I know if I am doing it properly?
- How do I learn through reflection?

Such questions reflect a technological approach – how can I know and do reflection? Important questions for the novice reflective practitioner to find the path. Whilst there are many frameworks available to practitioners to access reflection, it is vital that they see it only as a path and not the destination.

John Driscoll (2000) posits three reflective movements: What? So what? Now what? I used this approach recently in summing up the Toronto reflective practice conference in May 2008. I asked the audience –what has been happening during the conference? I then asked – what's been significant about what's been happening? And lastly I asked – what learning has taken place and how do we move forward from here as a consequence? The questions enabled a flow of thought that moved through the conference into an anticipated future.

Guarding against a prescriptive legacy

I am wary of cyclical or stage models such as Gibbs (1988) because they suggest that reflection is an orderly step-by-step progression. Reflection is not a neat movement between different stages or cycles. To view it in this way suggests a mechanical flow through discrete stages. Reflection is complex, whereby the mind engages all the stages. There may be some value of stage models for novice practitioners in helping them grasp the essence of reflection although I think the MSR does this adequately without the need for stages. My caution is that stage models immediately present reflection as some technical linear task. In a technological society, the risk exists that reflective models will be grasped as a technology and used in concrete ways. From a technological perspective (as opposed to a reflective perspective), the risk is that practitioners will fit their experience to the model of reflection rather than using the model creatively to guide them to see self within the context of the particular experience (I make the same point about models of nursing in Chapter 2).

I must emphasise that all models of reflection are merely devices to help the practitioner to access reflection, they are not a prescription of what reflection is. In other words, models are heuristic – a means toward an end, not an end in itself. From a reflective perspective, the practitioner will view all models for their value, rather than accepting the authority of the model on face value. Rather like the skilled craftsman, the practitioner will choose the tool that is most helpful.

Reflect on Rinpoche's words (1992:64-5):

> Largely because of our Western technological culture people tend to be absorbed by what I would call 'the technology of meditation' [reflection]. The modern world, after all, is fascinated by mechanisms and machines, and addicted to purely practical formulae. But by far the most important feature of meditation [reflection] is not the technique, but the spirit: the skilful, inspired, and creative way in which we practice [reflect], which could also be called the 'posture'.

The model for structured reflection (MSR)

Having warned against a prescriptive legacy, I now discuss the MSR that I designed as a guide to enable practitioners to access the depth and breadth of reflection necessary for learning through experience. I first designed the MSR in 1991 through analysing the patterns of dialogue that took place in guided reflection relationships framed within Strauss and Corbin's grounded theory paradigm model (Johns 1998a). Since then, the MSR design has been reflexively reviewed, culminating in the current 15A edition (Box 3.1). The cues within the MSR are arranged in a logical order, enabling a progression of thought through each cue. Remember – the cues are merely cues, a means towards gaining insight. With use, the reflective cues become embodied and shape the clinical gaze moment by moment in mindful attention. In constructing the 15th edition, I added the new cue '*What factors might constrain me responding in new ways?*'. I have also added '*What insights have I gained?*' alongside '*Am I more able to realise desirable work?*'.

Box 3.1   The Model for Structured Reflection (edition 15A)

Reflective cue
- Bring the mind home
- Focus on a description of an experience that seems significant in some way
- What issues are significant to pay attention to?
- How do I interpret the way people were feeling and why they felt that way?
- How was I feeling and what made me feel that way?
- What was I trying to achieve and did I respond effectively ? (aesthetic)
- What were the consequences of my actions on the patient, others and myself?
- What factors influence the way I was/am feeling, thinking and responding to this situation? (personal)
- What knowledge did or might have informed me? (empirical)
- To what extent did I act for the best and in tune with my values? (ethical)
- How does this situation connect with previous experiences? (personal)
- How might I reframe the situation and respond more effectively given this situation again? (reflexivity)
- What would be the consequences of alternative actions for the patient, others and myself?
- What factors might constrain me responding in new ways?
- How do I NOW feel about this experience?
- Am I more able to support myself and others better as a consequence?
- What insights have I gained?
- Am I more able to realise desirable practice? (framing perspectives)

Moving into dialogue with the text, I dwell with the text, asking it questions. This dialogue takes me into a reflective spiral – moving from perception (significance – what lies on the surface of the experience and what may seem obvious) to insights that lie enfolded within the text (enfolded within me).

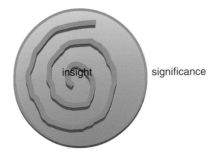

This is a journey into self to find meaning. As Van Manen (1990:58) notes:

> It is not a simple matter of etymological analysis or explication of the usage of the word. Rather, it is the construction of a way of life to live the language of our lives more deeply, to become more truly who we are when we refer to ourselves as doctors, nurses, therapists.

The MSR cues also have considerable value in developing clinical skills, as I highlight through my exploration of each cue.

Bringing the mind home

31 May 2008 – I am attending the reflective practice conference 'Refresh, Reflect, Renew' in Toronto that I have convened in collaboration with Centennial colleagues in Toronto. My birthday. Fran gives me a card in which he quotes Ram Dass: 'The quieter you become, the more you can hear'. Ah! So simple, so true! Bringing the mind home.

Bringing the mind home is not so much a reflective cue but a preparatory cue, to put the person in the best position to reflect. The idea of bringing the mind home was inspired by Sogyal Rinpoche (1992), in his book *The Tibetan book of living and dying*. He states:

> We are fragmented into so many different parts. We don't know who we really are, or what aspects of ourselves we should identify with or believe in. So many contradictory voices, dictates, and feelings fight for control over our inner lives that we find ourselves scattered everywhere, in all directions, leaving no one at home. *Reflection then helps to bring the mind home* (p59)[2]. ... Yet how hard it can be to turn our attention within! How easily we allow our old habits and set patterns to dominate us! Even though they bring us suffering, we accept them with almost fatalistic resignation, for we are so used to giving into them. (p31)

Do you recognise yourself in Rinpoche's words? The focus on bringing the mind home helps to shift the balance of seeing reflection as a cognitive activity to a more meditative

---

[2] Italics are my emphasis. I replaced 'meditation' with 'reflection'.

activity – a time of quiet contemplation to pay attention to the self – the way I think, feel and respond to situations, mindful of the gusts that will blow us off course and skilled to hold the rudder fast when the currents would take us elsewhere. Yet can we create this space within ourselves to bring the mind home?

> We must slow down or we will miss all that has meaning. Meaning is revealed only when you pause, when you stop, when you pay attention. Learn the lesson of the tribal people. Put your busy-ness on pause, eliminate distractions, and allow the meaning of life and living to return to you. Slow down in order to connect to the meaning of life. (Blackwolf and Jones 1996:90)

Taking time out to reflect sounds like easy advice, but when our lives are addicted to being busy, it may be hard to focus one's thoughts within rather than be scattered outside. Although Rinpoche is referring to meditation, reflection is a similar activity.

Susan Brooks (2004) writes:

> One of the most priceless skills learnt over the last 2 years is that of bringing home my mind – slipping out of the noose of anxiety, releasing all grasping and relaxing into my true nature (Rinpoche 1992). Rinpoche (1992) records that by relaxing in this uncontrived, open and natural state we obtain the blessing of aimless self-liberation of whatever arises. This has certainly been my experience and the joy of feeling able to distance myself from the daily pressures of work by bringing my mind home is immense and a practice that, I believe, will stay with me indefinitely. Hatha yoga has become an element of my daily practice as a means to bring my mind home and to promote my own physical and mental well-being in a meditative context. Such practice has revealed to me that *I* do matter as a person and am not simply a faceless cog in the healthcare organisation. How many times have I said or heard the comment, 'I am just a nurse'? Nurses generally have not trusted their own sense of self-importance enough and yet the fact that nurses do matter is a fundamental truth (Tschudin 1993). Bringing my mind home focuses me on me, underpins my own sense of self-importance but also emphasises my crucial need, as a transformative leader, to recognise and encourage the development of the personhood and thoughts of others. Reflective thought has become a pleasure rather than a threat and as I sit to review the period of this study and my journey so far, I am contentedly aware that my mind is unshackled by the contradictory voices, dictates and feelings that usually fight for control over our inner lives (Rinpoche 1992). Being available to self in this way has implications for my leadership, support and development of others since I would argue that unless I am truly available and knowing to self, transference of such availability would be problematic.

Calligraphy

Journal entry – On my birthday Fran Biley gave me the calligraphy he had painted in Japan on his recent visit. It was the Japanese symbol for the heart. He had used it in his evocative presentation at the Toronto conference. I was struck with the simplicity and beauty of his work. He talked about the meditative significance of such activity towards developing mindfulness, inspiring me to play with this idea in enabling mindfulness with therapists attending a two-day mindfulness workshop at the Christie Hospital. I give each member of the group a copy of the Japanese symbol for compassion (see overleaf).

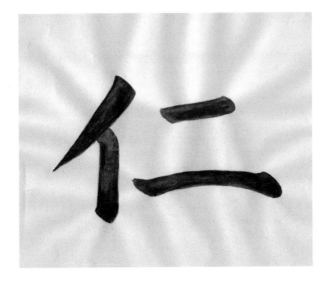

I asked them to carefully paint this symbol in black ink and to sign their name in red ink. Prior to this activity we had meditated for about 20 minutes using the breath to quieten the mind. The room is very still and for 30 minutes the group paint. I chose this particular symbol because compassion is healing energy. I sensed that doing this activity would nurture and stir the therapists' stillness and compassion. The results are profound.

Practical skills (1)

- Bringing self fully present to the moment
- Dealing with stress or anxiety
- Teaching patients to relax through the breath
- Sense of being in control
- Nurturing compassion

What issues are significant to pay attention to?

Standing back from the text, I ask myself – what is significant within the text? This may seem obvious as presumably I paid attention to the experience for a reason. Perhaps moved by a feeling or thought. Writing the description clarifies the thought or feeling, bringing it into focus together with all the other stuff that lies around it.

Standing back, looking more objectively, I can see the pattern within the whole and can begin to see the relationships between things. Dwelling with the text, I can pull out significance for exploration but never losing sight of its relationship within the whole of the experience.

So much seems significant within my text of Tom and Joan. My text feels like an exposé of nursing culture, as if I have lifted the edge of the curtain to reveal what goes on inside. I find myself inside struggling to reconcile my caring values with normal practice. The contradictions are stark and painful to experience. I feel my frustration yet temper it in a need not to appear overly critical, not to alienate myself. It is somewhere I want to return to, somewhere I might offer my expertise. Perhaps, as a consequence, my voice is muted. It suggests but does not condemn.

Also Tom and Joan's voices are significant. Are their voices heard and respected? I found myself advocating for their voices and yet urging them to find and express a voice that could be heard. The idea of advocating becomes significant. Does my advocating for these patients disempower them? By advocating, I sense I also wanted to open the eyes of the staff to see these people in their suffering and that we might better ease their suffering.

The unwitting carelessness of the staff is significant, as are my values that might judge such carelessness. I was frustrated with Marie. She was not mindful of her impact on Tom – like so much of care, it had become mundane and routine, as if these patients had become objects of care rather than engaged in care. What time would Tom liked to have bathed? Probably, given the choice, he would say whatever time is convenient to you. I know from previous experience that patients like Tom endeavour to fit in with nursing patterns, they want to be co-operative, they do not want to be a nuisance despite their suffering. Perhaps they have learnt from previous experience that it pays to fit in rather than be viewed as some difficult, dirty, demanding, old man. Perhaps Tom knows he will get more kindly attention if he fits in.

So the list goes on. I am certain that you can tease out many more issues that are significant for you …

Practical skills (2)

> - Paying attention and recognising significance within the unfolding situation
> - Developing the senses
> - Becoming aware of the person within the context of their life and the practice environment

31 October 2008 – I ask the speech and language therapists to identify what is significant in their written stories, encouraging them to look just under the surface or skin of the story to notice less obvious significances. Laura offers to share the experience she has written. I ask each of the other therapists to tell Laura one thing they feel is significant within her story. Such a rich feast of significances that expands Laura's own observation. I note that this is one way we can work in peer-guided reflection (see Chapter 16).

How were others feeling and what made them feel that way?

Without doubt, illness and admission to hospital create significant anxiety for people. How did Tom, Joan and Marie and others involved in my reflection feel? And why did they feel that way? Was Marie wrapped up in her own concerns with her mother and hence less available to give herself to Tom? I like to think so but I do not know Marie, and such ideas are speculative. I mustn't jump to hasty conclusions and label her as uncaring or careless. Tom's and Joan's feelings were worn on their sleeve for anyone to see if they glanced that way. They were in deep despair, fearful of uncertain futures. I was aware that Tom's needs (and his wife's needs) were not being met. Understanding how others are feeling strengthens my empathic inquiry – my ability to know and connect with the experience of the other person.

Practical skills (3)

- Developing empathic inquiry
- Catharsis

How was I feeling and what made me feel that way?

> We grow by being where we are and experiencing what our life is right now. We must experi-
> ence our anger, our sorrow, our failure, our apprehension; they can all be our teachers when
> we do not separate ourselves from them. When we escape from what is given, we cannot learn,
> we cannot grow. That's not hard to understand, just hard to do. Those who persist, however,
> will be those who will grow in understanding and compassion. How long is such practice
> required? Forever. (Beck 1989:124)

I was troubled by my experience with Tom and Joan at the hospital because of the contradiction I was experiencing between my values and the reality of the situation.

I felt frustrated with my colleagues. I do not state my frustration with Marie and the unit generally. I did write in my reflective journal 'why are we so blind to the patient's experience?'. I highlighted in Tom's notes key issues in his care, notably his distress and fears. I also shared this verbally with the unit sister, having no confidence that the notes were an effective form of communication. I hope my presence with Tom modelled a way of being with Tom that would influence Marie, but I doubt it. I doubt it because ways of being are deeply embodied. Yet she did note the difference in Tom even as she ratio-nalised that as male company.

I have often used this story in my teaching to prompt discussion. The story evokes much passion, guilt and outrage. Yet the same nurses who express such strong emotion seem to be chained by their inappropriate models, seemingly unable to break free although they know there are more congruent ways of responding to clinical practice. Perhaps that is the guilt – knowing that they too slip unwittingly into routines that dimin-ish personhood and inadvertently cause suffering. They live leading contradictory lives where the illusion of being a caring person barely papers over the cracks. In time, people who live contradictory lives become alienated from self in the struggle to maintain the illusion. Jourard (1971) says that people alienated from self are unable to use themselves in any therapeutic way and hence are no longer able to care beyond a perfunctory response to the other as an object. Blindness is the refuge of those in despair, masking the truth.

Undoubtedly, reflection is most often triggered by negative or uncomfortable feelings (Boyd and Fales 1983). It seems natural to focus on negative experiences because these situations present themselves to consciousness.

> Whenever we begin to feel frustrated in what we are doing, we should slow down and pay closer attention to it. Frustration takes us away from ourselves; we become alienated from our experience. When we feel this beginning to happen we need to pay more attention to our experience. (Paramananda 2001:58)

Some practitioners may find writing helps them work through their feelings but for others, writing about events, especially traumatic events, may lead to a sense of reliving the situation and cause distress. As Gray and Forsstrom (1991:360) note:

> The process of 'journalling' may sound simple and easy to execute, but at times it was extremely difficult. Mostly the incidents recorded were identified because there was an affective component. This may be related to feelings of personal inadequacy to cope with the demands of the situation. Alone, it was emotionally painful to journal events that were largely self-critical.

Writing about my feelings is cathartic, working out and converting negative feelings such as pity, frustration, anger and hatred into positive energy for taking action. Here the help of a guide may be invaluable. Given that so much of our work as healthcare practitioners is emotional, this is important work. This cue leads to deep insights into self and the development of therapeutic poise or equanimity.

As Beck (1989:42-3) says:

> For a time our life may feel worse than before, as what we have concealed becomes clear. But even as this occurs, we have a sense of growing sanity and understanding, of basic satisfaction. To continue practice through severe difficulties we must have patience, persistence and courage … we learn in our guts not just in our brains …

Our feelings give access to our inner world, often a negative feeling or sense of discomfort about something that has happened during the day. So write a description of your feelings in your journal, in the middle of the page …

> I feel frustrated
> I feel irritated
> I feel angry
> I feel satisfied

Now ask yourself some questions about the feelings. Why do I feel frustrated? Do I often feel angry in similar situations? Could I have not been angry? And so on.

Another approach is to simply write a story around the feeling.

30 April

> Today I felt angry at Jane, the junior nurse, because I asked her to help a patient wash, but she ignored me and went to help someone else. I was puzzled why she did this. It made me feel angry but I could not challenge her … I just didn't want a fuss … but it made me angry … and I'm still angry, at myself for letting her get away with it. Where does this anger come from? How should I act for the best?

I often suggest drawing a line down the middle of the page and writing the description in the left-hand column and asking questions of the text in the right-hand column – the questions flow naturally from the text yet are all grounded in the MSR cues.

Today I felt angry at Jane, the junior nurse because I asked her to help a patient wash, but she ignored me and went to help someone else. I was puzzled why she did this? It made me feel angry but I could not challenge her … I just didn't want a fuss … but it made me angry … and I'm still angry, at myself for letting her get away with it. I want to scream but it's bottled up inside me.	Why did Jane respond like that? How was she feeling? Does she normally respond like that? Was I sensitive enough in the way I asked her? Where does this anger come from? How can I shift this anger? When I see her tomorrow, how will I feel? What do I need to do? What theories might help me understand the pattern of communication between us?

Reflection is about coming to know 'who I am' so I can better use my self for therapeutic work. As George Elliot wrote in *Daniel Deronda*, 'There is a great deal of unmapped country within us which would have to be taken into account in an explanation of our gusts and storms'. Reflection is mapping, charting the unknown self, to better recognise, understand and control these gusts and storms. In his book *Awakenings*, Sacks (1976:15) says:

> In our study of our most complex sufferings and disorder of being, we are compelled to scrutinise the deepest, darkest, and most fearful parts of ourselves, the parts we strive to deny or not to see. The thoughts which are most difficult to grasp or express are those which awaken our strongest denials and our most profound intuitions.

Reading these words may give an impression that reflection is more like therapy. In Chapter 1 I note Rosenberg's (2004:145) words. They are worth repeating:

> We have been seeing our fear, for instance, as a huge boulder that stands in our way, but now we see that it is more like a cloud.

Through reflection we become aware of our fear and see the way it constrains our practice. As we reflect we begin to work through the fear. Perhaps we see the fear as huge and immovable as if it were a boulder. As we reflect, we can begin to accept the fear as our own rather than something that will destroy us. As we do so, the boulder seems to dissolve, loosen and fall away. We can learn to shift our images of fear and see fear as a cloud obscuring the blue sky. We can see that it is not permanent and will float away. Slowly our attachment to fear weakens and, as Rosenberg notes, '… little by little, we're not so enslaved to things' (p145). At every point, reflection is freedom to become who we desire to be.

However, the deeper we go, the more defended we are likely to be. I am reminded of the saying 'we don't know what we don't know' and it seems the deeper we go, the further we journey into uncharted territory. How would we know it? One reason why reflection needs to be expertly guided is to explore these depths within a secure relationship.

Journal entry – A first-year student nurse suggested that students always focused on negative experiences for two reasons: firstly, that was what teachers expected, and secondly, how can you reflect on a positive experience? He gave an example of a male patient thanking him for giving him a bath. 'What is there to reflect upon?'

For a moment I paused before this challenge and then a number of questions tumbled out.

- How did that make you feel?
- Is it important to feel like that?
- Why is it important to feel like that?
- How do you feel if patients don't thank you?
- Does it make you feel differently towards them (than those who do thank you)?
- If you feel negative towards the patient, are you less available?
- Do male patients like being bathed/touched by male nurses?
- How do you feel about bathing women patients?

These questions may seem obvious yet it is not a natural way to think. Such understanding suggests the need for guidance from another perceptive enough to pose these types of questions, especially for practitioners who lack reflective or clinical experience, who have yet to develop their connected or separate voices. Yet what a rich teaching opportunity stemming from one line – 'A male patient thanked me for helping him bath'. It is like getting into a groove, tuning into the experience that appears on the surface as unproblematic. Scratch the surface and see what lies underneath.

In general, practitioners are less likely to pay attention to experiences that do not arouse strong feelings simply because these experiences do not project into conscious thought. As practitioners become increasingly mindful of self within practice, then more experience becomes available for reflection. I have also noted a shift of pattern as practitioners become more reflective – they reflect less on situations that reflect themselves as problematic and more on experiences that are self-affirming. Perhaps you have noted that within your own reflection.

Practical skills (4)

> - Knowing your emotional self and learning to manage this therapeutically, thus becoming more available to the patient and less anxious
> - Developing sympathetic resonance and developing balance with empathic inquiry (see Chapter 6)

What was I trying to achieve and did I respond effectively?

This cue guides me to reflect on my responses and actions within the experience and whether my responses were effective in meeting my intended outcomes.

The idea of effective action can be viewed as four movements:

1. how I appreciated the situation
2. how I made clinical decisions (phronesis or practical wisdom)
3. my skilful response
4. my reflection on consequences.

Collectively these four movements are what Barbara Carper described as the *aesthetic* way of knowing (Carper 1978, Johns 1995): the way the practitioner grasps and envisages what is to be achieved (practical wisdom) and intentionally responds with skilful action (praxis) to meet intended outcomes.

The emphasis on aesthetics is significant because it implies beauty and performance – that practice *is* beauty and performance. Like a dancer, I move about the patient.

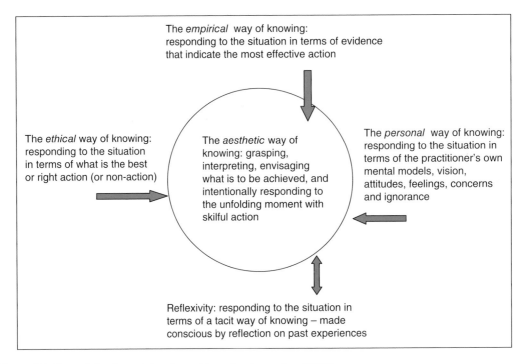

The *empirical* way of knowing: responding to the situation in terms of evidence that indicate the most effective action

The *ethical* way of knowing: responding to the situation in terms of what is the best or right action (or non-action)

The *aesthetic* way of knowing: grasping, interpreting, envisaging what is to be achieved, and intentionally responding to the unfolding moment with skilful action

The *personal* way of knowing: responding to the situation in terms of the practitioner's own mental models, vision, attitudes, feelings, concerns and ignorance

Reflexivity: responding to the situation in terms of a tacit way of knowing – made conscious by reflection on past experiences

Figure 3.2 Carper's fundamental pattern of knowing in nursing (1978).

Like a sculptor, I shape my practice. Like an actor, I play out the drama. Like a poet, I sense the poignancy within the unfolding moment.

Carper identified aesthetics as one of four fundamental ways of knowing in nursing. The other three ways are the *empirical*, the *ethical* and the *personal* patterns of knowing. In Figure 3.2, I set out the aesthetic as the core way of knowing informed and influenced by the other ways of knowing. In doing so, I identified another possible way of knowing that I term reflexivity – a pre-reflective knowing in the moment that can be partially known through reflection. I say 'partially known' simply because reflection can never capture its wholeness, only its partial memory trace. It is probably like tacit knowing – that knowing which manifests itself within the moment yet which is unable to be articulated in its wholeness (Polanyi 1958, Schön 1987).

Other theorists have postulated other ways of knowing. White (1995) suggested the sociopolitical ways of knowing to contextualise the ways of knowing within societal norms, whilst Munhall (1993) suggested 'unknowing' as a way of knowing, that influences the clinical response.

Configuring Carper's work led me to develop the Model for Reflective Inquiry (Fig. 3.3) which, in essence, is a rearrangement of the MSR. In this model I inquire 'Did I act effectively?'. This leads me to review the way I appreciated the situation, made clinical judgements, responded skilfully, and finally to consider if I was effective in meeting the patient's health needs.

I then inquire about the influence of the ethical, empirical and personal ways of knowing on my performance (as encapsulated within specific MSR cues).

I can then inquire 'what is significant about this experience?' and reveal any creative tension between what I intended (desirable practice) and my actual practice. As I do so, I work through any emotional tension.

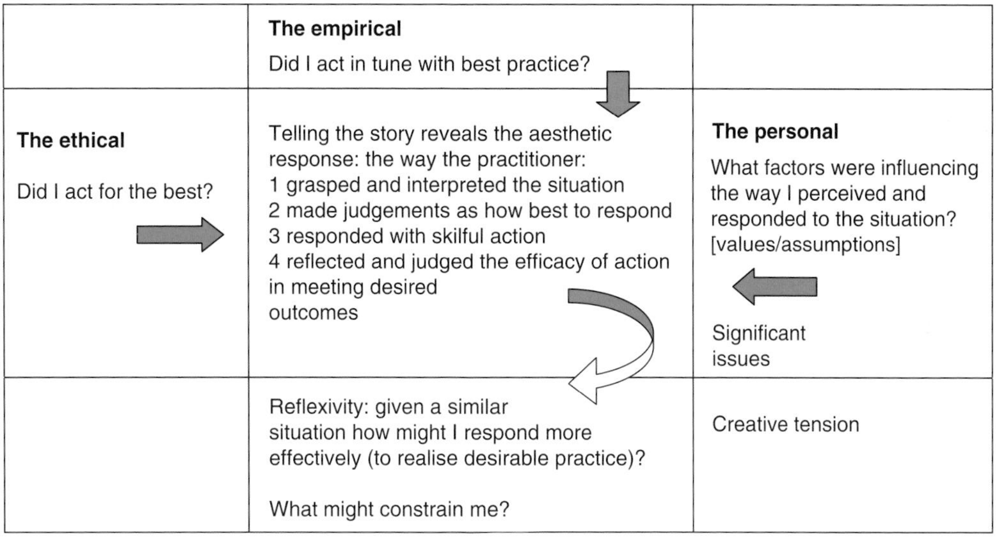

	The empirical Did I act in tune with best practice?	
The ethical Did I act for the best?	Telling the story reveals the aesthetic response: the way the practitioner: 1 grasped and interpreted the situation 2 made judgements as how best to respond 3 responded with skilful action 4 reflected and judged the efficacy of action in meeting desired outcomes	**The personal** What factors were influencing the way I perceived and responded to the situation? [values/assumptions] Significant issues
	Reflexivity: given a similar situation how might I respond more effectively (to realise desirable practice)? What might constrain me?	Creative tension

Figure 3.3 Model for Reflective Inquiry (Johns 2006).

I can then contemplate how I might respond 'more effectively' given the situation again (using the MSR 'looking forward' cues – see below).

The Model for Reflective Inquiry lends itself to a more objective reflective stance on the situation with less emphasis on the person. More looking out at the situation than looking in on self. Hence it may feel more clinical and less threatening. It offers a useful approach to clinical audit, answering the three questions at the core of quality assurance.

1. Did we act for the best?
2. Do we know what the best is?
3. What needs to change so we can act for the best? (see Chapter 13)

I use the Model for Reflective Inquiry to structure reflection on a portfolio module I have developed as a framework for developing clinical effectiveness (see Chapter 16).

Practical skills (5)

- The ability to reflect on efficacy of actions in context of patient needs
- Developing clinical judgement (phronesis)
- Ethics
- Developing praxis (assimilating theory and research within action)

What were the consequences of my actions on the patient, others and myself?

This cue guides the practitioner to contemplate the consequences of her actions for others and herself. The cue is deceptively deep. On the surface of things, the consequences of actions may be quite obvious, yet when we begin to pay attention we can see that often actions have far-reaching consequences, some of which are not anticipated or even known

Conforming to normal practice/ habit? The weight of tradition	Negative attitudes and prejudice? Racism?	Expectations from others? Need to be valued?
Limited skills/discomfort/confidence to act in new ways?		Fear of sanction? The weight of authority
Emotional entanglement/over-identification?	What factors influenced my decision making and actions?	Misplaced concern – loyalty to colleagues versus loyalty to patient? Anxious about ensuing conflict?
Personal stuff/baggage? Deeper psyche factors?		Knowledge to act in specific ways? The weight of theory
Wrapped up in self-concern? Pity? Stressed? Guilt? Frustration? Other feelings?	Time/priorities?	Expectations from self about 'how I should act' Doing what was felt to be right?

Figure 3.4 Influences grid (adapted from Johns 2004a: 24).

about. It is like throwing a pebble into a pond and seeing the ripples spread out. In the second edition of this book, I wrote 'All actions have consequences for which the practitioner accepts responsibility' and yet is this possible? Should I be able to perceive far-reaching consequences? If so, this requires me to be very careful about my actions and perceive as far as possible potential consequences.

On the surface, my responses to Tom and Joan seem therapeutic. Yet what might be the unintentional consequences?

Practical skills (6)

- Recognising the impact of actions, both intended and not intended
- Developing sensitivity and mindfulness

What factors influenced the way I was feeling, thinking or responding?

The cue is a gateway to knowing self – what makes me tick, what factors pull my strings? This cue is deceptively difficult to respond to because the self tends to view itself normatively. Influencing factors or mental models are deeply embodied and hence not easily perceived. To change ourselves, we have to access, appreciate and then shift our mental models.

The cue can feel scary because it leads the person deep within themselves, unearthing and revealing influences that stem from social and cultural practices or past experiences that have left a trace. These influencing factors can be threatening. Perhaps this is one reason why some people must turn away from the reflective mirror or *smudge the mirror* to distort the image of self being reflected back, to give a better impression. Patti Lather (1986a,b) describes this distortion as 'false consciousness'. This distortion is not done consciously; it is as if defence mechanisms are working to protect the threatened ego. As such, it is not easy for the practitioner to recognise distortion. A guide is needed to challenge the practitioner to pull away the masks of false consciousness and help the practitioner reveal and accept their true self (see Chapter 4 for exploration of guidance).

Through analysing practitioners' reflections, I have identified a number of common influencing factors (Fig. 3.4). These are grounded in issues of tradition, power/force and embodiment, issues that Fay (1987) identified as barriers to rational change. The weight of embodiment is heavy indeed. It reflects how I have come to be who I am through socialisation. To change who I am requires awareness and understanding of these influences so I can begin to let go of them and learn new patterns of being more congruent with desirable practice. As the motto goes, 'old habits die hard'. They need active and prolonged confrontation. It can be like hitting your head on a brick wall – what I term the hard wall of reality (see Framing perspectives, p77). Issues of force and tradition are evident within normal patterns of relating and again tend to be embodied. These too are hard to shift because they are 'normal' – to change requires changing others besides self. However, to begin to respond differently to someone will provoke a difference in their response (not necessarily one you would desire) so change is underway.

The practitioner can surf the influences grid to consider the impact of each influencing factor within the particular experience. You will be surprised just how many are relevant, reflecting a collective nursing consciousness of subordination and societal prejudice.

For example, issues surrounding racism continue to surface (Blackford 2003, Puzan 2003). Puzan notes:

> There is so much familiarity in talking about the alleged racial differences of non-white people in public discourse and so little familiarity in talking about those racial properties attached to being white, that the concept of whiteness (or a recognition of racial formation) has little resonance within nursing. While issues related to cultural difference are not ignored, they rarely include the difference specifically engendered by 'whiteness', which is structured to avoid and deflect interrogation or critical reflection. (p194)

Reflection then opens a space for such discourse.

So, what factors were influencing me at the community hospital that cold day in spring? I sense the tension between my expectations of self to speak out (integrity) versus (unspoken) expectations from others not to be critical. Linked to that, I sense the tension between speaking out for others (paternalism) and enabling others to speak for themselves (empowerment). I found myself absorbing the suffering of both Tom and Joan, identifying with them, pitying them to some extent. Being supernumary, I had more time to spend with them but I can imagine the strain on staff to find time to prioritise being with them in the demand to get through the work. I could feel this cultural strain ripple through the unit.

This cue inevitably explores the boundaries with therapy and highlights the vital need for self-development in human–human encounter work that espouses the intention to work with people from spiritual, psychological and emotional frames of reference.

Practical skills (7)

- Knowing self and developing the therapeutic self and self's impact on practice

What knowledge did or might have informed me?

Without doubt, the effective practitioner is an informed practitioner. This cue guides the practitioner to identify and access relevant theory or research, critique it for its value to inform the particular experience, and assimilate it within personal knowing to inform future practice, enabling the practitioner to develop *praxis* – informed moral practice.

Keeping informed is a mighty onus on the individual practitioner given the vast amount of 'knowledge' and 'evidence' out there. An organisational response is required, for example developing standards of care and protocols that have systematically and periodically reviewed research with clear guidelines to inform practice.

This cue enables the practitioner to respond meaningfully to the evidence-based practice agenda. However, it is important to caution against using such guidelines as prescriptions simply because all clinical situations are unique, they have never happened before. In medicine, NICE guidelines do prescribe specific responses to specific situations. However, this does risk turning practitioners into technicians to apply the prescription and patients into objects to be manipulated.

Consider my experience with Tom and Joan. What theory might inform my decisions and actions?

One example is the therapeutic of enabling people to retain control of their environment whilst in hospital, which is significant for self-esteem and maintenance of competence (Charmaz 1983).

Mapping

All theory can be mapped so the practitioner can position self within the theory. For example, in Chapter 7, I set out the four stereotypes of women map developed from the work of Ann Dickson – the practitioner can consider which stereotype descriptor best fits and which stereotype she would like to be within the particular situation being reflected on. The map can then be used over successive experiences to plot any developmental shift of position, offering a concrete way of monitoring development. Other examples are dotted through the chapters. Maps help theory come alive.

Practical skills (8)

> • Accessing, critiquing and assimilating relevant theory with practice (developing praxis)

To what extent did I act for the best and in tune with my values and beliefs?

The effective practitioner is an ethical practitioner. All action is ethical. Every story is a moral story concerning the practitioner's intention to act for the good. This cue has two inter-related issues: firstly, an ethical reflection on the 'best', and secondly, a review of my values and beliefs that constitute desirable practice. I have added beliefs to the MSR because people may view values and beliefs as different.

The *Compact Oxford English Dictionary* (2005) states:

> values – beliefs about what is right or wrong and what is important (p1149)
> belief – a feeling that something exists or is true, especially one without proof/a firmly held opinion (p81)

Ethics is enshrined within the Hippocratic oath that doctors should do good (beneficence) and not do harm (non-malevolence). Nurses similarly are informed by a code of professional ethics that sets out the nurse's responsibility to act ethically. However, the healthcare world has changed. The consumer movement demands the right for people to be involved in decision making about their healthcare. People are more informed: 'Google' any health condition and the internet will reveal a plethora of information.

Applying ethical principles in practice is not straightforward. Often ethical principles contradict each other. As such, *acting for the best* always needs to be interpreted within

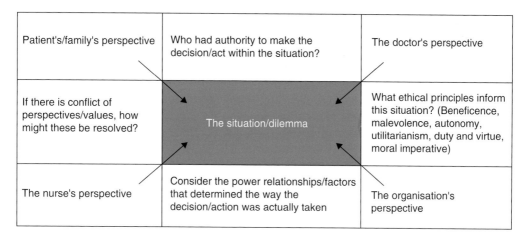

Figure 3.5 Ethical mapping (Johns 1998b).

each moment (Cooper 1991, Parker 1990). This may create difficulties within the team if practitioners have different values and personal agendas or demand compliance with authority.

To guide the practitioner to explore *acting for the best*, I developed ethical mapping (Fig. 3.5).

The ethical map trail
Frame the dilemma

Most ethical issues can be reduced to a dilemma (for example, should I confront Marie's approach to Tom or not? Should I walk Joan or not?).

Consider the perspective of different actors, commencing with your own perspectives

By considering the perspectives of people involved within the experience, the practitioner is challenged to see and understand other people's views and to confront her own partial perspective. It is rather like a fish bowl in that, depending on where you are coming from, you will see something different from other positions, so each perspective is a partial view. These perspectives are not necessarily motivated by what's best but by personal, professional or organisational interests. Ethical mapping encourages the practitioner to move from her own partial view to gain a global or helicopter view of the whole. Only then are we in a position to negotiate in terms of what is best. Understanding the perspectives of others will help me develop empathic skills, which is the basis for all therapeutic relationships.

Consider which ethical principles apply in terms of the best (ethically correct) decision

Professional autonomy ↔ Patient autonomy

Having gained an understanding of different and partial perspectives, I can consider the way ethical principles might inform the situation. The major ethical principles are those concerned with professional autonomy – beneficence and non-malevolence, patient autonomy; the idea that it is the patient's right to be self-determining is respected; the role of the professional is to enable the person or patient to make the best decision. Natural tension exists between professional and patient autonomy within which the practitioner needs always to position self.

From a holistic perspective I lean towards patient autonomy, However, it is not enough to respect autonomy. For vulnerable people such as Tom and Joan, I must create the space in which they can express their autonomy (Seedhouse 1988).

Another key ethical principle is utilitarianism – the idea that the needs of the individual are secondary to the needs of society as a whole. This principle involves the use of resources, justice and equity. Common issues are the use of time and appreciating priorities (see Janet and Michelle's story below).

From this perspective we can draw a tension along which many dilemmas can be plotted:

Needs of the individual ↔ Needs of society

A further ethical principle is the idea of virtue or duty; the way the practitioner should conduct self befitting of being a nurse. An obvious example of this is that a nurse should always act in a caring manner. This also means not causing suffering through careless action, for example failure to provide Joan with a plateguard when she is unable to use a knife and fork. A further ethical principle is Kant's moral imperative – 'do as you would be done for'. In other words, imposing your own values into the situation – 'if that were my mother …'. The problem with this principle is that the patient is not your mother and that imposing such values may be misguided.

Consider what conflict exists between perspectives/values and how these might be resolved

Having considered the different perspectives and ethical principles, the practitioner can consider whether conflict exists and if so, how it might be best resolved considering the ethical principles.

Consider who had the authority for making the decision/taking action

This part of ethical mapping challenges the practitioner to consider her autonomy, authority and accountability for making and acting on decisions. According to Batey and Lewis (1982), autonomy has two dimensions: legitimate autonomy as set out in the person's job description, and discriminant authority – the autonomy the person believes she has. However, job descriptions are often vague and working in bureaucratic organisations seems to diminish discriminant autonomy, especially for groups of workers, such as nurses, who may perceive themselves as a subordinate workforce, which may also distort their perception of responsibility. Reflection always seeks to empower practitioners to expand their field of autonomy and counter any sense of oppression.

Consider the power relationships/factors that determined the way the decision/action was actually taken

In the real world, decisions are not necessarily made in terms of what's best for the patient or family, but in terms of power and fear of sanction (see Cathy and the GPs story in Chapter 7). Within the learning organisation professionals need to dialogue and find the best solution in terms of the patient's best interests, including the patient as appropriate and casting aside personal agendas.

As you read the story of Mrs Denver, use the ethical map to reflect on ethical action.

Mrs Denver[3]

Michelle is a mature staff nurse on a 5-day surgical ward. She has been qualified 12 months. She shares her experience concerning Mrs Denver, a woman admitted for a breast biopsy, with Janet, the ward sister, in clinical supervision.

Michelle: She was a nurse, a pleasant lady. Next morning I was on an early shift doing the drugs. I asked her whether there was anything she needed? She said 'No … oh I do feel weepy' and then she burst into tears. I pulled the drug trolley over and pulled the curtains around her bed. She said her friends had been saying how scared they would be if it was them [having a breast biopsy] … she hadn't appreciated these feelings until now. She said 'Oh my husband and my children!'. It made me think – she's a nurse and she's so vulnerable. I don't know if I did any good.

Janet: Put yourself in her shoes … you spent half an hour with her. How would you have felt if a nurse did this for you? Nurses often underestimate the work they do with patients. Could you have done more?

Michelle: I made a conscious decision to blow the pills, no-one will come to any harm. It made me feel so vulnerable – what do you say?

Janet: Did you have to say anything? Nurses aren't very good at sitting and listening … it's OK giving out information and advice.

Michelle: The silence is difficult … it's keeping quiet I find the hardest. Did we give her the opportunity to chat? Did we keep away because she was a nurse? Are we frightened of being patronising? Should she be treated any differently?

Janet: You are the patient's named nurse and therefore it was appropriate for you to spend time with her. Finding someone to take over the drug trolley or even finding the named nurse if you hadn't been the named nurse would have lost the spontaneous moment for this lady. Did you discuss this with other staff?

Michelle: Yes … we are not as sensitive to these ladies with breast lumps as we could be. Would a counselling course help? I'm at a loss to know what to say to them – am I helping or hindering? It's such a sensitive issue. They look jolly and jovial outside but inside it's like a bombshell!

Janet: Did you use touch?

Michelle: I put my hand on her arm when she apologised for crying. Not knowing her well enough stopped me from holding her hand.

Janet: Could you have done anything differently?

Michelle: I could have been more available to her preoperatively. I couldn't have made it better for her … change what was wrong.

Janet: What would have happened if this had been a busier morning?

Michelle: I wouldn't have left her but I wouldn't have been so calm. I'd have been thinking more about other work that needed to be done, premeds, eye drops and things … thinking 'I wish you'd hurry up'. That's really wrong – how do we get over that?

---

[3] The data were collected as a part of a research project to monitor the impact of clinical supervision as a model for developing clinical leadership (Johns 2003a).

Janet: I don't really know. Perhaps as practitioners we need to be more prepared to defend our actions.

So, what do you conclude from this story about ethical action? Consider:

- How would you want a nurse to respond to you?
- Do you think Michelle responded for 'the best'?
- How would you know what 'the best' is? Don't leap too quickly to an emotional response – weigh it up carefully.

Finding an upset patient whilst doing the drug round is a common occurrence on hospital wards yet in this dialogue it takes on profound significance. Mrs Denver is no longer 'a task to do' but a suffering human being, a vulnerable woman who has undergone a breast biopsy and is waiting for her results.

On reflection, Michelle could express her own vulnerability and lack of ability and confidence to respond as she felt she ethically should. She could see the way she avoided the situation, until the moment Mrs Denver's suffering bubbled over and confronted Michelle. Michelle's caring instinct made her respond as best she could. It is a sobering thought to consider how many women suffer in silence and how many nurses are ill equipped to respond to suffering and as a consequence avoid it.

In Figure 3.6 I apply ethical mapping. As you can see, I do not entirely agree that Michelle acted for the best, even though her response was most caring. She was 'mopping up a mess' that might have been lessened by being more caring beforehand. It really does highlight the need for connection and relationship. Michelle needed to be more mindful of the impact of breast biopsy on Mrs Denver and other similar patients. Michelle's comment 'I could have been more available to her preoperatively' is very insightful; consider the Burford cues 'What meaning does this breast biopsy have for Mrs Denver?', 'How is Mrs Denver feeling about this procedure?', 'What factors are important to make her stay in hospital comfortable?' and 'How do I feel about Mrs Denver?'.

As Janet said, 'put yourself in her shoes' – what would you be thinking and feeling? Having a breast biopsy may be a minor surgical procedure but what does it mean to the woman? Reflect on Mrs Denver's fears – 'Oh my husband and my children!' – that reveal the threat of death. The literature indicates that this is a very distressing time. As Woodward and Webb (2001) note:

> The quality of life a woman experiences during the process of investigation and treatment for breast disorders is linked with the communication and support provided by others, and includes family members, friends and clinic personnel. Knopf (1994) recommends that nurses working with breast cancer can develop strategies to help patients clarify, interpret and process information: this needs to be extended to all breast disorders. Greater attention should be given to the emotional experiences of all women during the diagnostic phase of breast disease. A breast biopsy is not a benign experience (Northouse *et al* 1995).

There is a significant literature concerned with breast lumps that Michelle might explore to inform her practice, and which Janet might direct her to in responding to the MSR cue 'What knowledge did or could have informed my practice?'. If Michelle had known of this literature she might have been more sensitive to Mrs Denver's potential anxiety and emotional reaction. In other words, Mrs Denver's suffering and distress might have been lessened by a more proactive response. Butterfield (1990) describes this as 'upstream

Patient's/family's perspective/other patients	Who had authority to make the decision/act within the situation?	The doctor's perspective
Mrs Denver was visibly upset and needed care at that moment Other patients may be watching and expect nurses to be caring yet also know they are busy, and may also expect Michelle to give them their drugs first	We do not know if Michelle was the 'nurse in charge' or patterns of ward authority; Janet's response suggests that Michelle did have authority to respond as she felt best	Most likely to see Michelle's primary role as ensuring that all patients received medication on time
If there is conflict of perspectives/ values, how might these be resolved? Michelle experienced intrapersonal conflict, uncertain in her own mind what's best. Options: 1 Michelle could have spent less time with Mrs Denver 2 She could have gone back to Mrs Denver after the drug round 3 She could have got someone else to speak to her or to take over the drug round	*The situation/dilemma* Should Michelle stop the drug round or continue it?	*What ethical principles inform this situation?* Ethically, Michelle had to weigh up the needs of the individual against the needs of the whole Would other patients have come to harm? Virtue – what should a caring nurse do?
The nurse's perspective Michelle could not leave Mrs Denver suffering. However, she also felt she should continue with the drug round, that her colleagues would criticise her for leaving work undone	*Consider the power relationships/factors that determined the way the decision/action was actually taken* Michelle felt she should continue the drug round (socialised by medical power)	*The organisation's perspective* Anxious to avoid complaint from patients not receiving their drugs on time or medical angst about 'irresponsible' nurse behaviour Tasks are appealing because they reinforce the primary value of 'smooth running' of the organisation

Figure 3.6 Ethical mapping: should Michelle stop the drug round or continue it?

thinking' – responding to prevent people falling into the stream rather than having to rescue them once they have fallen in. Perhaps on a short-stay surgical unit that specialises in breast biopsy, such thinking should be second nature. Yet practitioners get so locked into a reactive culture, it is difficult to see ahead. We may need prompts to draw our attention to things.

In choosing to spend time with Mrs Denver, Michelle chose not to spend time with other patients. The juggling of priorities is ethical action. The reflective practitioner is an ethical practitioner, mindful of competing priorities and mindful of her values so they are not compromised. So Michelle might take Mrs Denver's hand and communicate her care and understanding. She might say 'I can see you are upset'. She might say 'I can't be with you at this moment' but because she has invested in creating a caring relationship, Mrs Denver knows that Michelle cares about her and will return at an appropriate time. Mrs Denver will feel Michelle's care even in that brief moment, and her suffering will be eased. In other words, if we reflect deeper on Michelle's experience we can see that the conditions for caring were problematic.

Michelle must be able to justify her decision to stop the drug round, to confront others' perceptions of priorities when these are misplaced, and to resist any blame as a consequence.

The drug round reflects a task approach to nursing – that all patients receive medications at uniform times, helped by routine drug administration in fixed time-patterns. The task is considered as an efficient way of ensuring work is delegated and completed. However, the routine administration of drugs may detract from seeing and responding to people's individual needs. Tasks break up the pattern of holistic care by fragmenting aspects of the whole and demanding conformity to the organisational pattern. It is as if the organisation sets the wavelength that patients must find and flow with or else be viewed as deviant and all the consequences that such labelling brings. A counter approach would be that nurses tailor drug administration to their individual patients, an approach in my view that takes no longer and yet creates a caring moment for being with the patient, *especially* on busy surgical wards, when being with the patient may seem like a premium. Again the question of values arises.

Unfortunately, the mindset is to get the task done and interruption is often viewed as a nuisance. From this perspective, the drug round was itself the problem. The solution would be to scrap the drug round and ask nurses to administer drugs on an individual basis.

Reflect on the routines and tasks of your day and consider whom they benefit. Is the routinisation of work through tasks arranged in a hierarchy of importance? In my research (Johns 1989) I identified a hierarchy of work priorities.

- Executing medical responses and physical care
- Complying with organisational demands, for example completing documentation
- Talking with patients (emotional, psychological and spiritual care)

When I fed back my interpretation to the staff, they felt uncomfortable because it shattered the illusion that they practised holistic nursing. The contradiction was stark. The hierarchical task approach to work was so deeply embodied and embedded within tradition that it could not easily be shrugged aside. Failure to comply to this hierarchy led to conflict amongst staff and with nurse managers whose interests were reflected in maintaining the hierarchy. The staff knew that the solution was to collapse the hierarchy into a new culture of professional responsibility and judgement based on the unit's holistic vision but could they actually achieve that? Even they doubted that possibility.

In a world of shrinking resources (although I wonder why, when the world seems richer and richer), practitioners are at great risk of role overload that inevitably squeezes the caring aspect and heightens the dilemma of managing priorities. Betz, O'Connell (1987) describe role overload as being responsible for more tasks than an individual could perform within shift time. They note that role overload is greater when associated with perceived 'low-level' tasks and paperwork. As Leslie noted, in his role as a primary nurse at Burford hospital, 'when I focus on patient care my stress goes down and when I focus on workload, interviews, case conferences, my stress goes up' (Johns 1998a).

One response to shrinking resources is to break down the 'shift-bound' culture and move to a new culture of role responsibility. When practitioners felt valued, felt they had a choice about issues and felt in control of their own time, they were less stressed and willing to use their own time to fulfil their perceived role responsibility. Otherwise they resisted and resented impositions on their own time (Johns 1998a). This understanding is significant in creating a culture of responsibility and support. The two must be in balance. However, such a culture is always open to abuse by unscrupulous organisations who do not value caring, and who see nursing as a prime target for resource savings.

How does this situation connect with previous experiences?

> If we don't stay connected and remember the lessons from the past, are we not doomed to repeat them? (Blackwolf and Jones 1996:78)

An experience is not an isolated moment in time. It is part of a continuous stream of unfolding experiences. This cue challenges the practitioner to consider if the experience being reflected on is linked to past experiences. How has the practitioner handled similar experiences in the past? Is there a pattern of response that locks the practitioner into a certain response?

It is a significant cue simply because the judgements and actions that practitioners take are largely determined by what they have done before, especially when what they have done before seems to work. As I suggested within the influences grid, practitioners also tend to carve out comfort grooves and then get stuck in them. Much of practice becomes habitualised, complacent and resistant to change, as if other ways of seeing the world and doing things threaten our security.

Practical skills (9)

> • Being mindful of the way previous experiences influence current practice and may not be the most effective ways of doing things

Looking forward cues

So far, the cues have tended to look backwards at the event or at self within the moment. As a consequence, the practitioner now has a reasonable appreciation of contradiction between my intention (to realise desirable practice) and his or her actual practice. I can now turn towards the future to consider ways in which the contradiction might be resolved given the situation again.

How might I respond more effectively given this situation again?

Linked to my tension between paternalism (speaking out for Tom and Joan) and enabling them – I can see I could have asked them if they would like me to speak for them. Of course, such a solution is so obvious but in the moment, perhaps due to my anxiety having absorbed their suffering, that option was obscured.

Perhaps I might have taken Marie aside and asked her to reflect more on what made Tom so happy this morning when he had been so miserable. Perhaps I would not have walked Joan, but contacted the physiotherapist directly, to come and see her. Walking her may have put her at some risk, again responding to our mutual frustration to do something. I would like to have been less frustrated. I feel certain my voice had a critical edge as I gave feedback to the senior nurse. I felt her slight recoil. Her defensive posture dilutes my message. I then become the problem rather than the actual issue.

I open to these possibilities. And this is the significant thing about this cue – the fuelling of inquiry and opening to other possibilities in the quest for effectiveness and professional responsibility.

Nothing is permanent

In this scenario I have been visiting Gill at home for the past 20 months, giving her reflexology since the beginning of her chemotherapy following mastectomy and breast reconstruction for breast cancer.

28 May 2004 – The wall I usually park my car against next door to Gill's house is being demolished. The neighbour is converting his front garden into a car park. Nothing is permanent. Gill makes tea and toast for Chloe who is still in bed at 10.00. Precious moments of mothering.

The operation itself went well although the circumstances of her hospital stay were more problematic. Gill recounts the ordeal; no bed, changing in the arrival lounge and going from there to theatre, and no sleep that night due to an admission of an elderly lady with her daughter.

Gill says: 'Eventually I sat in the corridor for some peace and quiet! Yet praise for all the nurses and doctors. I felt calm … it was the reflexology the day before that helped, I'm sure about that … I can now lift my right arm without feeling it's being clamped. Evidently the valve had to be cut out. The silicone implant was the wrong size. No information about wound care or rehabilitation exercise. No matter, I'm pleased the deed is done.'

But more bad news stalks her. 'My aunt in Ireland has been diagnosed with breast cancer. I wonder if my cancer is genetic, I've been worrying about the girls inheriting it from me.'

'Such fears are perhaps natural when relatives develop breast cancer.' I say this as a statement rather than as a question. Gill is silent. I add, 'It's nearly 2 years for you now.'

Gill's lip curls to contain her tears. 'I didn't expect to be here today … I really didn't. When I was told I thought that was that … it was a death sentence.'

I mention the wall next door. 'They were going to move but decided to stay. I spoke to them recently about the cancer for the first time. We have avoided talking for nearly 2 years.'

Cancer fills people with dread. It disrupts normal patterns of relating so nobody knows how to be normal any more. So it is avoided.

On deeper reflection I ponder my response to her words 'I've been worrying about the girls inheriting it from me'. My response was to acknowledge her fears as natural. I wonder if I had said something like 'What do you need to do about this fear?', would that have helped Gill to release her fear whereas my response may have dampened her fear? I sit and conjure up other responses if the situation was replayed, imagining the consequences of each. I sense that saying 'What do you need to do about this fear?' would have strengthened her fear at a time I wanted her to let go and relax. Hence normalising her fear, saying that is a natural response any mother would have, helped to weaken the fear. Perhaps I am nit-picking but when someone's life is at stake, the sensitivity and appropriateness of my responses are vital. Reflection helps me turn these stones over.

What would be the consequences of alternative actions for the patient, others and myself?

This cue follows on from the previous one, challenging me to consider the possible consequences of responding in different ways within the particular situation. It helps me weigh up my judgements (developing practical wisdom) rather than leaping to quick assumptions. Considering each possible way of responding is like planting seeds in my mind to germinate in similar future situations (Margolis 1993).

What factors might stop me from responding differently?

Weighing up possibilities and considering the consequences of each leads me to choose the preferred option. Then I return to the influences grid (Fig. 3.4) and do a re-run to consider if I can respond as I would like to in future situations. Remember the limits to rational action.

I know I am a conflict avoider and that is what might stop me from challenging the staff.

Practical skills (10)

- Appreciating new ways of responding within particular situations and their consequences
- Developing professional responsibility

How do I NOW feel about this experience?

This cue draws my attention to my feelings as a consequence of reflection. Am I left frustrated or angry or have I been able to work through my feelings in a positive way? Have I converted my negative energy into positive energy for taking action based on my insights?

As I look back through subsequent reflections, I sense the way my voice has grown … my ability to assert myself without the tinge of frustration by being tougher on issues and soft on people. I have learnt to address issues by asking others 'How do you think Tom feels?' rather than me saying 'Tom feels like this …'. It is opening up spaces rather than closing them down.

Practical skills (11)

- Acknowledging the negative emotional impact of work in particular situations and sensing the value of releasing emotional tension

Am I now more able to support myself and others better as a consequence?

This cue challenges me to review whether I am supported well enough within my clinical practice. Are effective support systems in place so that practitioners get the emotional support they need to be most available to their patients? It is our individual responsibility to keep ourselves in good shape so we are available for therapeutic work. Yet so many of us carry loads of residual stress on our backs, pulling us down, depleting our energy (see Chapter 7).

Practical skills (12)

> • Ensuring that support for self and others within practice is valued and available as necessary
> • Keeping self fully (emotionally) fit for practice (emotional intelligence)

Dwelling with the text and gaining insight

Having worked through the reflective cues, I seek to gain insights. As I become more experienced at reflection, I internalise the cues and find myself not using them so formally, more as a checklist, especially the influences grid and ethical mapping. Reflection becomes increasingly intuitive and creative.

However, for the novice reflective practitioner having worked through the MSR cues, take a pause and take a further step backwards from the text to see the bigger picture. At this stage it may be helpful to break the story text into single lines. In doing this, I open up the text, the spaces between the lines where meaning and insights are often found. Remember the saying 'reading between the lines'? I do this with my story of being with Tom and Joan.

After his wash, Tom cleans his own teeth.
He is normally shaven
using an electric razor
because the nurses feel clumsy with wet shaves
even though Tom likes a wet shave.
He appreciates the wet shave I give him.
I am mindful how this 'little thing' of shaving Tom makes a difference in caring.
I know this informs Tom of my concern for him.
By paying him attention, my concern is fed and grows.
I experience a mutuality in his response.
He begins to care for me.

Read these lines again, slowly. They are packed with significance as if, in these few words, the essence of caring is touched. What emerges for you from between the lines?

Breaking the description into single lines is like writing a prose poem. It is as if I am scrolling down the text into a new screen. I borrow the idea of scrolling down the screen from Jeanette Winterson. In *The Powerbook* (2001:20)[4] she writes:

There are so many lives packed into one.
The one life we think we know is only the window that is open on the screen.
The big window full of detail,
where the meaning is often lost among the facts.
If we can close that window,
on purpose or by chance,
what we find is another view.
This window is emptier.
The cross-references are cryptic.

---

[4] From *The Powerbook* by Jeanette Winterson, published by Jonathan Cape. Reprinted by permission of The Random House Group Ltd.

As we scroll down it, looking for something familiar,
we seem to be scrolling into another self –
one we recognise but cannot place.
The co-ordinates are missing,
or the co-ordinates pinpoint us outside the limits of our existence.
If we move further back,
through a smaller window that is really a gateway,
there is less and less to measure ourselves by.
We are coming into a dark region.
A single word might appear.
An icon.

These icons are often the genesis of insights. This is an imaginative, intuitive and creative process – rich qualities to nurture for any practitioner. Tuffnell and Crickmay (2004:119) note that:

> Imagination is not a separate faculty, rather it engages all parts of the mind and intelligence – fusing or bringing together often surprising aspects of what we feel or know, imagination expands our seeing

… and yet our imaginations have been trimmed:

> Of course, the sad thing, the tragic thing, is that many of us do get trimmed. We all start off with real heads full of space and imagination, but slowly, somewhere along the path that we call growing up, our heads get trimmed. We become caught up in the doings of this world, the realities of adult life, and we get cut down to size … without imagination the world loses its mystery and sense of depth in which we can find meaning. (Paramananda 2001:71)

Reflection is opening to our imagination, expanding our seeing. Scrolling down the text, I dwell within the text, what I call creative play, inspired by Ben Okri (1997:21):

> Creativity, it would appear, should be approached in the spirit of play, of foreplay, of dalliance, doodling, messing around – and then, bit by bit, you somehow get deeper into the matter. But if you go in there with a businessman's solemnity or the fanaticism of some artistic types you are likely to be rewarded with a stiff response, a joyless dribble, strained originality, ideas that come out all strapped up and strangled by too much effort.

The idea of dallying suggests giving the mind free rein to explore, allowing the imagination to wander and accept anything that comes up. Keeping the censor at bay!

In dwelling with the text, I am patient, as if going deeper cannot be rushed. Dwelling within the text can be described as contemplation, the sharpening of the intellect. It is a way of knowing that perceives everything with precision and clarity; open to possibility, such knowing does not judge or even compare. As Fremantle notes (2003:118), 'it is like watching a play'.

Being mindful of reflection, the practitioner keeps the mirror clean of the 'dirt' of ignorance and confusion in order to see things with clarity. A guide may be helpful to clean the mirror until we can keep the mirror clean ourselves. So, as we dwell, we are curious, contemplative, compassionate and discriminating, moving within the hermeneutic cycle, letting go of attachment to ideas to allow the imagination and creativity to flow until tentative insights emerge, taking root. I put the text aside and then later, a new idea will dawn, perhaps as I sleep or walk or during meditation, or indeed at any time of the day. It is as if the idea is germinating in my head and then, suddenly, the root blossoms.

> When we concentrate on individual moments or fragments of experience, we see only chaos. But if we stand back and look at what is taking shape, we see order. Order always displays itself as patterns that develop over time. (Wheatley 1999:118)

Dwelling within my text of Tom and Joan, I perceive how the nurse's gaze was caught up in doing tasks in contrast with being with these patients and so that prevented her seeing Tom's crisis. He was seen as a collection of problems rather than as a whole, and yet his 'whole' screamed with suffering. I wrote in my reflective journal – why are we so blind?

I explore my own meanings that I give to holistic practice, notably the core therapeutic of acknowledging his humanness, that he is a worthwhile person with a positive future. This is not to give hope but to repattern the future as meaningful. In doing so, I seek to lift him out of an oppressive or life-destroying relationship unwittingly created by nurses. I say unwitting, because such ways of being had become normal and were viewed by the nurses as caring. They did not know they were being oppressive.

In response I become mindful of modelling to Marie and other nurses and domestics *being with* patients, a way of being grounded in the patients' concerns rather than my own (for example, in completing specific task at certain times). These insights deepen my previous understandings of holistic practice and in deepening, I live them more, I become more holistic, more confident of who I am and more assertive to challenge non-caring. Yet I do not impose my values – 'this is what you must believe!'. When I asked the nurses, they too shared similar values. Of course, how could they not? Anything less is inhuman. They did not know that they lived a contradiction.

In the following example, Janet Heywood (2006:23-5) illustrates how she used the idea of the 'left-hand column' to position emerging significance and potential insights against the text (Box 3.2). She writes:

> The cues in the MSR are used to challenge the text for meaning and insights. They are not intended to be used sequentially, but have a natural and logical flow: no model is designed to be used prescriptively but rather should be seen as a guide (Johns 2002). I find I sometimes use cues in the order presented in the model, though frequently I use them as the narrative demands. I often return to a cue as a new insight develops. The following example demonstrates the importance of using these cues flexibly.
>
> Saw V again today, still very tearful and anxious about breastfeeding. Positioning and attachment [of baby onto breast] much better, but nipples red and cracked, and strong evidence of deep breast thrush in her and oral thrush in baby. Has seen GP as I suggested last week – he has prescribed for baby but says he 'does not believe' in deep breast thrush and refuses to prescribe. V refuses to see another GP and says she does not want to make trouble or waste their time … so how will things ever change? Am frustrated and annoyed … have prescribed a topical antifungal. It's not the best treatment but all I can do. Why do people pander to GPs like this?
>
> It was after this experience that I began to experiment with the 'left-hand column' principle (though I prefer to use a right-hand one) that Senge (1990) suggests as a strategy for challenging and revealing how mental models operate to distort and manipulate reality (Box 3.2). I write on one side of a page, using the other to respond to cue questions from the MSR (Johns 2002) to reveal deeper meaning.

Box 3.2   Strategy for revealing how mental models operate

The written, explicit narrative	The unwritten, implicit narrative
Saw V again today	V is taking up a lot of my time
Doctor does not believe in deep breast thrush	My diagnosis is being questioned, which makes me look and feel foolish
V refuses to seek another opinion and does not want to make trouble	V senses the tension between me and the doctors
V does not want to waste the doctor's time	V values my time less than that of the doctors
How will things ever change?	I feel powerless to change things myself
I prescribe a less efficacious treatment	I feel forced to compromise my professional integrity by the doctor
I am frustrated and annoyed	I am not in control of the situation
Why do people pander to doctors like this?	I want to avoid a confrontation with the doctors, and want V to do it on my behalf

In this experience, the cue 'what issues seem significant to pay attention to?' raised my awareness of my need for status and recognition, while 'to what extent did I act for the best?' prompted an ethical consideration of my prescribing decision, and V's right to act autonomously. Finally, 'what factors influenced the way I was feeling, thinking or responding?' and 'how do I *now* feel about this experience?' highlighted my conflict avoidance and need for control. This reflection revealed a sorry state of affairs and even as I return to it now, I gather new insights from it, as I look at it with my changed perspective through the intervening experiences. My competitiveness with the doctors shines through my words.

Framing perspectives

Insights are inchoate, tentative. They impact on future practice and in doing so are transformed in response. They are not easy to articulate and certainly not predictive of how I will respond in future situations, even as they open the door to new ways of being and responding.

So, how might insights be framed? My approach was to develop the framing perspectives grid that represents the dimensions of learning necessary for being and becoming an effective practitioner (Fig. 3.7). Issues of role and vision frame every experience. As I have noted, vision is at the heart of reflection, whilst understanding the nature of one's current reality can only be viewed from the context of one's role responsibility. Role responsibility is both diffuse and complex, its primary focus contentious depending on where different people are coming from, each one invested with power dynamics. There are at least six sources of responsibility: being responsible to:

1. the patient and family, to help them meet their health needs and support them through the medical response
2. self, to act with integrity according to beliefs and values and to ensure self-effectiveness
3. society, to fulfil and enhance societal expectations of nursing
4. the organisation, to fulfil role responsibility as set out in a job description
5. the profession, to justify actions within the guidelines of the UKCC Code of Conduct
6. peers, to work in collaboration and mutually supportive ways to ensure patients and families receive congruent, consistent and effective care.

Philosophical framing	Role framing	Theoretical framing/mapping:
How has this experience enabled me to confront and clarify my beliefs and values that constitute desirable practice?	*How has this experience enabled me to* clarify my role boundaries and authority within my role, and my power relationships with others?	*How has this experience enabled me to* draw on extant theory and research in order to help me make sense of my knowing in practice, and to juxtapose and assimilate theory/research findings with personal knowing?
Developmental framing *How has this experience enabled me to* frame becoming a more effective practitioner within valid and appropriate theoretical frameworks/learning outcomes?	Insights	Reality perspective framing *How has this experience enabled me to* understand the barrier of reality whilst helping me to become empowered to act in more congruent ways?
Parallel process framing *How has this experience enabled me to* make connections between learning processes within my supervision process and my clinical practice?	Temporal framing *How has this experience enabled me to* draw patterns with past experiences whilst anticipating how I might respond in similar situations in new ways?	Problem framing *How has this experience enabled me to* focus problem identification and resolution within the experience?

Figure 3.7 Framing perspectives grid.

Developmental framing

As I suggested, theory can be mapped in ways that enable the practitioner to position self within the theory. In the Tom and Joan story I utilised Halldorsdottir's modes of being typology (1991) to map my own and Marie's mode of being with Tom. Halldórsdóttir worked with different groups of patients and women experiencing childbirth and cancer. Experiences of cancer were characterised by uncertainty, vulnerability, a sense of isolation, discomfort and redefinition. Because patients expect nurses to be caring, when they are not they often experience non-caring, characterised by lack of interest, coldness and inhumanity, that led to a decreased sense of well-being for the patient. Patients and relatives need to feel cared for at a time of high anxiety. Besides Halldorsdottir's work, other studies (Larson 1987, Mayer 1986, Reiman 1986) are particularly significant in identifying the perceptions of both nurses and patients regarding caring and non-caring encounters.

Did Marie and I ease Tom's suffering or did we contribute to it? Halldórsdóttir (1991) constructed a typology of modes of being with another that ranged from life giving to life destroying (Box 3.3), that offers a powerful reflective lens to consider our respective modes of being with Tom. The realisation that practitioners, through their attitudes and actions, can be uncaring and contribute to, rather than ease, suffering is profound.

In my view, Marie's mode of being with Tom was life restraining, yet she would be horrified to view herself as such. Tom rationalised this approach as 'these poor girls'

Box 3.3 Modes of being with another (adapted from Halldórsdóttir 1991)

Life giving (biogenic)	A mode of being where one affirms the personhood of the other by connecting with the true centre of the other in a life-giving way. It relieves the vulnerability of the other and makes the other stronger, and enhances growth, restores, reforms, and potentiates learning and healing
Life sustaining (bioactive)	A mode of being where one acknowledges the personhood of the other, supports, encourages, and reassures the other. It gives security and comfort. It positively affects the life of the other
Neutral (biopassive)	A mode of being where one does not affect the life in the other
Life restraining (biostatic)	A mode of being where one is insensitive or indifferent to the other and detached from the true centre of the other. It causes discouragement and develops uneasiness in the other. It negatively affects existing life in the other
Life destroying (biocidic)	A mode of being where one depersonalises the other, destroys life and increases the other's vulnerability. It causes distress and despair and hurts and deforms the other. It is transference of negative energy

(having to look after someone like me). Marie's response to Tom had become routinised. As a consequence, she had become desensitised to his suffering. Her care of Tom had become depersonalised, focused around maintaining his physical needs as a tolerant mother might be with a child. In contrast, my own mode of being was life giving, connecting with him at the core of his own being and affirming his personhood.

Whilst developmental framing using frameworks such as the modes of being with another enables the practitioner to focus on their development of expertise within a particular aspect of their practice, it does not offer a global framework for monitoring the whole of desirable practice.

So how might desirable practice be known? I could not find any adequate solutions to this challenge within the literature and so I developed the 'being available template', based on the core therapeutic of the practitioner being available to work with the person (patient, client) to enable the person to find meaning in their experience, to make best decisions about their health, and to assist them as necessary to meet their health needs. I explore the template in Chapters 6 and 7.

Conclusion

In this chapter I have described the basic scheme for reflection as movement through six dialogical movements. I have then set out the first two movements, concerned with the fundamental skills of journalling and reflection on experience, leading towards gaining tentative insights and the way insights might be mapped within the framing perspectives.

In Chapter 4, I explore the third and fourth dialogical movements.

Chapter 4

The third and fourth dialogical movements

In Chapter 3 I explored the first two dialogical movements within narrative construction that guide the practitioner to draw and hold tentative insights. In this chapter I explore the third and fourth dialogical movements that can guide reflective practitioners to substantiate their insights.

The third dialogical movement: the dance with Sophia

In the third dialogical movement, holding the tentative insights gained from the second dialogical movement, I turn to dialogue with a diverse literature to inform and deepen these insights. As Dewey (1933) notes:

> Reflective action entails active and persistent consideration of any belief or supposed form of knowledge in the light of the grounds that support it and the consequences to which it leads.

My tentative insights inform my practical wisdom or phronesis – the knowing I use in making clinical decisions and considering the consequences of my intended actions in terms of what is the right thing to do.

> Phronesis in Aristotle's *Nicomachean Ethics* is the virtue of moral thought, usually translated as 'practical wisdom', sometimes as 'prudence'.
> Aristotle distinguishes between two intellectual virtues: *sophia* and *phronesis*. *Sophia* (usually translated 'wisdom') is the ability to think well about the nature of the world, to discern why the world is the way it is (this is sometimes equated with science); *sophia* involves deliberation concerning universal truths. *Phronesis* is the capability to consider the mode of action in order to deliver change, especially to enhance the quality of life. Aristotle says that *phronesis* is not simply a skill, however, as it involves not only the ability to decide how to achieve a certain end, but also the ability to reflect upon and determine that end (this latter point is denied by some commentators, who contend that Aristotle considers the desired end, *eudaimonia*, to be given, such that *phronesis* is merely the ability to achieve that end). *Phronesis* is concerned with particulars, because it is concerned with how to act in particular situations. One can learn the principles of action, but applying them in the real world, in situations one could not have foreseen, requires experience of the world. For example, if one knows that one should be honest, one might act in certain situations in ways that cause pain and offense; knowing how to apply honesty in balance with other considerations and in specific contexts requires experience. Wikipedia.[1]

---

[1] http://en.wikipedia.org/wiki/Phronesis

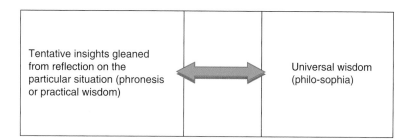

Figure 4.1 The dance with Sophia.

Put another way, phronesis is the basis for the moral life. However, all insights are only partial, gleaned from the particular situation, even though I have experienced many similar situations. Holding these insights I can now dialogue with the wider diverse universal wisdom: what I call the dance with Sophia.

Philosophy represents truths that are generally held as universal reflecting the nature of life and, as such, intends to guide the way people go about things, for example the nature of the caring relationship. At this level of dialogue, I accept I am not alone in the world but am situated within a community that shares common ideas and values as the basis for social and cultural life. At this level of dialogue I dwell critically within these ideas, problematising both my insights and the wisdom literature for its potential to inform my insights. As Trihn (1991:157) says:

> Experience, discourse, and self-understanding collide against larger cultural assumptions concerning race, ethnicity, nationality, gender, class, and age.
> Collide, rub against, grate … words of friction that scrape and open up the surface of insights. Words that capture something of the tension. Then reflection becomes exciting in the quest to know and transform self. I punch my skinny fist towards the sky.

Trihn states *concerning race, ethnicity, gender class and age* – reflecting the autoethnographic agenda of liberation from oppressed states that dominates this literature in the USA. Shades of a critical social science more grounded in liberation from political systems. I might add professional and managerial domination that suppresses nursing from realising its therapeutic potential. Perhaps this is gender.

And yet, in my experience, healthcare practitioners rarely engage with philosophy.

- Why is this?
- Do you?
- What philosophical and theoretical literature informs your practice?
- Do you think you should be more engaged on a philosophical level?
- If not, why not?

Is the non-engagement with philosophy itself a form of self-oppression, that nursing is about doing not being or even thinking too deeply? As I suggested earlier, I suspect it is because nursing and therapy are defined more in terms of what they do rather than what they value. Doing rather than being, epistemology rather than ontology. Reflection confronts this attitude. It demands that the practitioner focuses or refocuses on a values-based foundation to clinical practice. Ask yourself, what does it mean to be a nurse or indeed any other healthcare identity? These are vital questions that this third dialogical movement grapples with.

When I first read theory, it is 'out there' in a space that my mind grapples with. Gradually, as I dialogue with the theory within the context of my particular experience, I absorb and assimilate the theory as my own. It becomes part of me and begins to influence the way I see and respond to the world.

D. Soyini Madison (1999:109) captures this unity:

> Performance helps me live a truth while theory helps me name it – or maybe it is the other way around. My mind and body are locked together in a nice little divine kind of unity: the theory knows and feels, and the performance feels and unlearns. I know I am a un/learning body in the process of feeling. You too.

There is no gap between theory and practice, between the mind and the body, no dualism, just the tension that reading theory opens up against the landscape of performance. It is creative play. I do not look at theory just once, but again and again through repeated performances, making myself anew as I engage and dialogue with it within the context of my particular experience or performance. Indeed, this whole book reflects a dialogue with all sources of knowing – theory, theology, philosophy, science, ancient wisdom and the rest – as I move to embody ideas and transform myself through my performance as an educator and clinician, enabling myself and those with whom I work towards self-realisation to become more fully human, whatever that might mean for the individual and for society.

Consider the way I weave ideas between the lines of my story concerning Michael's wife. *Michael's wife* is a story taken from my narrative in *Engaging reflection in practice* where it was just 14 lines long (p139) and little more than a footnote to Linda's story (p132–41), in which I suggest that caring is intimate and mindful. I have developed the text, breaking it down line by line into what might be described as *prose poetry*, expanding it to reflect its deep significance *in passing people by* and the way I process attention.

When I perform, I read it slowly, pausing, emphasising key moments, dwelling on the immense poignancy and vulnerability within the moment. I give out the four readings to members of the audience as indicated in the text to deepen the emphasis on meaning, positioning my tentative insights into a wider philosophy and, more significantly, drawing the audience deeper into the brief text with their participation.

There is no Powerpoint background to this performance. I prefer to sit alone centre stage, reading from my journal.

Michael's wife

Holding my blue wooden box of essential oils
I wait in the corridor outside the door to her single room
for Linda to return from the bathroom.
I glance across the corridor and catch her eye;
Michael's wife.
She sits alone by Michael's bed in vigil.
Perhaps she smelt the fragrances seeping from the box
and looked up to catch my eye?
We had met last week,

the only time we have conversed.
Then I had given him reflexology,
then smiles and easy talk.
Now I give a sad smile and truncated wave
and look away.
I feel her deep despair drift across the space to where I wait.
I feel the pang of contradiction
that to look away adds to her suffering
when my vision is to ease it.
I know I cannot pass her by.
I move across the corridor into the room
and ask how are things.
Now Michael is not doing so well.
She says, '*It will be a sweet release when he "goes" for both of us.
It's hard to watch him struggle*'.
She looks down.
I touch her arm.
Just a light touch as if sensing the boundary between us,
feeling for the trace of our previous intimacy
not assumed but heart-felt.
She looks up. Her eyes meet mine;
eyes so full of suffering.
I am aware of my breath and beating heart,
I am mindful of her eyes,
Mindful not to pass her by
even as my mind waits for Linda's return
and a host of other demands logged into the mind system.
So many competing voices demand
none more so than my own in response to the ethical demand
to care for this life put into my hands.
to stay and dwell in the moment ...
for this moment is itself a lifetime.
Logstrup's words reverberate.

"by our very attitude to one another we help to shape one another's world. By our attitude to the other person we help to determine the scope and hue of his or her world; we make it large and small, bright or drab, rich or dull, threatening or secure. We help to shape his or her world not by theories and views but by our very attitude toward him or her. Herein lies the unarticulated and one might say anonymous demand that we take care of the life which trust has placed into our hands." (Logstrup 1997:18)

The demand to care.
Perhaps that is why some practitioners must turn their eyes away,
fearful of the emotional work to be sprung,
or anxious at being caught up when another task is yet undone.
Aching with self-concern, they avoid the other's plight.
A few words pass between Michael's wife and me
I feel more the silence between the words
I sense that words are merely attempts to fill the silence
that bring us face to face with the reality of Michael's dying.

"At best our cry for meaning, for serenity, is answered by a greater silence, the silence that makes us seek higher reconciliation. I think we need more of the wordless in our lives.

We need more stillness, more of a sense of wonder, a feeling for the mystery of life. We need more love, more silence, more deep listening, more deep giving." (Okri 1997)

In the silence I wonder
What does she think, what does she feel?
My empathic inquiry to connect with her
as we sit alongside his broken body.
Finding pattern in the chaos of this experience.
As Margaret Wheatley says: "Pattern recognition requires that we sit together reflectively and patiently."
Some things cannot be rushed.
I can never pretend to know.

Tears spill down her cheeks
I feel her ache within mine,
my sympathetic resonance to share her grief
so she is no longer alone.
I feel her aloneness in the world as death pulls her apart
and in the quietness of the fading light we dwell,
the room a sacred space infused with grace.

Joseph Rael (1993:29,88–9) says that there is energy that comes to all of us from the sacred place, the vibrations of an ancient past, wisdom we would come to find one day. Once the sacred place is discovered, we begin to open to the wisdom. It descends upon us just as it did when the beings from the spirit of life brought spirit to the people. What is interesting about this lifting energy is that when it happens to us, it also happens to other people who are also being lifted to the next level [and] when we began to lift ourselves from we were before to a higher place, something dramatic happens in our lives.

This is a powerful image.
Tuning into this healing energy
Lifting myself and people beyond suffering with wisdom and compassion
The Bodhisattva ideal;
I imagine Avalokiteshvara's thousand arms spread to embrace suffering.
The image guides me in my practice.

Linda waves at me from the open door,
the spell is broken.
Michael's wife places her small hand over mine and thanks me for my time.
it seems that time had ceased in this brief moment.
Without doubt practice is a mystery I must tread with care.
Care *is* being mindful, being fully present in corridor moments
even with those we barely know.
For in the moment, if I am mindful enough,
I know better now than to look away and pass people by.
Presence opens a glimmer of possibility within her darkness
where she had felt hopeless.
In the face of compassion suffering is lightened.
The circumstance has now changed, it now seems less hopeless.
Her suffering is recognised and validated, and to some extent transformed.
I do not seek to fix her suffering but to enable her to ease within it.
And we can see that to know caring unfolding is mindfulness – sensed through reflection
and nurtured within the unbroken reflexive spiral of creation;
liberation uncoiling into space.

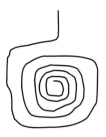

The text contains four short readings that strongly influence my therapeutic approach. First, consider Logstrup's idea of the ethical demand.

> Herein lies the unarticulated and one might say anonymous demand that we take care of the life which trust has placed into our hands.

Read these words again slowly ... sense what the ethical demand might mean for yourself as a healthcare practitioner. Think about these words when you are next with a patient. Trust is the very core of relationship. If you take Logstrup's words seriously they must radically influence the way you perceive the therapeutic relationship with the patient. Think about it. As Arthur Frank (2002:13) says:

> Caring is one of those activities that people know only when they are involved in it. From within, and only from within, caring makes sense. To try and explain care leads to the circularity expressed in statements such as 'caring for this person requires doing this, and I do this because I care for this person'. Philosophy teaches that, for some activities, there is only practice.

It follows that if we accept Frank's position, caring is only relational and that is only known within the relation as it unfolds. Caring is therefore not a thing that can be known as an abstract idea. The practitioner knows themselves as caring only within the moment. As such, caring is a mystery drama unfolding. The reflective practitioner, mindful of self within the moment, is aware of and curious about this drama unfolding, seeking to know it and shape it as it unfolds.

As a Buddhist, I am influenced by Buddhist philosophy or doctrine that permeates through the text like a soft stream. Ideas such as the Bodhisattva ideal symbolises myself as caring – a beacon to work towards. The Bodhisattva, with deep compassion and wisdom, dedicates self to alleviating suffering wherever it is found. It is a powerful idea. Suffering, the causes of suffering, cessation of suffering and the path that leads from suffering – the four noble truths – go to the very heart of Buddhist philosophy and to my own practice. The gate to the path is vision and then the path leads me to help ease suffering in the person.

Reflection only really works when the practitioner approaches it seriously with the commitment and intention to be authentic. Only then can the practitioner really come to know and become self as caring.

Consider Joseph Rael's words within the text. Joseph Rael is a Native American and his wisdom may be hard to swallow for the rational Western mind. And yet, such wisdom is my truth. I feel it vibrate through me like a soft healing wind. As a therapist, open to the possibility, Rael speaks a universal truth that is so obvious to me. And so when I dialogue with these words, I touch my energy. My energy is a continuous insight unfolding. It is not something new yet it is inchoate, always being formed, always being known through successive experiences in its subtlety. I am integral to the patient's environment. Hence my energy impacts on the person, creating a healing environment or sacred space (Quinn 1992, 1997).

This energy is life giving and as I open to it, so those I work with, both patients and staff, are also opened to it. It radiates through people. It is available to everyone as a potent healing power. You know this for yourself. You know from your own experience how some people lift you whilst others drain you. When you pay attention to this idea and cultivate 'lifting energy' then it becomes a powerful therapeutic energy.

Ben Okri's words on *silence* help me pay attention, to quieten so as to be fully present within the moment and to see that moment as with a sense of *stillness and reverence*. It is a gateway to being with someone, not just as they face death but with any potentially healing encounter. His words remind me to be still in the midst of apparent chaos.

The idea of order within chaos reverberates through Margaret Wheatley's words; that if I can somehow let go of my need to control situations and go with the flow, things work out fine as long as I keep my vision in mind.

The fourth dialogical movement: dialogue with peers and guides

I dialogue with guides and peers to check out, confront, inform, deepen and affirm my tentative insights, even generating new insights as the dialogue unfolds.

The need for guidance

Boud *et al.* (1985) observed how their model of reflection was something the student could do for themselves, but noted that 'the learning process can be considerably accelerated by appropriate support' (p36) – the idea of guided reflection. For a number of reasons[2] reflection *may* benefit from guidance to maximise its learning potential. I say *may* because the context of guidance is very significant. I pick this point up later in the chapter.

- To enable the practitioner to take responsibility for their own performance in guided reflection and clinical practice (preparing the ground).
- To gain insights into self, one's vision and one's reality.
- To hold the practitioner along this journey.
- To remoralise the demoralised practitioner.
- To gain insight into new ways of being and responding congruently.
- To co-create meaning.
- To infuse the practitioner with resolve (courage) to take action as necessary. (Adapted from Johns 2004a, 2006)

Preparing the ground

For the practitioner to enter into guided reflection is a serious matter. It requires commitment and responsibility. Yet many practitioners struggle to keep a reflective journal

---

[2]This list has been adapted and summarised from the 2nd edition.

(Johns 2002, p17). They are tired at the end of the day, they want to switch off, they don't see the value, they don't have the discipline, they don't find it meaningful. I am sure you can add to the list! They might benefit from some encouragement.

Karen was an associate nurse at Burford. She noted the flowering of her commitment to her practice and reflection.

> Sessions 1–6 were very much led by my supervisor, but in session 7 we had a sudden break-through and I took control. From then on I felt I was growing through supervision – I remember telling Chris I felt like a seedling in spring which has felt the sun and is now growing big and strong into a tree. (Johns 1998a)

The growth of commitment to herself and to her practice was an emotional and revelatory experience for Karen. She noted how she increasingly looked forward to her sessions: 'I knew how much I benefited, but I also knew how much energy it took and I often felt drained afterwards' (Johns 1998a).

Initially Karen felt ambivalent about supervision not just because of the effort of reflection, but because she felt threatened that her lack of competence would be exposed and that she would be judged as a poor nurse. She was anxious to demonstrate her competence after qualifying with a nursing degree. As such, at the time when she most needed support, she resisted it because she wanted to show she was competent.

An ironic twist, yet seemingly a common response from newly qualified practitioners (Cherniss 1980). This is one reason why reflection needs to be meaningfully embedded within professional pre-registration programmes so that both reflection and guidance become second nature for the newly qualified professional.

Once she had accepted responsibility for her performance and grasped the nature of guided reflection, Karen valued guidance because it gave her such positive feedback about practice and helped her resolve difficult situations and emotions.[3]

Practitioners simply need guidance to get going so they can actually sense the point for themselves. It is no good saying research says reflection is good for you. You must feel this for youself. So you need time to sense the point. Imagine sitting with a patient who has just been told his cancer can no longer be treated. He needs to talk and share his story. He needs to find meaning and find a way to move forward. You are his guide. Your guide works in a similar way ... to help you find meaning in the experience, to draw insight and move forward positively, more knowingly into an uncertain future.

Gaining insights into self, one's vision and one's reality

Cox *et al* (1991:285) note that:

> Reflection in isolation is difficult to sustain because of the difficulty in surfacing and transcending our own distorted self understandings, asking ourselves difficult, often self-exposing questions, facing difficult answers to such questions, and, perhaps most particularly, keeping our vision directed toward new possibilities for understanding and action.

However, if people distort their reality they do so for reasons that are, in themselves, a significant focus for reflection. All stories are full of bias, contradictions and uniqueness (Remen 1996) and hence any firm grasp on reality is always tenuous. Perhaps the most

---

[3] See exemplar of guided reflection involving Karen in Johns 2004a, pp131–44.

significant aspect of guidance is to help practitioners pull away the masks that distort seeing self and reality for what they really are. Lather (1986b) terms this 'false consciousness'. Only then can the practitioner gain true insight and change the nature of their reality. It is like cleaning the reflective mirror of smudges that have accumulated over the years until a thick greasy dust obscures and distorts the view. We have become who we are through years of socialisation, through years of self-neglect, taken ourselves for granted, learning to fit in as best we can to societal demand and defend ourselves from anxiety. As mentioned, the forces of authority and tradition have shaped us, until we have embodied a way of being that is not easily amenable to change.

So transformation is not a given. It has to be worked at with commitment, discipline and a sense of play to lift the load when it seems arduous. It also requires vision. As such, guidance helps the practitioner to clarify the vision, learn the discipline and techniques as appropriate, prop up the hard times, encourage the play, be patient when frustrated. The guide helps the practitioner touch the breadth and depth, the subtlety of each MSR cue, becoming more aware, more proprioceptive of one's thinking and being. It is all too easy to scrape along the surface of these cues and miss the point. The guide points the finger.

On the basis for knowing one's reality, the guide then helps the practitioner to view self and practice in line with their desired vision even as self and the vision are constantly shifting through understanding. My intention is to enable the practitioner to see other ways of being and responding in situations, as if opening shutters that had been closed, confronting attitudes that had been partial and prejudiced, nurturing and developing personal power so the practitioner can feel empowered and take action congruent with their vision, reinforcing integrity and self-worth. At times, I may open the doors for the practitioner as they grope about in the dark, but I always do this cautiously, mindful of not imposing a particular way.

Holding

Inevitably, exploring self creates anxiety, as those deeper parts of self become exposed. The guide helps the practitioner to face up to anxiety rather than to defend against it. In this respect the guide becomes part of the practitioner's defence system, a supportive hand across Schön's metaphoric swamplands (1987) until firmer ground is felt. I have already noted the significance of reflection as energy work. The guide is a catalyst to convert negative energy into positive energy.

The guide must be mindful and comfortable about being with the practitioner in this way. In my experience, this is not a big deal, a big psychotherapeutic drama. It is more a natural, mindful, caring way of being in dialogue whereby I am non-attached to the other yet caring deeply for them, connected to them yet separate from them.

Most significantly, it models the holistic way of being-in-relationship within the liminal space between one experience and another. In this sense all experience is liminal, at the threshold of becoming.

Remoralisation

Listening to the practitioner: their stories of joy, suffering, affirmation, doubt, ignorance, yearning, caring, effectiveness. I accept the stories unconditionally even as I probe and explore them, picking up cues that lead the story forward to where insights lie buried. Being heard, the practitioner is remoralised (Frank 2002); a self that has often become demoralised through loss of care, both the care they give and the care they receive. This is why concern for the practitioner is vital, care in the sense of enabling the other to grow (Mayeroff 1971). Concern might also be described as compassion or simply care. And of course, it is the same care the practitioner has for those she cares for.

Co-constructing meaning

As I listen to the practitioner's experience, I refrain from imposing meaning on it. I encourage the practitioner to dwell within the experience, slowly turning it over to see it for what it is; seeing self within it in relationship with others. Slowly insights spin out, tentatively held yet gathering substance and conviction with each turn of the wheel. I pick up cues that I sense are significant and ask questions. I may then offer my own tentative insights yet without imposing any authority onto what the experience might mean. It is holding back, not crowding the reflective space, not cramping the practitioner as she endeavours to expand her consciousness. Through dialogue we shape meaning, crafting insight, fusing our horizons, whereby our perspectives are transcended in reaching new perspectives (Gadamer 1975). In other words, reflection is mutual growth. As I listen, I also reflect, challenging my own understandings, being open to possibilities, developing my own insights. This is the nature of dialogue.

Horizon is another way of describing context. It includes everything of which one is not immediately aware and which one must in fact remain unaware of if there is to be a focus for attention; but one's horizon is also the context in terms of which the object of attention is understood. This horizon can be called life or world but must always be conceived as mobile, fluid and temporal. As opposed to the objective world of natural science, the life world is 'the world in which we live in the natural attitude which never as such becomes objective for us but on the contrary represents the pre-given ground of all experience' (Weinsheimer 1985:157). Our own horizon is constantly in the process of formation, not least through our encounters with the past.

Insights into new ways of being and doing

Guidance helps practitioners see the pattern of their practice … the way they are locked into habitual ways of perceiving and responding to situations, challenging them to think about things differently, opening and exploring their mental models that govern the way they feel, think and respond to situations.

In guided reflection with me, Lisa, a Macmillan support nurse, noted:

> I felt that being challenged is an essential element of guidance, providing you feel comfortable in your environment and at ease with your guide. The challenge element encouraged me to think further than I had been and to deal with issues in a way I would not have considered before.

In challenging, I am planting and watering seeds of doubt (Margolis 1993). The mind learns to become mindful, paying attention to its thoughts, no longer taking things for granted, lifting the mundane into something significant moment by moment. The practitioner's curiosity and responsibility aroused, she learns to challenge self, to become her own judge. She develops critical consciousness. Margolis considers that new ideas compete with existing ideas. The success of adopting new ideas depends on the robustness of existing ones and the force of argument available to support the new idea. The guide's role is to help plant these seeds of doubt in tune with desirable practice and to water them so the seeds grow and blossom, whilst weeding away old ideas that are no longer tenable.

Accepting the new idea is just the beginning; the ensuing congruent action cannot be guaranteed. As I have discussed, practitioners do not change their responses simply on a rational basis (Fay 1987). This point highlights the folly of imposing liberating structures such as supervision on people, in that practitioners, such as nurses, who have been socialised to be powerless and subordinate are unable to respond to liberating opportunities when they present themselves. The emphasis must be on the practitioner coming to realise a new reality for themselves, rather than having this reality explained to them. For example, all shared experiences concerned with conflict have a fundamental power inequality at their root which manifests itself through different attitudes, beliefs and behaviours. This is not difficult to see or understand providing it is sought, and not just taken for granted as part of the 'natural' background of the experience. All understanding is cast against the practitioner's background while at the same time, the naturalness of social arrangements is challenged so that the practitioner and the guide become cognisant of both the restraints and the potential to change the situation so that the seeds of doubt will flourish and blossom.

Through the continuity of guidance, new ideas can quickly be put into practice and subsequently reflected on. If the seeds don't take because the soil is stony, then the stone is chipped away slowly, until the moment when the new seed takes hold. Change is a social process (Ottaway 1978) that requires patience, persistence and passion, and perhaps freedom from persecution.

Resolving creative tension

Holding creative tension is one thing, acting to resolve it is quite another when pinned against the cold face of reality. To take action often involves challenging the barriers that constrain us – barriers of tradition, authority and embodiment. It is as if the practitioner has shed her socialised skin and is growing another one. Yet between skins she is most vulnerable. Hence the need for challenge to shed the skin and support to hold her until her new skin grows. We are all snakes.

Without adequate challenge the practitioner may rationalise the contradiction and decide to let matters lie, particularly where she is fearful of consequences. She may fear disapproval and sanction. Smyth (1987:40) notes:

> Most of us, unless we feel uncomfortable, shaken, or forced to look at ourselves, are unlikely to change. It is far easier to accept our current conditions and adopt the least line of resistance.

Lieberman (1989:88) notes that:

> Working in bureaucratic settings has taught everyone to be compliant, to be rule governed, not to ask questions, seek alternatives or deal with competing values.

In response, Day (1993) asserts that reflection will bring the practitioner into tension with prevailing dominant organisational values, suggesting that reflection will struggle to make an impact unless the organisation is sympathetic to more collaborative ways of working. The participants in Kieffer's (1984) study of empowerment of grassroots community leaders in the USA referred with great emotional intensity to the importance of the external enabler to support their struggle against more powerful others who were motivated to maintain the status quo. The practitioner connects with her guide or supervisor as a representative of the wider community, the gatekeeper and guide to this new world. In order to do this, the guide must connect with the practitioner in terms of her existing reality and, simultaneously, in terms of a potential new reality. Fay (1987:265–6) puts it like this:

> Coming to a radically new self-conception is hardly ever a process that occurs simply by reading some theoretical work; rather it requires an environment of trust and support in which one's own preconceptions and feeling can be properly made conscious to oneself, in which one can think through one's experiences in terms of a radically new vocabulary which expresses a fundamentally different conceptualisation of the world in which one can see the particular and concrete ways that one unwittingly collaborates in producing one's own misery and in which one can gain emotional strength to accept and act on one's new insights.

Clearly the attitudes of both practitioner and supervisor are important. Yet I meet few practitioners who are happy with their 'lot'. It is a tough world working within the NHS and practitioners are tired and frustrated. I get this message time and time again through the stories practitioners disclose to me. It is not easy to see nurses suffer because of lack of caring. It becomes an ethical issue to urge them to take action and watch them stumble and fall against the hard edge of reality. Maybe it is easier to say 'OK this is beyond you' and such judgements need to made sensibly.

Carl Rogers (1969) noted how people were ambivalent about learning because any significant learning involves a certain amount of pain, either pain connected with learning itself or giving up previous learning. He notes that the first type of ambivalence is illustrated by the small child who is learning to walk. He stumbles, he falls, he hurts himself. It is a painful process. Yet the satisfaction of developing his potential far outweighs the bumps and bruises. Or in the immortal words of CS Lewis spoken by Anthony Hopkins in the film *Shadowlands* – 'I've just come up against a bit of experience. Experience is a brutal teacher but by God you learn ... you learn'.

But you learn more with support and challenge with an appropriate guide. So practitioners – choose your guides with care and take control of the supervision agenda – it is *your* practice!

Reflection may create a sense of crisis of confidence and even identity as one's 'old ways' are challenged. The practitioner is caught between defending self from this anxiety and opening self to new possibilities. However, in exploring new, more congruent ways, the practitioner may experience a crisis of isolation or separateness (Isaacs 1993) whereby group norms and ways of relating must shift. This may overflow into personal lives as practitioners find their voices and speak out. Isaacs notes:

> Such loosening of rigid thought patterns frees energy that now permits new levels of intelligence and creativity. (p38)

The voice of freedom is a powerful cry and may be resisted by those affected by the practitioner's new ways of thinking, feeling and responding to situations. Through dialogue the practitioner can emerge transformed into a new dawn, ever mindful. She becomes remoralised, reconnected to caring.

But we do need to choose our guides carefully.

The nature of guidance

Guidance is a therapeutic relationship that, in many respects, mirrors the practitioner's clinical relationships. As such, the guide can model ways of being that are congruent with therapeutic practice.[4] The most obvious is dialogue itself as an enabling and empowering process. As the guide seeks to *be available* to the practitioner so the practitioner seeks to *be available* to the people she works with.

Being available has six dimensions:

- a shared vision of guided reflection
- concern for/commitment to the practitioner
- knowing the practitioner
- skilled and ethical guidance
- knowing self
- creating the conditions for effective guidance.

Being available is the core therapeutic of holistic practice – enabling the practitioner to find meaning and insight into their experience, and on that basis to make best decisions and take necessary action to realise their vision of practice as a lived reality. The basis for all therapeutic relationships is commitment and trust based on a mutual appreciation of the relationship and characterised by high challenge/high support.[5]

As a guide, it may help to write your own vision statement to give to practitioners as a form of contract. Perhaps something like this:

> Through your stories I guide you to draw insights from your story to inform your future practice. In doing so, I commit myself to this relationship, to challenge and broaden your horizons to see things for what they are and other ways of being and doing. I help you to awaken your senses, arouse your passion from its slumber, to open your mind to possibility, and help you cleanse your being of toxic ways of being that contaminate your practice and distort the view. I hold you when you stumble against the hard wall of reality. I help you become free in joyful harmony within a community of inquiry where we co-create and learn through our mutual stories.

A cautionary note

However, guidance is not unproblematic. It is contextual and clearly strongly influenced by the relationship between the guide and practitioner, notably in situations where embodied patterns of relationship have led to traditional subordinate relationships. For example, the guide may view themselves as an authority and demand compliance, vet the practitioner's agenda, and even determine what insights the practitioner has gained.

---

[4] The idea of being available from a clinical perspective is explored in Chapters 6 and 7.
[5] See also Chapter 16.

As with all helping or mentoring relationships, it is open to abuse from its collaborative intent. These issues are explored more deeply in Chapter 16 in relation to clinical supervision.

Conclusion

In this chapter I have set out the third and fourth dialogical movements concerned with substantiating tentative insights. In doing so, I open up the idea of guided reflection as a helping relationship and the significance of engaging with philosophical ideas. Like wisdom itself, we learn to be patient and dwell with the insights. These movements cannot be rushed … the deepening is a maturing … getting the point, developing the posture.

Chapter 5

The fifth and sixth dialogical movements: weaving the narrative

The narrative is woven from the first four dialogical movements into a coherent and reflexive form that adequately plots the unfolding journey in such a way that is open to further dialogue between the narrative writer and the narrative reader.

In Figure 3.1, I set out the six dialogical movements within the hermeneutic circle. By this I mean there is a constant movement within the whole towards greater understanding and gaining insight through the dialogical movements. At times, diverse aspects of experience are looked at with a view to deepening meaning within the perspective of the whole experience – we 'foreground' perceived significances against a canvass of the whole particular experience which is itself a microcosm of our whole total experience.

What started as 'doodles in my journal' or *story text* was first developed into *reflective text* and is now developed or woven into *narrative text*. Eventually, when shared with others, it develops into a *substantive text* through dialogue with others.

'Substantive' seems an appropriate word to capture the idea of dialogue reflecting consensus towards a better world, that through dialogue the insights and meanings within the narrative ripple outwards, changing people, changing the world.

Narrative always serves two purposes:

- to inform the reader of the author's reflexive journey
- to open a space for the reader to reflect on their own experiences, so opening the possibility of dialogue and developing the substantive text.

In shifting from story to reflective text, the description is investigated to reveal significance and develop insights. These insights are then explored with literature and with guides, deepening and shifting them. The narrative is written around these insights, transforming the original descriptive text into a coherent and reflexive narrative that adequately plots the journey of realising one's vision as a lived reality, revealing those factors that have constrained this realisation and ways they have been confronted and hopefully shifted.

In weaving the narrative, the reflective practitioner draws on her imagination and creativity, using metaphor, writing poetry, images, art, dramatic prose, photographs, nature, music, performance, film and dance to capture her insights. These different forms give richness and texture to the narrative.

Box 5.1 Development of text

Story text	Reflective text	Narrative text	Substantive text
Dialogical movement 1	Dialogical movements 2, 3 and 4	Dialogical movement 5	Dialogical movement 6

Reflection as art

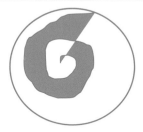

The koru is a Maori image inspired by the uncurling fern frond. It represents peace, tranquillity, personal growth, positive change and awakening, new life and harmony. I discovered this image when visiting New Zealand and now wear the koru, made from green stone or pounamu, as the symbol for my reflective practice. Each time I draw the koru it is different, again representing that each experience is different although the basic pattern is familiar. As Tuffnell and Crickmay (2004:41) poetically put it:

> An image evokes a world, a solar system of connections and meanings, of associations, qualities, *textures* and memories ... an image forms a bridge between what's inside us and what is outside ... it brings us more fully into a felt relationship with the world.

The neglected right side of the brain is like the dark side of the hill tucked away out of view, out of touch. The left side whirs away in its rational cognitive way, imposing logic over intuition, reason over imagination, observation over perception, technique over creativity.

Dwelling with the text, opening the lines, opening the imagination, we seek metaphors, icons and images which better capture our experience and meaning than words. Breaking the text into lines immediately opens the door to writing a prose poem.

There are a number of poems scattered through this book that capture the poignancy and intimacy of the moment, that express the self beyond a rational or cognitive level of knowing. Writing a poem is a release of tension, an expression of compassion, that honours self and other and the connection between you.

As I read back through my past narratives, I am struck by the power of the poems – the way poems hold meaning and insight in their poignancy and beauty.

Four poems are set out below. I am tempted to explain the insights within them but refrain – you can always read the narratives in which they are situated. I wrote *The heron and the tree* and *The waiting room. Blue ... for Greta* was written by Christine, a staff nurse at the hospice. She was deeply moved and distressed by Greta's father's death. I suggested she try and write a poem that somehow captured her feelings. It was a deeply cathartic and transformative experience – a narrative in itself.

The poem *The river of tears* was written following a clinical supervision with a ward sister who was very distressed throughout the 1-hour session.

The heron and the tree (Johns 2006: 86)

Each day we dwelt beneath the small tree
That stood outside your window
to witness the change of colour
From green to yellows and reds
And then brown to mark the leaf's descent into the earth.

Each day fewer leaves
were attached to the tree's life
Reflecting Autumn's time for death
Within the cycle of life.

In the shade of the tree sat heron
as if a guide who waited patiently
To guide your journey
From this dimension of life to the next.

I know heron brought you comfort
Even a sense of stillness
In those poignant moments
When fear gripped the raw edge of emotion.

Some days heron would catch a leaf
Or two as it fell from the tired tree
Damp with rain the leaf held fast
As if reluctant to let go.

The leaves are a symbol of life
Each day a few less leaves
Until the last time I sat with you
just one or two clung tenaciously to life,

Reluctant to let go.
As if each leaf falling was a countdown
To that inevitable moment
when your breath would cease.

Yet you did let go
In peace
surrounded by your family
to melt into the divine light.

Blue ... for Greta (Johns 2006:105)

The moment had come ...
But, you were unaware of what was unfolding,
The bewilderment in your beautiful eyes told me that.
Eyes of the same vivid blue as your dad,
So startling,
So trusting,
So sad.

You could see mummy crying,
You could feel her sadness
As she held you tightly,
Kissing you, stroking your hair,
Softly speaking,
Softly crying,
Softly, softly ...

She held daddy to her, reluctant to let him go
Knowing there were no more options;
She was losing him,
The battle was being lost,
He was going,
He did not want to,
He had no choice ...

Through my own tears
I was aware of yours
As you looked from mummy to daddy;
You had your thumb in your mouth,
You touched your mummy's hand;
She did not notice.
She could not help it,
She was oblivious ...

For the briefest moment,
She was aware only of him,
She went with him to the brink

But could go no further;
This was now his solo voyage.
Breathing together,
Breathing for him,
Breathing alone.

Then she looked up into big blue eyes,
Your blue eyes,
His blue eyes,
His legacy to her
And held you close to her.

The waiting room (Johns 2006:152)

We all wait ...
Expectant
Waiting for the last breath.
Searching for the signs of departure
Of death's train

We all wait ...
Crowded into the waiting room
Finding some shelter from the gusts
Of death's wind

Waiting marks the social death
A void where we falter
In knowing what to say unable to move on
Or retreat.

Waiting ... I hold your hand
You smile and gaze into my eyes
I feel your soul glow through your gaze
In the stillness of what is ...
You also wait
And comfort those who tremble.

Waiting is hard
For those who gather about
Whose souls shout
For tender release
Grasping for the sign
Seeking some closure.

We all wait
For the train to depart
The track ahead is not yet clear
The red light shines
Yet your death is certain
Only when..
Until then we wait ...

The river of tears (Johns 2004a:86)

This space between us
A river of tears
Where your tears flow,
The flow of pain
Hurt to the quick.

This river of tears
Where once your passion flowed
And where your passion will flow again
When the storm has passed
And the sun shines again.

And when I gaze across at you
I feel the touch of my concern
My gaze as an eagle's wing
That gently touches
the blue mood of despair.

The dark woman has broken
I feel her tears flow
Into the dark river that flows between
No words spoken
A clear winter's day within shadow.

I feel the swarm of bees about me
And the song of the bee about me
The dark woman stung
My words a balm
To loosen the binds that bound.

Tears like dewdrops
Sweep across the soft lids
Eyes glisten as the smile breaks through
Her anguished cry stops
In the soft dawn of hope.

Within each tear spilt
I sensed your hopes and fears
Your sense of being betrayed
The machine says 'tilt'
No longer can you play.

Nerve shredded along the raw edge
Cut to the quick
You recoil hurt and vulnerable
Frailty exposed along the ledge
Take my hand.

I meet you in this space
Where we can move beyond
With energy renewed for the task
The past already a blur
We have learnt from.

And on another day
and in another place
We can look back
And bathe in this river of tears
Where the demons drowned.

Often, having written a poem, practitioners say that they do not know where their words have come from. Many are astonished that they can write poetry, as if it is some untapped, latent potential within us all. It seems that in a technology-driven world, the artist is trimmed. Yet the latent artist lives within each of us ... just needs to be woken up and injected with some spirit. One risk of introducing models of reflection to structure writing is that it will stifle the spontaneous flow of words. It is easy to get locked into the technology of reflection – 'how to do it'– simply because we live in a technological world that demands explanatory models. Poetry is like taking a short cut to the unconscious, bypassing the cognitive realm. As such, aesthetic expression balances the more cognitive approaches to reflection, a more holistic approach that draws on and uses all the senses and taps the deep pool of tacit knowing (Polanyi 1958).

Undoubtedly caring is a form of aesthetic expression (Wainwright 2000) that both reflects and nurtures caring. Art opens up a creative possibility although the practitioner may need a guiding hand to move beyond barriers that portray art as soft and flaky.

A number of studies have used art and poetry to help practitioners find meaning in their experiences of being with suffering patients (Begley 1996, Brodersen 2001,

Eifried *et al* 2000, Parker 2002, Vaught-Alexander 1994). Of course, this is no surprise, because it is the essence of art therapy (Mayo 1996, Tyler 1998). These studies reflect the way humanities can open a space where practitioners can dwell safely with their own vulnerability, where expressions of vulnerability can be expressed in whatever form and learnt from. As McNiff (1992) eloquently puts it, 'Whenever illness is associated with a loss of soul, the arts emerge spontaneously as remedies'. Put another way – whenever activity is related to the soul, the arts emerge spontaneously as soul food.

Wagner (1999) interviewed 18 nurses for their reflections of family impact on the dying experience. She then reduced these experiences into a set of categories using fragments of the nurses' reflections to justify each category. In doing so, I felt she lost the meaning in these nurses' stories. However, Wagner then re-interpreted the nurses' words into poetry, as a way of knowing subjectively and inter-subjectively the fullest meaning of the data (p21). Her poetry reflects a deeper level of interpretation beyond cognition; in my mind, it heals the story and makes it possible to connect with the experience because it is whole, it is felt rather than read.

Perhaps the words flow from deeper consciousness, shaped into a beautiful creation. It is this sense of creativity that softens suffering and enables people to learn through reflection. As Parker (2002:104) writes: 'Art and aesthetic expression unite us and contribute to our wholeness. They are essential means of communication and move us all toward increased well being'.

In one workshop, I painted a reflection on my feelings after the death of Iris, a patient I had given reflexology over 2 years. The painting was simply the six colours painted horizontally that represented each of the major chakras I balance as part of reflexology. In the middle of the painting I portrayed a gaping dark grey hole that represented the disruption of the energy fields with Iris's death and my sense of loss. Inside the hole, I spread the shavings from sharpening the colour pencils, each shaving representing the fragments of Iris's life ... the memories of being with her collected together. I wrote the poem *Shavings* to accompany the painting.

Shavings

I sense the black hole
Blown open inside
Its angst leaking out
Across the anguished soul

I sense the shavings of your life
Fragments of wholeness
Reflecting all the different colours
that flow within

Like broken bits they float
about; unconnected
like bits of self
now lost

Yet I see your colours bright
that surround the gloom
my hand connects you
to sense your beauty.

Recent work by Cameron *et al* (2008), Gaydos (2008), Fordham (2008) and Jarrett (2008) stunningly illuminates the way these practitioners and lecturers use art in their narratives and guide students through reflective art to tell their clinical stories. Art workshops are vital within the curriculum to open the imaginative and creative right brain and fuel the reflective endeavour (see Chapter 18).

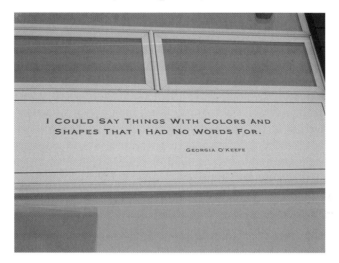

I photographed these words on a building in Boulder, Colorado.

Being playful, being disciplined

I have suggested that the writer stands back from the text in order to dwell within it, as if reading the text like a play. Ben Okri (1997: 22) says 'the artist should never lose the spirit of play'. Let us dwell with such words and sense their significance as we begin to craft our narratives. Play reminds me of children in the sand, being imaginative, finding the flow of creative life without censor. Play should be fun! Yet there are rules to play the game.

Again, Ben Okri puts the ideas of play and discipline into balance:

> An ideal creative genius would be one who knew how to consciously initiate great play, as well as how to harness great discipline, towards the most sublime endeavours ... with smile in the soul. (p22–3)

Ben Okri has most inspired my approach to narrative. Interpreting his work, I can set out some basic guidelines for narrative:

- that narrative should plant seeds in the reader's mind
- that narrative should be both enchanting and challenging, where beauty and horror lie side by side
- that narrative should be transgressive, always challenging the taken for granted, the complacent, the oppressive state of affairs
- that narrative should always be transformational
- that the reader does half the work.

Picking up the point that the reader does half the work, Okri asserts (1997:41):

> the writer ... does one half of the work, but the reader does the other. The reader's mind becomes the screen, the place, the era. To a large extent, readers create the world from words, they invent the reality they read. Reading, therefore, is a co-production between writer and reader.

I wonder about the extent to which such claims hold good for narrative written as self-inquiry and transformation. Okri asks that writers should serve truth, be humble, and finely craft their words arrowed to the deepest points of the reader's hearts and minds –then they should be silent, leave the stage and let the imagination of the world give sanctuary (p42).

To serve truth is an utter requirement even if the narrative is fiction, a finely crafted fiction based on insights. Perhaps this is necessary when the words are too sharp, arrowed at oppressive systems which may take strident offence if they can detect the author. The ethics of narrative are a swampy field.

Gadamer (1975) asks that the reader not take offence, not project meanings into the text but read it with an open mind in order to enter into the text and learn from it. Okri asks that readers bring the best of themselves to meet the best in the writer's work (p42). Noble sentiments. If only we were all so open-minded and concerned for the truth. When the status quo of the dominant is threatened then such pleas fall on closed ears. So I disguise names and places even within the narratives. I speak my own truth through my stories but am careful not to hurt. Where I criticise, I intend it to be moral and constructive. People dying should always be at the centre of best care. There is no compromise. No contradictions can be tolerated.

Yet, how our censors pull us back and impose their own rules. I return as I so often do to the words of Virginia Woolf (1945:105):

> So long as you write what you wish to write that is all that matters; and whether it matters for ages or only for a few hours, nobody can say. But to sacrifice a hair of the head of your vision, a shade of its colour, in deference to some ... professor with a measuring rod up his sleeve is the most abject treachery.

I read second-year nursing students a story of my complementary therapy practice. I ask them how they feel about the story. They say they wish they could write like that but cannot because they know they would fail the examination, get comment back that it is too descriptive. They would fail. They value reflection but are frustrated by these professors who impose rules – use a model of reflection as if that is the end-game. Perhaps then my own narratives are not good exemplars of reflective writing?

Remember, the narrative has a point – to plot the practitioner's reflexive journey towards realising desirable practice. It is a plot of being and becoming structured around insights gained through reflection on experiences. Reflexivity – looking back and seeing self as emerging towards realising desirable practice – requires a congruent framework whereby this can be seen. This is why I developed the being available template so practitioners could know themselves as holistic practitioners and yet always testing the framework for its adequacy to mark the journey of transformation. All theory can be mapped to mark the transformation journey.

Narratives are always process focused, not outcome focused: they are not to be judged in terms of whether desirable practice has or has not been achieved. It is the moment-to-moment unfolding that is vital in narrative, the mindful excursion through experience. It can simply be a single experience lasting only a few minutes, as some of my own narratives testify, because, if I am mindful enough, I am gaining and applying insight moment by moment. Such brief narratives as Michael's wife are themselves part of a continuous narrative of experience.

Autoethnography

Whilst Okri sets out some criteria against which the adequacy of narrative might be judged, developing guided reflection or narrative with Masters and doctoral students demands a more thorough appreciation of what constitutes adequate narrative. Autoethnography seemed a natural fit with its emphasis on self-inquiry, if less so with transformation. This is not the space to develop these ideas – they are discussed in the second edition of *Guided reflection: advancing practice* (Johns 2002), dedicated as it is to guided reflection as a research process.

Ellis (2004) and Bochner and Ellis (2002) initially inspired my first immersion in autoethnograhy and its fit with guided reflection as self-inquiry and transformation. In considering the criteria for coherent narrative, I can dialogue with Ellis (in italics), drawing on the work of Clough (2000), Bochner (2000), and Denzin and Lincoln (2000:252).

Does the narrative have the possibility for changing the world?

In response, influenced by Okri, I view narrative as always transgressive in enabling people to become who they desire to be. In nursing this always seem to be against an oppressive gradient, both internalised and realised within the natural pattern of relationships. Narrative is a liberating structure for reflexive self-inquiry and expression, and as a liberating structure its form must be determined by the writer.

Good autoethnographic writing should motivate cultural criticism

In response I view narrative as 'critical' – that in order to change self then the nature of reality must be clearly understood in the way it limits potential for realising desirable practice and that the nature of desirable practice itself must be critiqued – that it shouldn't simply be an ideal but grounded in social purpose.

Narratives must be hopeful, well-written and well-plotted stories that show memorable characters and unforgettable scenes

In response I view narrative as being articulate, focused and memorable in that it draws the reader into the text, as if they were present within the scenario, feeling it as well as thinking it; leaving indelible marks and planted seeds to explode at later moments in terms of their own experiences.

Conclusion

Constructing narrative cannot be prescribed beyond its coherent and reflexive demand. Like experience itself, it can never be formulaic even as we seek to impose order on the world. However, in the demand for scholarly work and rigorous research, reflection represented as narrative or as performance poses challenges to the idea of coherence, whereby reflexivity becomes coherence. In Chapter 19 I explore these ideas. In Chapter 6, I explore the 'being available template' as a coherent approach to marking the reflexive development of realising holistic practice within narrative.

Chapter 6
Being available

I go to help Tony get up for lunch. He is 53 and has a primary lung cancer with liver metastases. He is in the hospice for respite care. He has been here just 4 days and he wants to go home. In his words, 'Not that it's unpleasant in here but …'. Unspoken words but I sensed he didn't like the reminder of his forthcoming death that the hospice seemed to represent. Neither did he like being a patient. He had always been a very independent man and now he rebelled against the disease that was sucking way his energy and his life.

I see the hand-drawn cards blue-tacked to the bedroom wall.

I gaze at Tony. I sense his life is in crisis; what does he think and feel about this cruel twist of fate that threatens his life? I seek to connect with him but he keeps me at a distance. But then we have not met before. I am another stranger he stumbles on along this rocky path.

I ask 'How are you?', the ubiquitous greeting. Almost banal when I can see his suffering etched across his brow. He doesn't answer. I sense his irritation with me. Does he want me to go? Words unvoiced … but then messages do not need words. Body language says it all.

I wonder if I should accept his dismissal of me or assert my authority to be his helper whether he likes it or not. To be a good patient, he should conform to my authority, and what potential anarchy if we accepted that all patients had the right to choose which nurses cared for them.

So I reject his unspoken dismissal, which I rationalise as an expression of his suffering, his existential angst which he projected into me. Yet I am anxious. So I hang around him, communicating my availability to help him if he wishes it. In the morning report I was told that Tony struggled to co-ordinate himself; that he needed but didn't want help.

I pick up his ambivalence and feel uncomfortable; I do not want to irritate him further but recognise his need for help. I am trying hard to be open and positive to create a space in which we can work together even as I struggle to tune into his wavelength. Perhaps he wants Susan, whom he knows and feels comfortable with. Yet, he doesn't say that … at least not in words. In his shoes I would prefer Susan.

He conforms and takes off his pyjamas. His nakedness exposed to this clumsy stranger. I hold him steady as he moves into and out of the shower. No resistance. Slowly he dresses. I help him with his socks and shoes. I have now been with him an hour.

I ask, 'Do you have any pain?'

'No.' His pain is well controlled but in writing I chide myself – 'why are nurses so focused on pain?'. Perhaps *we* understand, feel comfortable with, feel more useful with such concrete issues as symptom management than with responding meaningfully to his sense of irritation and search for meaning. Distance work. Safer territory.

'Who made the cards?'

'My grand-daughter.' He becomes animated talking about her and I sense she is very special to him, adding to his sadness and restlessness. Things that make us happy also make us sad. As Benner and Wrubel (1989) note, the things we care about are the things that make us vulnerable. Caring and vulnerability – two sides of the same coin and yet paradoxically, the more I care, the less vulnerable I am, as if in caring I forget myself, I leave myself and my ego concerns behind me. And yet at times I feel exposed, as if caught on the edge.

I have opened a door to connect with Tony – talking about the one thing that he cares most deeply for and grieves its forthcoming loss. We talk about his grand-daughter, about schooling, about my two children. We talk about his work – he had been a plumber; he knows he is not going to work any more and accepts this. All the while I sense his irritation. It makes me uncomfortable with him. Do I let him know I sense this? 'Am I bothering you?' Such confrontation might prick the tension I am feeling and yet it might embarrass him. I would be acting for my benefit rather than his. But why should I feel comfortable? And why shouldn't he be irritated? I might also be wrong, that his irritation is not directed at me, that I am simply absorbing it as if it was. The consequence of my anxiety … distorting the signs?

I ask, 'You seem irritated being here?'

He poignantly says as if I have pressed a button, 'I want to be at home'.

'I know …' Acknowledging this need, feeding back my empathy, understanding and acceptance of his predicament. 'So why are you here?'

'I have no choice about going home because my daughter is away for the week and I need her support.'

He relaxes. He has expressed his irritation – a seemingly complex angry cocktail at the hospice, at me, at himself, at the cancer, at his daughter, that he may die, at the world at large. He relaxes more when I confess I am an academic, as if he can accept my being here more easily, rather than me being a new nurse he has never met before with the need to churn through it all again – the effort of making a relationship. In my experience some patients like to tell their story over and over, and others prefer their own solitude. Tony is one of the latter. Yet he is intrigued by my academic role at the hospice.

He moves out of the cancer shadow to enter into a relationship with me. He needs to know me, frame more clearly who I am, put me into context in order to accept my presence as more than just a 'visiting nurse'.

Even though it is true that I am a 'visiting nurse', it is a conservative truth. I visit often. The hospice is where I develop my palliative care skills and the stories I teach through. I ask myself, 'Why should he be pestered by an inquisitive *visiting nurse* when he is contemplating his own death and the loss of his relationship with his grand-daughter? For whose benefit was the pestering? Did I pretend I was helping him? Does the need to be useful or, even worse, the need to fix his problems for him become a mentality that threatens to reduce him to the status of some curious object?'

I know I didn't feel like that, but perhaps Tony feels that way? This is a vital insight.

We get to lunch in the communal dining room. Everybody else has gone. He invites me to join him for lunch. I stay with him until he has finished. There is something normalising about having a chat outside the immediate care environment and having a meal with someone. He had been a keen cyclist which gives us something concrete and interesting to chat about. By the time we finish I feel as if I am on his wavelength and sense his ease. I am also easier, having worked through the discomfort that blocked me being fully present or available to Tony. Turning my flight from anxiety into fight to let go of my concerns.

On reflection, it had been an uncomfortable 90 minutes where I struggled to manage my ambivalent feelings towards this man, even as he struggled to manage his ambivalent feelings towards me. In this experience I sense the way feelings are reciprocated. It highlights for me the fundamental need to know people in order to respond appropriately to them on a level that is meaningful. This reflects a deep concern that Tony matters to me, a concern that was threatened by his barely concealed hostility, and my ability to manage my feelings of rejection so as not to poison the possibilities. It also requires a mutuality – that it takes two to tango and dance well. As long as Tony resisted me, no therapeutic relationship was possible. We got there but it took an immense effort. Should I have bothered? Perhaps I should have said to Susan 'this man needs you' and walked away. Did I hang in there because of my own need not to fail? This is a profound question because we need to recognise that we are not omnipotent and cannot impose our idea of relationship or help everyone all the time. The very nature of suffering, dying and human relationship must always make relationship precarious. In getting to know someone who is dying and suffering loss, we must trip along a fine edge of raw emotion.

Whilst I could have simply (simply?) connected superficially with him by helping him to wash, dress, escort him to lunch, administer and monitor his pain medication and other symptom relief, this was not the level of help he really needed. On a deeper level he was in spiritual crisis. I could read that but that was my difficulty. I could not respond easily to the superficial caring issues outside that deeper context. Hence helping him wash and dress became difficult once I had looked into his eyes and touched his suffering. He also knew that and perhaps resisted me because he needed to protect himself from this intruding stranger. On the other hand, he might have preferred my superficial attention. As it was, I did feel intrusive, as if my caring ethic had trapped me. Although he eventually accommodated me, I felt as if I had pushed his limits and challenged his control of the situation.

Later, holding this dilemma, I share this experience with Susan. She affirms my experience, acknowledging Tony's struggle in facing his death. She also acknowledges my difficulty in tuning into him. She feels I shouldn't worry unduly about that as Tony is 'difficult'. So, *ipso facto*, my experience is normal. Sensitivity flattened in order to cope with the stresses of the day.

Susan's concern for me is genuine. But I am struck, yet again, that it is the patient who has the problem rather than the nurse being unskilful. Undoubtedly practice is very messy at times. Writing has helped me through some issues that I had been conscious of within the moment but which are now clearer. Now I feel positive toward Tony. My compassion for him has been fed and grown. I feel no sense of pity toward him despite his impending loss. Indeed, I look forward to picking up my relationship with him although it is unlikely we will meet again.

Being available

In Tony's story I made reference to my *being available* to him. Being available is not an abstract concept; it is always being available towards enabling the other in some way. In terms of my vision it is being available to ease Tony's suffering and help him to grow through his health-illness. It is being available to work with the person in order to enable him or her to find meaning in the health-illness experience, to make best decisions and to take appropriate action to meet their life needs. Gadow (1980) describes this as existential advocacy, contrasting it with a parental type of advocacy characterised by taking action in the other's best interests. Hence it is essentially a *working with* rather *than doing for* relationship. Being available is one of the explicit assumptions of the Burford reflective model (see p40).

The extent to which I can be available is determined by the weaving of six inter-related *influences* moment by moment: holding and intending to realise a vision, knowing the person, concern for the person, aesthetic response, poise, and creating an environment where being available is possible (Table 6.1). The first five influences concern the therapeutic relationship. The sixth influence positions the therapeutic relationship within the caring environment.

These six influences were appreciated by analysing over 500 experiences reflected on and shared within guided reflection relationships over a 4-year research period that involved 15 practitioners in seven clinical practices (Johns 1998a). The aim of the research was to understand the impact of guided reflection in enabling practitioners to realise desirable practice, resulting in the construction of the being available template as

Table 6.1 The being available template (adapted from Johns 2004a)

The practitioner's ability to be available is influenced by:	Brief significance of each factor
holding and intending to realise a vision	From the perspective of my own clinical practice this means being mindful of easing the other's suffering and nurturing their growth through the health-illness experience. Such vision gives meaning and direction to practice. It nurtures wisdom and focuses compassion.
the extent to which the practitioner knows the other	Through empathic inquiry the practitioner appreciates the pattern of the person's wholeness and the meanings they give to health. It is tuning in and flowing with the unfolding pattern of the person's experience.
the extent to which the practitioner is concerned for the other	Concern for the other and compassion is caring energy. Concern creates possibility within the caring relationship. The greater the concern I have for you, the more available I am for you.
the extent to which the practitioner can grasp and interpret the clinical moment and respond with appropriate skilful action (the aesthetic response)	The aesthetic response is reflected in the practitioner's performance and expertise. It is being aware of my own limitations and taking responsibility for ensuring I am most skilful in my response to ease suffering.
poise – the extent to which the practitioner knows and manages self within relationship	Being mindful of my own stuff so that it does not interfere with being fully available to the person. It involves dealing with any resistance to the person so I am fully present to them.
the extent to which the practitioner can create and sustain an environment where being available is possible	Ensuring I work in assertive and collaborative ways with my colleagues towards realising a shared vision and can act politically to maximise available resources for caring.

the core therapeutic of realising holistic practice together with an appreciation of the pattern of effective guidance in enabling practitioners to become available.

In constructing the template, I was keen to avoid a simple reduction. Hence the core therapeutic of being available is essentially irreducible. The being available template offers the reflective practitioner a way to *know* holistic practice. Of course, it is only a representation. It is not holistic practice itself but it does give the practitioner a measure against which to judge self.

I shall review each of the first five dimensions in more depth to create stronger images of what each means in light of Tony's story. Creating an environment where being available is possible is explored in Chapter 7.

Holding and intending to realise a vision

My intention is to ease Tony's suffering and, in doing so, to enable him to grow through this experience. By holding the intention moment to moment, it is more likely I will realise it. Intention is a reflection of mindfulness. It shapes the moment and gives focus to my compassion. It reminds me 'who I am' and 'what I am meant to be doing being here with Tony'. It is the antidote to the resistance I felt towards Tony.

The extent to which the practitioner knows the other

To reiterate the words of Hall (1964:150):

> There is nothing simple about patients who are complex human beings, or a nurse who is also complex and who finds herself involved in the complexities of disease and health processes in a complex helping relationship.

I repeat this because it is imperative to appreciate the complexity of the caring moment. Caring is not simply a stimulus–response event. It is not reactive although at times we are caught by surprise given the mystery and unpredictability of the human situation.

So, who is Tony? It is a significant question if I am to care for him. What does it mean to know a person? I can never pretend to know Tony. I catch glimpses of him as the situation unfolds. I can open spaces in our talk for him to reveal himself but first I must reveal something of myself so he can begin to trust me. Not easy, as the text reflects.

Always I am making interpretations, drawing assumptions and then checking them out. Trying to make sense in order to respond appropriately and therapeutically. I endeavour to tune into his wavelength and appreciate the pattern of his life so I can flow, journey with him as necessary and appropriate to help him meet his health needs.

The *Burford NDU Model: caring in practice* sets out a pattern of cues to guide the practitioner to tune into the person within the context of her holistic values (see p36, Chapter 2) and gather information to nurse the person.

- Who is this person?
- What meaning does this illness/health event have for the person?
- How is this person feeling?
- How has this event affected their usual life patterns and roles?
- How do I feel about this person?

- How can I help this person?
- What is important for this person to make their stay within the healthcare setting comfortable?
- What support does this person have in life?
- How does this person view the future for themselves and others?

The first cue – 'Who is this person?' – challenges me to see Tony as a unique 'whole' person in the context of his world. His family and culture are brought into focus and scope of care. The cue encourages me to see *him* and counters any tendency to see him primarily in terms of his symptoms and diagnosis, as significant as these things are. Of course, humanness is a reciprocal thing. If the practitioner sees the other's humanness she is more likely to see and respond from her own. The cue also reminds me to be mindful and curious – who *is* this person that I endeavour to connect with?

Empathic inquiry

The second cue – 'What meaning does this health event have for the person?' – focuses me to listen and be empathic to Tony's experience. What does this health event *really* mean for him? I emphasise *really* because so often I can read the surface signs and I can assume what it might mean. The reflective practitioner holds the space to inquire, dig a little deeper below the skin. Tuning into Tony opens these doors to knowing him and for him to know himself, so he can make sense of his bewildering experience.

Empathic inquiry is compassionate and intentional listening to connect with what the other is experiencing. Yet I can never really know Tony's experience. I must guard against jumping to hasty assumptions, being patient in dwelling with Tony, mindful to check out any assumptions. It is the practitioner's greatest skill for it sets up possibility.

Pattern appreciation

I prefer the term 'pattern appreciation' (Cowling 2000) to 'assessment'. It better represents the complex interplay of the signs I need to pay attention to in order to know the other person; reading the person's life pattern as a complex whole – a pattern continually shifting moment to moment along the person's health-illness journey. This is achieved by reading the signs on the person's surface, for example pain, anxiety, high blood pressure, sadness in the eyes, and pursuing these signs into the deeper self as appropriate. Pattern is always shifting in light of unfolding events. Only when the practitioner is in tune with the person can she understand and respond appropriately to the person's unfolding needs.

Margaret Newman (1994:13) writes:

> The new paradigm of health, essential to nursing, embraces a unitary pattern of changing relationships. It is developmental. The task is not to try to change another person's pattern but to recognise it as information that depicts the whole and relate to it as it unfolds.

Wavelength theory

Tuning into wavelength is only the beginning. The practitioner must then flow with the other's wavelength as it unfolds. Newman describes this as synchronicity, a rhythm of

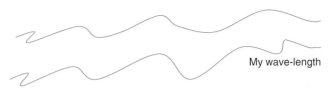

Figure 6.1 Tony's wavelength.

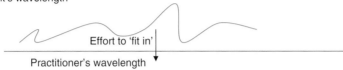

Figure 6.2 The patient trying to fit in.

relating in a paradigm of wholeness. This movement along the wavelength can be viewed as a dance (Johns 2001b, Younger 1995), each step a caring movement sometimes led by the practitioner and sometimes by the other as appropriate.

I capture flowing with Tony on his wavelength in graphic form (Figs 6.1 and 6.2).

When people like Tony experience crisis in their lives, their wave patterns are likely to become chaotic; descents to ever greater depths as suffering and despair take hold, zigzagged with moments of hope and salvation. By flowing with them, I am most available to them. When practitioners lose sight of the person, they expect the person to fit into the wavelength of the 'good patient', a symbolic straight line that literally flattens humanness. The patient (diminished person) tries to 'fit in' to be accepted and cared for. Failure to 'fit in' often leads to censure as characterised by the image of the 'unpopular patient'.[1]

Blackwolf and Jones (1996:185) capture the sense of wavelength in their portrayal of an eagle.

> Look up and see Eagle ride the invisible. Up and down, coasting, then back up and down again. With deliberate intent, she manoeuvres her wings in order to catch the next current, rising to a new height. Levelling and riding a straight course, she gains new sights. Then, accepting the inevitable downward drift, she surrenders to each experience. Invisibly changing and unpredictable, the air currents carry Eagle to the places she must go. Eagle understands the dance of life and accepts the downward as naturally as she accepts the upward.

As my experience with Tony illustrates, it is not necessarily easy to tune into the other's wavelength or to flow with the other on the pitch and roll of their journey. It may feel like surfing! To stay on the other's wavelength, the practitioner must be mindful of the pitch and roll and manage any resistance she may have toward the patient. Of course, sometimes this can be difficult when, like Tony, the person is resistant, angry, unco-operative.

Understanding Tony's experience opens up the possibility for me to tune into and synchronise with his wavelength and to flow with him on the ebb and flow of his health-

---

[1]For example, see Johnson and Webb (1995), Kelly and May (1982), Stockwell (1972).

illness experience, helping him find a new, more harmonious wavelength in tune with well-being. The dialogue between us establishes the caring relationship based on mutual understanding where his involvement in his healthcare process is honoured and actively facilitated. If I view him at a distance and make assumptions, then the risk of misunderstanding is great.

The third cue – 'How is this person feeling?' – guides me to inquire into Tony's particular concerns and anxieties. Tony is angry, resentful, sad. These feelings ripple through him, bubbling to the surface in his manner. I trip along this cue cautiously, gently probing his resistance, not wanting to intrude inappropriately into his private world.

The fourth cue – 'How has this event affected their usual life pattern and roles?' – prompts me to appreciate Tony's lifestyle pattern. I guide him and his family, as appropriate, to review their lifestyle, reading the pattern for deeper underlying factors that may have influenced the current situation. Often serious illness can prompt a radical reassessment of lifestyle and the values people consider significant within their lives. It focuses caring as both a health promotion and illness prevention activity.

I could utilise a checklist to consider aspects of lifestyle, rather like the Roper, Logan and Tierney activities of living, or any other reductionist scheme. If you were to construct a checklist, what would it include? Obvious issues are work, leisure, daily living, and religious activities. Related to this are issues which affect these activities, such as mobility, fatigue, sleep, personal self-care, nutrition, pain, mood, bowels, etc. and social factors, such as support, attitudes, finance, etc. These aspects of daily living might be self-assessed as appropriate. In the narrative I mentioned pain, but it seemed irrelevant to pursue other issues at that particular time.

Sympathetic resonance

The fifth cue – 'How do I feel about this person'? – prompts me to pay attention to my own feelings, thoughts, concerns ad prejudices that may influence the way I see and respond to Tony, especially as he arouses strong feelings in me due to the expression of his suffering. As such, the cue acknowledges the 'who' of the practitioner and the uniqueness of the human–human encounter with its mystery, intimacy and vulnerability. Sympathy is differentiated from empathy (Morse *et al* 1992), sympathy being an emotional response to the experience of the other as a result of absorbing the other's suffering to some extent. In contrast, empathy is an objective view – a dispassionate glance yet motivated by deep concern for the other.

The sixth cue – 'How can I help this person?' – prompts me to pause and consider the information gained, to feed back understanding and begin to plan with the person (as they are able), and other healthcare practitioners, the best ways to respond to meet the person's health-illness needs. In doing so, I process the first five cues, creating a clearing where Tony and I can dialogue and negotiate care, both short term, in view of presenting issues, and more long term through anticipating future need.

The seventh cue – 'What is important for this person to make their stay in the hospice comfortable?' – prompts me to acknowledge that admission into the hospice is a disruption to normal lifestyle and may raise many issues of comfort and control, especially those 'little things' that make a significant difference to the person's comfort and perception of being cared for (Macleod 1994). Attending to this cue gives a strong message of affirming the person's individuality.

The eighth cue – 'What support does this person have in life?' – draws my attention to any ongoing care outside the immediate care environment by framing Tony more explicitly within his social and cultural world. I draw any family, friends and community into the caring gaze to explore the meaning of this event in terms of the future. At the time, I did not explore the support Tony had in life except to note that his stay in the hospice was for his daughter's holiday. I did not know the daughter.

The ninth cue – 'How does this person view the future?' –prompts me to dialogue with the person/family to explore what the future might hold, especially fears of dying and death and what support resources exist within the person's life and toward mobilising and developing resources to support the person's future. As with the previous cue, such dialogue may raise many difficult issues and feelings, such as the possibility of dying, disability, losing one's home, etc. Both cues are vital to focus care towards successful exit of the care relationship or transition of care across healthcare boundaries.

The extent to which the practitioner is concerned for the other

Simply put, the more concerned I am for Tony, the more available I am to him. Being concerned for him, he matters more to me. I pay him more attention as a person. Concern opens up the caring space. It engenders trust if I am patient enough.

If I am wrapped up in my own concerns then I matter more for myself. Then Tony would be at risk of being reduced to an object of care to do things to (rather like Tom in Chapter 3, when staff are more concerned with doing the task and getting through the work, anxious about the clock ticking). They become an object of care rather than a suffering human being. Then caring is not possible.

The idea of concern for the person resonates with Logstrup's idea of the ethical demand I noted on p83. To reiterate (Logstrup 1997:18):

> By our very attitude to one another we help to shape one another's world. By our attitude to the other person we help to determine the scope and hue of his or her world; we make it large and small, bright or drab, rich or dull, threatening or secure. We help to shape his or her world not by theories and views but by our very attitude toward him or her. Herein lies the unarticulated and one might say anonymous demand that we take care of the life which trust has placed into our hands.

Logstrup's words are compelling, *demanding*, illuminating how our visions of caring can be informed by philosophy. Tony did not articulate a demand, it was unspoken. Yet, being in the hospice, Tony put his life into my hands and the hands of all the care workers so what does it mean to take care of the life which trust has placed into my/our hands? It means that, as a nurse, I accept and honour this demand with grace.

Whereas my concern opens a clearing, my compassion fills it with a loving presence. Simone Roach (1992:58) describes compassion as:

> A way of living born out of an awareness of one's relationship to all living creatures; engendering a response of participation in the experience of another; a sensitivity to the pain and brokenness of the other; a quality of presence which allows one to share with and make room for the other.

Compassion is a nebulous concept, difficult to grasp and certainly difficult to talk about and teach. Yet it is the heart of caring.

> Love invests itself for itself. Love, although other-conscious, is also self-serving. As we love, we feed our love within … love enters into dark places and showers them with light. Love colours the experience with a free flow of energy. (Blackwolf and Jones 1996:66–7).

Yet compassion isn't a skill. It is always heartfelt. It isn't a technique to apply. I know Tony would sense if my compassion was false. Ask yourself – how would I know if I am compassionate? How would I know when my compassion is diluted? These are vital inquiries if compassion *is* caring. And yet, at every turn, my compassion is under threat in a world where compassion is strained.

John O'Donohue (1997:26) also uses the love word:

> When love awakens in your life, in the night of your heart, it is like the dawn breaking within you. When before there was anonymity, now there is intimacy; where before there was fear, now there is courage; where before in your life there was awkwardness, now there is a rhythm of grace and gracefulness; where before you were jagged, now you are elegant and in rhythm with yourself. When love awakens in your life, it is like a rebirth, a new beginning.

Powerful words for every healthcare practitioner to reflect on. Do we who purport to care have a responsibility to develop our compassion if compassion is a vital ingredient of caring? Do we fail our patients and ourselves if we lack compassion?

The bodhisattva ideal

Easing suffering lies at the heart of Buddhism, reflected in the Four Noble Truths. In easing suffering I am inspired by the image of the bodhisattva, an image that complements the being available template in terms of the being or posture of the holistic practitioner, expanding the idea of the compassionate person.

In my story of Michael's wife (Chapter 4, p82), I wrote '… and for a brief moment I imagine Avalokiteshvara, the Bodhisattva of compassion, wrapping us in his arms. Such a beautiful image and feeling'. Avalokiteshvara is known as the Bodhisattva of compassion. Bodhisattvas give themselves unconditionally to ease the suffering of others with deep compassion and wisdom.

> I bend with you to ease your suffering
> As the reed bends with the wind
> In graceful dance and harmony
> It bends but does not break
> So I too must learn.

Paramananda (2001) suggests that in growing up, our imagination has been trimmed, as if we have been cut down to size to conform to a professional image, as if there is a grey jealous fish trapped by a weir in our heart. The fish represents all that constrains our compassion. Through reflection, we can paint the heart and help the jealous fish jump over the weir into the wide ocean, freeing our imagination and compassion.

Get out your box of crayons and begin to colour in your vision of your heart.

Take care of the child within, just as you would your own child. The only two things you must give your child are life and love. Discover ways to nurture yourself, to honour the child within; come to recognise the need to keep the colours of your child eternally vibrant. (Blackwolf and Jones 1996:72–4).

The extent to which the practitioner can grasp and interpret the clinical moment and respond with appropriate skilful action (the aesthetic response)

The aesthetic response is lifted from Carper's (1978) fundamental patterns of knowing in nursing (see Fig. 3.2, p60). Essentially aesthetics is the quality and the beauty of my performance.

So, did I appreciate the situation well enough with Tony? Did I make good clinical judgements? Did I respond with skilful and ethical action? Was I effective in meeting Tony's need?

As Carper (1978) indicated, there are various influences that impact on my judgement:

- forces that are likely to influence my judgement: who I am as a person, my concerns, prejudices, attitudes, stress levels, values, my feelings at the time
- current research and theory that I am aware of that might inform my judgement
- knowing what is ethically the right thing to do
- past experience – knowing what worked well and what didn't work so well in past similar situations, what interventions I am skilled at and feel comfortable with using
- expectations from others about what I should be doing.

The narrative reveals the way my performance/response is centred on Tony's feelings, notably his anguish at anticipating the loss of relationship with his 4-year-old grand-daughter. It seemed to hang like a dark cloud over him. In terms of helping him, I could not lift the gloom. There were no off-the-shelf remedies to apply.

My skill was to gradually open the therapeutic space and use cathartic and catalytic responses to help him express his feelings and thoughts (Heron 1975). The key was asking him, almost confronting him with, the 'why are you here?'. This enabled him to express his pent-up ambivalent anger towards his daughter.

Poise – the extent to which the practitioner knows and manages self within relationship

To be available to Tony, I need to be available to myself, to be fully present within the unfolding moment. Previously I described poise as 'knowing and managing self within relationship'. I also used the word 'equanimity' but prefer poise because it suggests fine balance.

Opening the *Compact Oxford English Dictionary* (2005:785), I read that poise is:

A graceful and elegant way of holding the body
Calmness and confidence
Ready and prepared to do something

Fine words that need no further explanation or justification. Poise involves going deep into self in order to know and use self mindfully. Thomas Moore (1992:235) writes:

> Day by day we live emotions and themes that have deep roots, but our reflections on these experiences tend to be superficial ... not only are our reflections often insufficient to account for intense feelings, but we may have been living from a place that is too rational and dispassionate.

Rainer Maria Rilke advises the young poet to 'go deep into yourself and see how deep the place is from which your life flows'. We could all take note of this advice, go deep into ourselves and discover the source of our everyday lives.

To know Tony in the moments I was with him, I did need to go deep within me, to tune into him on a more intuitive level, on the level of spirit. How do we know things? How do I know myself?

Blackwolf and Jones (1996:4–35) help me feel the significance of knowing self.

> Watch the birds. Are the sparrows merely the colors of their feathers? Are they the songs they sing? Or are they the movement of their wings? The experience of their flight? Are sparrows the hunger and fulfilment they feel inside or the winds they ride? Are they what we see and experience them to be, or what they see and experience? Are sparrows all of this? None of this? More than this? Only a sparrow knows what it is to be a sparrow ... like the sparrow that only knows sparrow, only you know who you are.

Blackwolf's message is for ourselves, for we can only know the other in relationship to ourselves.

Tony struggled to find meaning. He is on an emotional roller-coaster. To flow with him I must both know and melt any resistance I have to him. I mustn't become entangled within him (Morse 1991). Ramos (1992) identified embodied impasses or resistance factors within the practitioner that limited the practitioner's ability to connect with the other. The first impasse was emotional involvement which reflected the nurse's failure to draw boundaries between self and other. The second impasse was the nurse's need to control the patient's experience in order to protect the patient and to manage her own anxiety. Therefore I must resist absorbing Tony's suffering or having pity for him, or needing to fix it for him as if fixing myself.

Stephen Levine (1986:168) writes:

> When you meet the pain of another with fear, it is often called pity. When you're motivated by pity, you're motivated by a dense self-interest. When you're motivated by pity, you're acting on the aversion you have to experiencing someone else's predicament. You want to alleviate their discomfort as a means to alleviating your own. Pity creates more fear and aversion. When love touches the pain of the other, it is called compassion. Compassion is just space. Whatever the other is experiencing, you have room for it in your heart. It becomes work on yourself – to let go, to stay open. To feel that being within you.

I play out the tension between pity and compassion. I seek to cultivate compassion and dispel aversion to the other suffering. It is a constant play.

Patience

To be poised is to be patient. 'Patience is a virtue' and in the mad rush to get things done it can easily be lost. Patience is tuning into, listening to and flowing at the person's own pace. Yet how hard it is to really listen if our mind is full of other stuff, if our heads are turned in other directions. To be empathic, practitioners need to juggle a space in their minds to give the person undivided attention.

Stress and coping with work

Stress accumulates without realising it. Neck and shoulder muscles ache, creating headaches and sapping energy to unbalance the body. I have felt so many practitioners' shoulders where their muscles are taut, knotted, aching. We can be stressed for many reasons. Stress leaves us feeling heavy and drained. With our energy depleted, we are not available to our patients. Anxiety kills and in the survival effort, we sacrifice the patient to save ourselves. Imagine instead finishing each workshift feeling light and fluffy.

Write down the reasons for your own stress. Look deeply because they are covered up with defence systems that also use your precious caring energy to balance the stress.

What did you come up with? No wonder we groan and moan under such a burden.

Interestingly, practitioners seem to suffer more with organisational issues and conflict than they do in relation to patient care (Vachon 1988). Is this observation true for you? Perhaps practitioners feel stress with caring when they are more burnt out and have lost their connection to caring (Benner and Wrubel 1989).

Taylor (1992) noted a theme within the literature of how nurses have been dispossessed 'of their essential humanness as human beings and as people, by emphasising their professional roles and responsibilities' (p1042). Taylor draws attention to the fact that nurses are human too and, as such, are vulnerable to the same issues that face their patients and families. The lack of recognition of humanness in nursing through a focus on roles and responsibilities has led practitioners to strive to be something they were clearly struggling to cope with. Taylor (1992) noted that practitioners didn't recognise or understand their own ordinariness as human beings. Consequently, they become alienated from themselves in their efforts to cope with and live with the contradictions in their lives. Jourard (1971) noted that such striving damages 'the self' and reinforces the need to cope in a vicious downward spiral of self-destruction towards burnout and a state of anomie.

Ironically, being patient centred may perpetuate a denial of self and reinforce contradiction and ultimate self-destruction. As Jade, one of the primary nurses at Burford Hospital, said, she didn't come to work dressed in protective armour (Johns 1993). Dewey (1933:30) observed:

Unconscious fears also drive us into purely defensive attitudes that operate like coats of armour – not only to shut out new conceptions but even to prevent us from making new observations.

Dewey believed that anxiety limited the practitioner's ability to learn through experience. The professional is closed to protect self rather than open to possibility. 'Armour' is akin to professional detachment.

The water butt theory of stress

To reiterate more of Hall's words (from Chapter 1):

Anxiety over an extended period is stressful to all the organ functions. It prepares people to fight or flight. In our culture, however, it is brutal to fight and cowardly to flee, so we stew in our own juices and cook up malfunction.

'Stewing in our own juices, we cook up malfunction' – people are unable to express or work out their anxiety, so they continue until, unable to contain any more stress, they 'blow their top'. Like a full water butt, I must spill over. Yet spilling over or more dramatically blowing my top creates a mess that others will feel uncomfortable with. No-one likes such overt displays of anger or despair – people clear the mess up and pretend it didn't happen, characteristic of the 'harmonious team' that sweeps up and brushes emotional mess under the carpet and pretends that everything is OK on the surface, that we, superficially at least, get on well together (see Hank's complaint later in this chapter).

Blowing my top, my stress levels drop to a manageable level and then slowly, drip, drip, drip, it fills up again, because the cause of the dripping has not been addressed. Sometimes a violent storm fills my water butt quickly and like lightening itself, I snap and blow my top and rage at events or people (Parker 1990, Pike 1991, Wilkinson 1988). Pike (1991:351) notes:

> Moral outrage ensues when the nurse's attempts to operationalize a choice is thwarted by constraints. The outrage intensifies when these constraints not only block action, but also force a course of action that violates the nurse's moral tenets.

I'm sure many practitioners wear this T-shirt. However, the water butt does have a drainage tap. The practitioner can learn to be aware of her stress levels, drain stress off and convert the stress into positive energy necessary to take appropriate action to resolve the sources of stress. Likewise, the gardener draws water from the water butt to water the flowers and nourish their growth. However, the tap might be blocked, requiring help to unblock it – the value of guided reflection. The water butt is a powerful metaphor for learning through experience.

The risk of burnout

Failure to realise desirable work or manage anxiety in constructive ways leads inexorably to burnout. Cherniss (1980) describes burnout as a process in which 'the professional's attitudes and behaviours change in negative ways in response to job strain' (p5). Maslach (1976) suggested that the major negative change in those experiencing burnout in people-centred work was 'the loss of concern for the client and a tendency to treat clients in a detached, mechanical fashion' (p6).

Not good news then.

McNeely (1983) observed that when practitioners felt they had lost the intrinsic satisfaction of caring, they became focused on the conditions of work, for example, off-duty rosters and workload issues, characteristic of bureaucratic models of organisation. McNeely believes that bureaucratic conditions are antithetical to human service work and strongly advocated that such organisations needed to move to collegial ways of working in order to offset the risks of burnout.

Benner and Wrubel (1989) believe that the answer to stress and burnout is not the development of an adequate personal detachment, as advocated by Menzies-Lyth (1988), but the reconnection of the self with caring. Burnout is a descent into a black hole when the caring self has been scraped away on the uncaring sharp edges of systems, despite rhetoric to the contrary. The contradictions are no longer tenable. The bonds that contain snap. It is as if nurses are dispensable. There is little organisational sensitivity to the profound nature of journeying with another person to help ease that person's suffering. There is lack of recognition of emotional labour (Bolton 2000, James 1989) – that somehow emotional work is natural women's work and therefore is unskilled, doesn't need to be taught, and is not valued, when emotional work is the greatest gift nurses can offer patients. Yet if the organisation doesn't seem to care, why should I? Quick route to burnout.

Yet burnout can be viewed as a healing space, whereby the nurse can descend into herself and discover her self. It may be dark, lonely and painful but it can still be a healing space. Such healing is a journey to discover, rather than recover, self because recovery suggests returning to what she was before … a self hurt only for the hurting to start all over again.

Creating caring environments requires leaders who appreciate the need to create practice environments in which practitioners can be available. Yet human systems can be shifted by individuals with determined political action simply by modelling caring behaviour – in the way the practitioner works with patients, in the way she talks and writes about her patients, in the way she responds to her colleagues, by keeping her integrity intact, others will notice and respond. It will ripple like the soft breeze of a butterfly's wings in flight – vulnerable, beautiful and yet tough to withstand the storm, not torn apart by conflict but embracing conflict with the intention of unifying her colleagues towards a better world.

Feeling fluffy–feeling drained scale

To help practitioners reflect on their stress, I designed the 'Feeling fluffy–feeling drained' scale. This consists of a visual analogue scale (VAS) 10 cm long on which the practitioner marks the extent to which they feel either fluffy or drained at the end of their workshift. The scale then poses three questions:

1. What factors contribute to your sense of feeling drained?
2. What factors contribute to your sense of feeling light and fluffy?
3. What can you do to go home feeling more fluffy and less drained?

Feeling fluffy is a feeling of lightness at the end of the day where one's energy remains full whereas feeling drained is having no energy. I am sure every reader has experienced both feelings at the end of the day.

At the end of the workday, the practitioner scores the extent to which they feel either fluffy or drained and explores contributing factors and what they can realistically do to improve their fluffy score by acknowledging and enhancing feel-good experiences and working at neutralising energy-draining situations. As with all reflective activity, it is first necessary to become aware of and pay attention to these experiences. Only then is change possible based on a realistic appreciation of the situation, perhaps requiring guidance given the practitioner's embodied responses to stressful stimuli within 'normal' patterns of relationships.

The practitioner can use the scale daily over a period of time (giving structure to a reflective journal) to monitor the (intended) improvement in 'fluffiness'.

In Figure 6.3, I give an example of one practitioner's score. Her normal score was around 7, suggesting a relatively high residual level of stress. On a very good day this might drop to 5. In the example, her score is 10, due entirely to an altercation with a patient's relative despite its successful resolution. Such was the stressful nature of the situation that it submerged her feeling fluffy factors. In clinical supervision, she was able to explore the situation in more depth, her response to it and ways of resolving it, so if

Week commencing 20th May 2002
Day – Wednesday

Please score on the scale the extent you feel light and fluffy or drained at the end of the workday

I go home feeling light and fluffy	← ——————————→ /	I go home feeling totally drained
What factors contribute to your sense of feeling drained?	*Arrived in the morning to a horrible phone call from a patient's relative who held me personally responsible for his wife's wait in A&E when I had already advised him that there were no beds in the hospital.*	
What factors contribute to your sense of feeling light and fluffy?	*Did teaching session - I always enjoy teaching. Also put together a bid for further training in the hospital, Didn't think I would be able to do it this quickly.*	
What can you do to go home feeling more fluffy and less drained?	*I confronted the relative and listened to his worries. He apologised to me for being rude. Problem resolved.*	

Figure 6.3 Feeling fluffy – feeling drained scale.

she faced a similar situation her energy would not be so drained. Imagine what better shape she would be in, if her average score was 3 rather than 7?

The sacred quiver

I often use Blackwolf and Jones' *sacred quiver* to enable therapists to develop their poise. The sacred quiver contains the arrows of change (Fig. 6.4). Blackwolf and Jones (1995) note:

> The sacred quiver carries two types of arrows: the straight and the crooked. Both arrows represent the movement that is inside us as the sun rises and sets … crooked arrows can be our teachers if we open our eyes to the target they direct us toward. They teach of consequences. Of pain. They take us off course, as they veer into dark forests of danger. (p146)
>
> Straight arrows are made of the strong shafts of ain-dah-ing. They pierce with sharp tips of awareness and they fly with the feathers of the spirit world. Fill your quiver with these straight arrows. They will bring you to the bliss of the spirit world. With them, you will travel the sacred hoop of joy. (p157)

The straight arrows (Fig. 6.5) can be seen as a path, where one straight arrow leads before we are able to give the gift of unconditional self to others, fundamental for all healers. The crooked arrows might be viewed as boulders along the transformative path that must be shifted to progress. In the workshop the therapists identify their crooked and straight arrows. I suggest they construct a warshield decorated with their straight arrows as protection against the crooked arrows. In doing so they become mindful of their crooked arrows and their straight path. It is a powerful and novel approach to knowing self and gaining poise.

> The fact that you have identified old patterns is a significant step in healing any emotional scars left behind … if some painful imprints of trodden paths continue to negatively affect

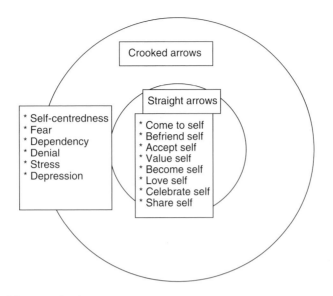

Figure 6.4 Contents of the sacred quiver.

your life's direction, first attend to your wound by gifting yourself forgiveness and heal with the help of another. (Blackwolf and Jones 1996:72)

In one warshield I painted, I used the Native American word *namaji* to represent my path. The green background (reproduced in this book as grey) represents the heart chakra.

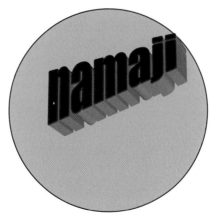

Namaji means respect, honor, dignity and pride. It is the highest of all Anishinaabe life principles. They are the gifts of a true connection to the spirit world. (Blackwolf and Jones 1995: 129).

In a more recent workshop, I painted a new warshield. The inner circle is blue to represent my throat chakra – where I must learn to speak my truth; this is the greatest defence – to be true to self. The outer circle is a mixture of other chakra colours emphasising wholeness, balance and energy, representing the eight levels of self that can be actively nurtured and developed through reflection when we find the balance between reflection on our strengths and reflection on our weaknesses.

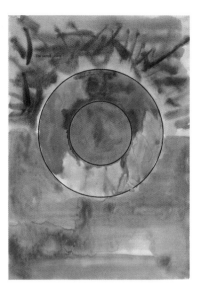

- Come to self – to open my eyes, wake up and see myself for who I truly am
- Befriend self – to see that I am a good person
- Accept self – to be a person in my own right
- Value self – to see myself as worthy
- Become self – to be authentic within my relationships with others
- Love self – only when I can love myself can I give love to another
- Celebrate self – opening a spiral of affirmation and self-esteem
- Share self – the giving of myself unconditionally within therapeutic relationships is to realise myself as caring.

Figure 6.5 The straight arrows.

The brown represents being grounded in the earth and the blue represents the freedom to fly and spread my wings. The black marks against the sky are the crooked arrows continuously flying towards me. Reading through Blackwolf and Jones' descriptions of these crooked arrows, they are all present to some extent. They all threaten my energy and sense of well-being. And yet, acknowledging them helps me begin to dissipate the negative energy tied up with them, helps me pull free from their destructive force, especially when I keep in mind my vision of easing suffering. This eases my own suffering, helping me pull free of the jungle into a healing space, where I can be more whole and more available.

The outer circle also represents mindfulness, like a protective layer to enable me to see and recognise the crooked arrows for what they are – to accept them and learn through them, converting them into positive energy rather than use my energy to resist them. Energy is a precious commodity to fuel my caring.

Learn to use your shield to warn others that you will not tolerate abuse in any form. Like the rattle snake, assertively communicate your intolerance for disrespect. Be open, honest, direct, calm, and specific as you communicate your intentions. (Blackwolf and Jones 1996:107)

Using the sacred quiver to know and nurture self is an imaginative approach to developing poise, illuminating reflective practice as creative endeavour. Learning becomes playful as the therapists bend over tables or lie on the floor with their paints and crayons.

Conclusion

The being available template enables nurses to know themselves as holistic practitioners. The first five dimensions of being available: holding and intending a vision, concern for the person, knowing the person, the aesthetic response, and poise, are concerned with the therapeutic relationship between the practitioner and the person requiring nursing.

In Chapter 7, I explore the sixth dimension of being available – creating and sustaining an environment where being available is possible.

Chapter 7

Creating an environment where being available is possible

In this chapter, I explore the potential of reflective practice to create an environment where practitioners can be available to work in desirable ways with the patient and family. The extent to which the practitioner is available to the patient and family is influenced by the conditions of practice. In an ideal world, there would simply be the relationship between the patient and the practitioner. However, there is no ideal world; the world is shaped by forces of power and tradition that lead to learnt ways of being that pattern normal patterns of working life. These ways are not easily shifted despite intention and the rationality of better ways of being.

I do not consider the physical environment, such as the colour of walls, the use of plants, noise and smell, opportunities for privacy, etc. Neither do I specificaly consider resource issues such as staffing numbers, staffing mix, shift patterns, equipment – all those things that make it more possible to be available to patients. However, many of these issues emerge within the narratives and all become the focus for the practitioner to take action. To take action, the practitioner has to realise her power.

Cathy and the GPs

Cathy is a district nursing sister who had approached me for clinical supervision. In one session she shared her experience with Brenda:

Cathy: I want to talk about Brenda. She is an 84-year-old woman I have been visiting each week since last summer. I knew her from before when her husband had been ill. She has had stomach cancer for which she has had massive surgery. She initially made a good recovery but then had a blockage that resulted in a stent being inserted. She was a deeply religious lady. Three weeks ago I was talking to her … she seemed a bit 'lost' … there was something about her … I couldn't put my finger on it … perhaps it was the up before the major down. We were chatting about things we normally talk about. I said something like 'See you next week Brenda'. She put a hand on my shoulder and said just as I as leaving, 'Yes, if God's willing'. She gave me that look. She died later that week after being admitted to hospital. She wouldn't have wanted that.

CJ: Were there other signs you could pick up on?

Cathy: She was more relaxed. She had talked about two of her friends who had died recently … she was quite a brave lady … she didn't like tablets and she had pain in her back. We had tried different painkillers that had hardly touched her. I did notice that the lines she had around her eyes had gone … her eyes looked bright, I thought.

CJ: Intuitively you knew what she was saying to you? That she knew she was dying?

Cathy: Yes

CJ: Could you have responded differently at that moment?

Cathy: I didn't because I didn't know what to say … I had a cry in the car for her.

CJ: She was saying good-bye. I suspect she didn't want any fuss about that. Did you go to her funeral?

Cathy: No … other things that needed to be done.

Cathy cries. I pick up on her tears and suggest that perhaps these are tears she might have shed at the funeral. I name the various emotions I sense she's feeling: guilt at failing Brenda and her family; anger at the GP for admitting Brenda to hospital against her wishes; sadness at Brenda's death. A cocktail of emotions that bend her low to the ground.

    Cathy (wipes away her tears): I know …

    I help Cathy visualise a 'space' between us where she could place these feelings in order to view and understand them for what they were, to feel more comfortable and consider what to do as a consequence. I emphasise my role is not to 'fix it' for her but to challenge and support her to resolve her troubled mind.

CJ: What if you have responded to her cue?

Cathy (uncertain): How do you respond to someone like that? Maybe I could have asked Brenda if she thought she was dying … and if so to hold her and say good-bye … it's such a difficult scenario to contemplate how I might have responded differently because I feel so emotional.

CJ: Is closing important for you?

Cathy: Yes … (She continues) I didn't attend the funeral because of a management meeting I was expected to attend.

CJ: Could you have prioritised differently? Could you have said to the GPs 'Can you please re-schedule this meeting so I can attend the funeral?' or simply given your apologies for not attending the practice meeting? Would the GPs have appreciated your dilemma?

Our supervision time is finished. We leave these questions spinning for Cathy to contemplate.

    Later, as I write the session notes, I add two further questions for Cathy:

- Brenda had wanted to die at home. If you had picked up the cue, could you have planned to keep Brenda at home rather than be admitted to hospital or alternatively arranged hospice admission?
- Did you not pick up the cue because you wanted to avoid uncomfortable feelings?

When we met for our next session 3 weeks later, I draw Cathy's attention to the notes.

CJ: Did you miss the opportunity to help Brenda manage her death appropriately?

Cathy: Brenda definitely didn't want to go into the hospice. Her husband had died there. We had discussed this. She said 'The hospice is a lovely place but I don't want to go in there because it brings back such memories'. She wanted to die at home … she did have a strong family and friends network around her.

CJ: What were the conditions of her admission to hospital?

Cathy: The GP was a bit vague. He admitted her on the grounds of a range of deteriorating symptoms … breathlessness. I was thinking of what you said about the 'gap' on the Burford model study day about accepting the inevitable as inevitable, and the way the GP had felt obliged to arrange her admission to hospital rather than accept she was dying.

The 'gap' (Fig. 7.1) exists when there is a mismatch of shared expectation between care staff in accepting the inevitability that the patient will die and that further treatment would be futile. The 'gap' represents the potential for conflict.

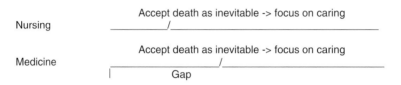

Figure 7.1 The gap.

Cathy: Yes … that's how it was … I acknowledged the inevitability of Brenda's dying before the medical team did. I intuitively felt this and our role was to help Brenda die in comfort. The GP also intuitively knew the inevitability of Brenda's dying yet within the moment he could not accept this 'failure'. So, in response to her symptoms, he arranged for her to go to hospital where she was admitted for treatment, as futile as that was, rather than arranging management of Brenda's death at home.

CJ: His learnt reaction, it does suggest how the 'cure' mindset works. Of course, he may have taken the easiest way out. The consequence was that the patient's best interests were disregarded and she died in circumstances she would not have chosen for herself … were there other ways of dealing with this situation?

Cathy: Brenda was a strong character but she would have complied with what the GP said.

CJ: How can you respond now?

Cathy: I don't know … the damage is done … what do you think?

CJ: Well, it might be useful to debrief with the GPs. Perhaps you can insist on being called if a similar situation arises so you and your team could have managed her at home. Issues of communication within the care team? I know in the emotional moment it was tough for you to respond to the cue she gave you, but we can see how circumstances unfolded that were not in Brenda's best interests, not in your best interests, and an expensive alternative for the NHS – the difference between being proactive and reactive?

Cathy: We are commencing a new series of meetings on Monday to improve our communication! The idea is to have 'team care plans' where everybody knows what the other is doing.

Brenda and Brenda's family perspective	Who has authority to make decisions?	The GPs' perspective
Is there conflict?	Should Cathy attend Brenda's funeral or the GPs' management meeting?	Ethical principles
Cathy's perspective	How was the decision actually made?	Organisation's perspective

Figure 7.2 Posing the ethical dilemma within ethical mapping.

CJ: So, the ethical dilemma – should you have attended Brenda's funeral or the GPs' practice meeting?

Cathy: For me, the funeral was my priority. In future I would be assertive about going to the funeral and say I would come to the meeting afterwards.

CJ: Closing seems such important work. Can you find some literature to support that? Knowing the 'evidence' may help you assert your priorities with the GPs – talking the language of the rational mind rather than the emotional mind. Consider, how might the GPs respond if you were to inform them that you were going to the funeral and not to their meeting? Let's use ethical mapping.

In the dilemma box I write 'Should Cathy attend Brenda's funeral or attend the GPs management meeting?' (see Fig. 7.2). I then explored with Cathy the perspectives of the different players within the situation. Before I set these out, ask yourself – what would be your own perspective? How would you ethically justify your perspective?

In terms of utilitarianism or greatest good, we could see a tension between Cathy responding to the needs of the individual versus the meeting, resulting in benefit for the wider community. However, we thought this was a weak argument to support the GPs' insistence that Cathy attend the meeting. In terms of virtue we could see another tension between Cathy acting on her holistic values and responsibility to the family against the values of the GPs who gave greater value to the smooth running of their practice. As Friedson (1970) noted, the principal aim of the bureaucratic organisation is its own smooth running despite the rhetoric of 'patients first'. Presumably, the GPs could easily debrief anything significant arising from the meeting at a later time. However, to do that, they would have needed to respect Cathy's demand to attend the funeral.

Different perspectives

Cathy felt that attending Brenda's funeral was the greater need but she wondered, was this just an emotional reaction? She felt she had failed Brenda and Brenda's family, which distressed her – feelings she had yet to resolve. She felt the family would have wanted her and benefited from her being at the funeral. She could see the GPs' perspective and that their response was both typical and arrogant. They assumed leadership of the team and expected compliance even though Cathy was not directly employed by them. Cathy felt the organisation would expect her to conform to the GPs' demand so as not to rock the boat, reinforcing her subordination to medical dominance.

Ethical principles

We framed the dilemma in terms of a tension between Cathy and the GPs' right to assert their professional autonomy. Could Cathy assert her autonomy to make her own decisions based on her professional judgement of what was the right thing to do? Interestingly, this mirrors the tension to respect Brenda's autonomy to stay at home, overridden by the GPs' decision to (mistakenly) act in her best interests or benevolence. Yet what was the right thing to do?

Conflict

We then considered 'Is there conflict of values? How might conflict be resolved?'. The answer was clearly 'yes, there is a conflict'. We could see that conflict manifested itself in terms of conflict of values, failed communication and power interests. Simply put, Cathy perceived that the GPs had the power to insist on her attendance. Cathy's authority to act reflected the way she perceived power relationships between herself and the GPs. She perceived that she didn't have the authority to resist the expectation that she attend the meeting and anticipated conflict with the GPs if she did resist. As a consequence she accommodated their request rather than risk the anticipated consequences.

We then used the influences grid (see Table 7.1) to reveal the factors that had influenced and constrained Cathy in making her decision to accommodate the GPs demand.

Patriarchy

Cathy's decision to attend the GP meeting rather than Brenda's funeral represents a triumph of patriarchal power. One discourse of power relationships is to view nursing and caring as feminine struggling against a dominant patriarchal view of medicine and managerialism. Gilligan (1982) makes the distinction that men and women differ in ethical priorities; women lean towards an ethic in which the primary responsibility is caring, whereas men lean towards an ethic of justice whereby primary responsibility is to ensure order (Fig. 7.3).

The 'team' meeting is a ritual of power flexing and control where the dominant voice of the patriarchy (both male and female doctors) and power pattern of relationships with

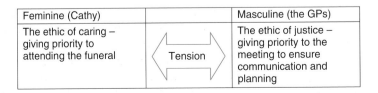

Figure 7.3 Power relationships.

Table 7.1 Influence grid for Cathy's dilemma

Influence	Significance
Expectations from self about how I should act	Cathy felt her expectations of how she should act were fundamental to her dilemma.
Conforming to normal practice	Cathy's normal practice would have been both to attend the GP meeting and to go to Brenda's funeral.
Expectations from others to act in certain ways	Cathy certainly felt the GPs expected her to be compliant with their wishes and 'know her place' within the 'team'.
Need to be valued by others	Cathy said she did not need to be valued by GPs but on reflection, she realised she did like positive feedback and did wanted to be valued by the GPs, and that this might have been a subtle influence she did not want to acknowledge.
Doing what was felt to be right	Cathy felt that attending the funeral would have been the right thing to do – more so than attending the GP meeting – even though both were 'right'.
Misplaced concern	Cathy felt 'forced' to be loyal to her GP colleagues rather than
Loyalty to staff versus loyalty to patient/family	Brenda and her family although in her heart her primary loyalty was to her patients.
Emotional entanglement/ over-identification	Cathy had a strong involvement with the patient and family. Indeed, she might have been accused of being too emotionally involved
Negative attitude towards the patient/family	which blurred her perception of what's best. In exploring this influence Cathy revealed her unresolved distress about her father's death. As a consequence Cathy felt she became entangled in the suffering of dying patients although she did not experience this as conflict. On the contrary she felt this made her more sensitive to the needs of her patients and families whilst recognising she still had some grief work to do for herself.
Limited skills/discomfort to act in other ways	Cathy admitted she was not very assertive and felt she would have been humiliated if she had challenged the GPs more strongly.
Lack of confidence	She recognised herself as someone who avoided or accommodated conflict.
Time/priorities	Cathy's NHS trust had significantly reduced the number of district nursing sisters (G grade), forcing her into a team leader role to manage more junior staff that had reduced her direct care role contact. Hence managing priorities and role conflict had become an increasing dilemma for her.
Anxious about ensuing conflict	Cathy's fear of sanction was the crux of her dilemma – what
Fear of sanction	sanction might ensue if she defied the GPs' demands? She recognised that she had internalised a sense of subordination and fear that saw challenging the GPs as a very uncomfortable prospect. She knew that they would probably report her to her managers.
Information/theory/research to act in a certain sort of way	Cathy was unable to make a good argument to support her decision to attend the funeral rather than the GP meeting.

subordinates is reinforced, providing subordinates attend. Not attending the meeting to attend a funeral may seem an innocuous event in itself, yet from a power perspective the decision is a symbolic challenge to the status quo. Cathy is making choices, which if tolerated, undermine the patriarchal dominance. The power game is to diminish her perceived autonomy to act on her own judgement. Batey and Lewis (1982) describe this type of autonomy as discriminatory autonomy, i.e. the degree of autonomy the practitioner believes herself to have. Roles overlap and there is always a degree of competition to 'own' the overlapping ground, a competition that nurses are ill equipped to win because of their internalised sense of subordination.

Watson (1990:62) noted that patriarchy presents a potent barrier to nursing's realisation of its holistic vision:

> Caring as a core value cannot be forthcoming until we uncover the broader, more fundamental politic of the male-oriented worldview at work in our lives and the lives of people we serve.

Reverby (1987) explored the way caring has been viewed as an extension of being a woman; indeed, as a woman's duty in contrast to her work. Reverby asserted that nurses' lack of power stems from this relationship between womanhood and caring and the subordinate relationship of nurses to doctors.

Lawler (1991) and James (1989) both note how caring in nursing is largely invisible, often devalued by nurses themselves, and seen as largely unskilled, being the natural extension of woman's social roles. Lawler's research, entitled *Behind the screens*, was concerned with bodywork whilst James' work, entitled *Emotional labour*, was concerned with emotional work. Perhaps then it is not surprising that nurses have tended to delegate this work to unqualified staff, valuing instead more medical type tasks as they seek recognition and acceptance into the dominant class (Roberts 1983).

Lou writes in her journal:[1]

> In the situation with Ruth, it wasn't until I was questioned by Chris – 'why did I find it difficult to challenge the diagnosis of the doctor?' – that I began to appreciate the subordinate role I was taking, reinforcing the stereotype that doctors exert power over nurses (Daiski 2004) and my hesitancy in dealing with issues of authority and power in my everyday relationships. Yet the medical team were asking for my opinion, recognising my authority and specialist knowledge. Reviewing this incident enables me to see more clearly my role, and how I relate to others and their perceptions of me.

Buckenham and McGrath (1983) highlighted how nurses have been socialised into a passive, subordinate and powerless perception of self *vis-à-vis* medicine, a perception that renders them incapable of fulfilling their self-perceived role of patient advocate. Nurses rationalised their compliance with medical domination because of the need to be valued. It is natural for dominant professions such as medicine to reinforce subordinate behaviour in other healthcare professions, such as nursing (Oakley 1984). In other words, doctors are always motivated to maintain the status quo and resist any rivalry for power.

Chapman (1983) suggested that doctors reinforced nurses' subordination through humiliation techniques that become a normative pattern of relating. The aim of the game is to keep nurses 'in their place'. Stein (1978) illuminated the nature of the doctor–nurse game whereby the nurse suggests to the doctor what to do in such a way that the doctor can claim credit for the idea. The point of the game is to ensure the doctor does not lose face. The game also reinforces the nurse's subordination. The game is also important for the doctor to play because he or she realises the significance of the nurse's knowledge. The pay-off for the nurse is the doctor's patronage or 'doughnuts'. Stein argues that failure to play the game is 'hell to pay'. Cathy knew that sanctions would be taken against her.

---

[1]Lou is a PhD student using narrative as a journey of self-inquiry and transformation towards realising her vision of practice as a spasticity nurse. See Jarrett 2008 (pp59–72) and Jarrett and Johns 2005 (pp162–79).

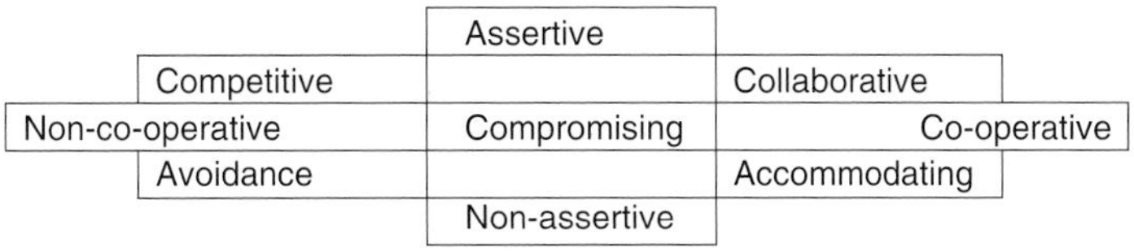

	Assertive		
Competitive		Collaborative	
Non-co-operative	Compromising		Co-operative
Avoidance		Accommodating	
	Non-assertive		

Figure 7.4 Thomas and Kilmann conflict mode instrument.

Perhaps the situation has changed since 1978 but then you, the reader, will know these things for yourself.

Power within bureaucratic systems such as the NHS has a typical authoritative pattern to ensure a docile and competent workforce (Foucault 1979), docile to the extent that its subordinates do not disrupt its smooth running.

Managing conflict styles

CJ: Cathy, what sort of relationships would you like with the GPs?

Cathy: More collaborative-type relationships where we value and respect each other … at the moment I don't think they respect nurses. It makes working difficult.

CJ: Let's look at Thomas and Kilmann's conflict mode instrument to consider the style you use and the style you would prefer.

I show and explain to Cathy the Thomas and Kilmann (1974) conflict mode instrument (Fig. 7.4).[2] It is designed along two axes: *assertive* – the degree to which individuals satisfy their own concerns; *co-operation* – the degree to which individuals attempt to satisfy the concerns of others.

I talk Cathy through each of the five styles.

- *Accommodating* is essentially a co-operative interaction but one in which the practitioner is not assertive, prepared to give up their own needs for the sake of maintaining harmonious relationships and their need to be accepted by others – 'apologetic'.
- *Avoidance* is characterised by negation of the issues and a rationalisation that attempts to challenge the behaviour of another are futile.
- *Collaboration* involves an effort to seek effective problem solving, to work towards a mutually satisfying conclusion, a win/win situation, i.e. concerned with the needs of self and others. Openly discussing issues surrounding conflict and attempting to find suitable means to resolve it.
- *Competitive* is pursuing his/her own needs to the exclusion of others – usually through open confrontation (results in win/lose situations).
- *Compromising* is realising that in conflict situations, not every party can be fully satisfied.

CJ: So what mode of managing conflict do you tend to use?

Cathy: With the doctors I tend to be accommodating … I don't like conflict at the best of times so I guess I generally try to avoid it.

---

[2] www.kilmann.com/conflict.html

CJ: Cavanagh (1991), using the Thomas and Kilmann instrument, researched the conflict mode styles of nurses and nurse managers. He found that avoidance was the most common mode followed by accommodation, compromise, collaboration and then competition. I suspect nurses avoid competition because they fear they will lose ... so you're not alone.

Cathy (laughs): That's some relief.

CJ: What style would you like to use?

Cathy: Compromise or collaboration.

CJ: If you want to be collaborative and you are accommodating or avoiding – how can you move from one to the other?

Cathy (laughs again, more nervously): I can't imagine that's possible ... I would need to be more assertive, less fearful.

CJ: We can rehearse being assertive. We can also use this map with each experience you reflect on and plot your journey moving from avoidance/accommodation to collaboration. How does that sound?

Cathy: OK ... it is something I have got to work on if I am ever going to feel confident at work with the GPs.

CJ: Cathy, can you let go of fear that the GPs will punish you?

Cathy: No, not easily ...

Becoming assertive

The Thomas and Kilmann conflict mode instrument gave Cathy a vision of collaborative relationships with the GPs – something to work towards. Whilst she recognised her inability to assert her perspective with the GPs, she also recognised that to realise desirable work, in this case attending Brenda's funeral, she needed to assert her perspective in ways that would be heard and respected by the GPs. As she said, it takes two to tango.

CJ: What do you need to do now about this situation?

Cathy: I don't like the idea of confronting the GPs ...

CJ: But you did say you would assert going to the funeral if the situation arose again?

Cathy: Yes, that's true ... but whether I could assert myself is another issue.

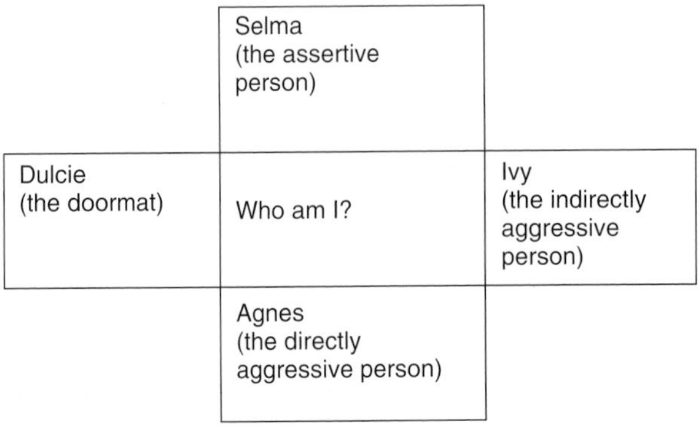

Figure 7.5 Dickson's four stereotypes of women.

Right	Score 1–10
I have the right to state my own needs and set my own priorities as a person independent of any roles that I may assume in my life	
I have the right to be treated with respect as an intelligent, capable and equal human being	
I have the right to express my feelings	
I have the right to express my opinions	
I have the right to say 'yes' or 'no' for myself	
I have the right to make mistakes	
I have the right to change my mind	
I have the right to say I don't understand	
I have the right to ask for what I want	
I have the right to decline responsibility for other people	
I have the right to deal with others without being dependent on them for approval	

Figure 7.6 Rights of women scale (Dickson 1982).

I asked Cathy to position herself within the assertiveness stereotype map comprising four stereotypes of women (Fig. 7.5) (Dickson 1982).

Instinctively Cathy says 'I am 'Dulcie …'. She laughs. 'The GPs walk all over me.'

CJ: Who would you like to be?

Cathy: I would want to be 'Selma'. I could never be like 'Agnes', it isn't my personality. I can see the risk of being an 'Ivy', bitching and back-biting. I know people like this, even at the surgery and know how destructive these people are.

CJ: So, Cathy, how do you move from being 'Dulcie' to becoming 'Selma'?

Cathy: I need to believe in myself more, be more assertive.

CJ: Cathy, the most vital point is to assert your right to be treated with respect and to assert your point of view. These two points are included within Dickson's (1982) 11 'rights of women', which offers a tool to reflect on your self … score yourself out of 10 for each point (Fig. 7.6). The higher the score, the greater your sense of self. You can re-score at later times to review your progress.

Cathy did not score herself. She felt she wouldn't score very high if she did. The scale made her feel inadequate. It was painful for her to look at herself like this because she felt, by and large, that she was a competent practitioner who got on well enough with the GPs. She didn't want to make a mountain out of a molehill and rock the boat, she would soon get over it and move on. The 'rights' scale had rocked her confidence. It was too challenging so we had to back-pedal to a safer place. So I introduced her to the assertive action ladder.

The assertive action ladder

I designed the assertive action ladder (Fig. 7.7) by analysing the pattern of becoming assertive with practitioners over many years in clinical supervision. This was vital work as so many of the experiences practitioners were sharing with me in supervision or on

10	Being able to tread the 'fine line' of pushing an issue and yielding	The controlled self
9	Keeping self and other in 'adult' mode	The managed self
8	Being adept at counter-coercive tactics against more powerful others	The empowered self
7	Being adept at interaction skills	The skill to assert self
6	'Taking the plunge'	The resolve to assert self
5	Creating the optimum conditions to maximise effectiveness	The scheming self
4	Being able to make a good argument	The knowledge to assert self
3	Understanding the boundaries of autonomy and authority in role	The right to assert self
2	Having a focused vision for practice	The ethic to assert self
1	Having felt the need to assert self	The motivational self

Figure 7.7 The assertive action ladder (Johns 2004a).

educational programmes were grounded in conflict, giving credence to the idea that practice is primarily concerned with managing conflict. It became very apparent that nurses were not equipped to manage conflict positively, leading to a huge wastage of energy and a low sense of self-esteem. It is true to say that the effective practitioner is an assertive practitioner and yet, in a culture where nurses are not expected to be assertive, this may itself cause conflict.

The ladder consists of ten rungs, each rung a sequential step for realising effective assertive action.

Applying the assertive action ladder to Cathy's experience, we obtain the following.

1. Having felt the need to assert self (the motivational self)

Cathy felt a strong responsibility to Brenda to attend the funeral and guilt when she did not attend. She knew this was an unsatisfactory state of affairs that reflected a pattern of working with the GPs that could no longer be tolerated.

2. Having a focused vision for practice (the ethic to assert self)

Cathy held a strong vision of holistic practice in which attending the funeral was significant in terms of her relationship to Brenda and responsibility to support the family.

3. Understanding the boundaries of autonomy and authority in role (the right to assert self)

Cathy was helped to see that she had the authority to decide to attend the funeral – she was not employed by the GPs, although she did perceive that the GPs had authority over her, and was helped to redefine the nature of this relationship. Her attitude was confronted as inappropriate although fear remained that if she upset them then she would 'pay for it'.

We explored how best to tackle the GPs given the situation again: a more proactive approach might be to take the initiative and think upstream and inform the GPs that she will be attending the funeral.

4. Being able to make a good argument (the knowledge to assert self)

This is the crux issue – how can Cathy convince the GPs that attending the funeral was more important work than their meeting, in language they would accept? Two key theoretical points need to be emphasised: firstly, the significance of closure within the therapeutic relationship and secondly, the support for the family. Is there research to support these points?

5. Creating the optimum conditions to maximise effectiveness (the scheming self)

Whether Cathy should see the GPs as a group or single them out individually? Whether to see them at a meeting or in the normal course of the day? During the morning or afternoon?

6. 'Taking the plunge' (the resolve to assert self)

Cathy has now thought the issue through and come up with her plan of action but can she carry it through? The coaching role was to reinforce her sense of responsibility for taking action, infuse her with courage, and deflate any sense of fear.

7. Being adept at interaction skills (the skill to assert self)

Cathy is now in the midst of asserting herself and needs to be skilled in communicating her message, for example being adept at using Heron's six-category intervention analysis.

8. Being adept at counter-coercive tactics against more powerful others (the empowered self)

Possible tactics might include the following.

- Cathy needs to be in collaborative mode for managing conflict – trying to keep the situation on the issues rather than conflict becoming a battle of wills. Hence, think 'we' – 'we' have a problem (see Fig 7.4).
- To confront the GPs with their caring values. It is often the organisation's Achilles heel to be revealed as uncaring - what I term as 'taking the moral high ground'.
- To give the GPs' behaviour back to them if they assert power over Cathy – 'asserting your power does not help solve the problem'.
- To reduce their power by visualising them as bully boys trying to get their own way.

9. Keeping self and other in 'adult' mode (the managed self)

To stay in adult mode, Cathy must be aware of and manage her own anxiety, especially the urge to flee into child mode in order to cope with the parental onslaught of being viewed as difficult and irresponsible. The key is to keep the issue in focus rather than let it degenerate into competitive mode and a win/lose battle that she is ill-equipped to win. It is vital that Cathy is not afraid of any threat of sanction or loss of reward.

10. Being able to tread the 'fine line' of pushing an issue and yielding (the controlled self)

The mindful practitioner will sense this line and realise that to overstep it may risk being marginalised as difficult or actually being punished in some way. Cathy may need to yield because the GPs are more powerful than her and refuse to accept her perspective. She could still exercise her authority and go against the GPs' wishes.

As we ascended the ladder rung by rung I felt a shift within Cathy, as if climbing the ladder was infusing her with a new confidence.

Cathy (smiles): That was so helpful, maybe I can be more assertive than I imagined.
CJ: Only time will tell … when we meet next time bring some new experiences that involve conflict with doctors. However, if you can't assert yourself as you wish, that's OK – you can choose to yield … remind yourself about the quality of yielding.

Yielding

Yielding is retreating with dignity, with one's integrity intact.

> Learn to yield. Yielding is not being passive. It is being sensitive to energy flows and extending wisdom. Allow the winds of change to flow through you rather than against you. Be flexible with what is happening today. Yield to the circumstance, yet rooted with who you are. (Blackwolf and Jones 1996:281).

Yielding to the situation is a strength. It is not a weakness. To fight when you cannot 'win' is to exhaust yourself and feel a failure. Some situations cannot be won. Perhaps at the time Cathy could not 'win' the battle against the GPs. If she had been more mindful she might have made this judgement and decided to yield, sparing herself angst. However, the decision must be made with integrity otherwise it becomes a lame excuse for not acting. This is why guided reflection is so valuable, because Cathy can develop insight to prepare herself for the next situation she finds herself in with the GPs. Maybe next time she can act more assertively.

Realising our power

Imagine standing at the doorway of a room full of people you usually find intimidating. How do you feel? Now measure your personal power by positioning your hands at a point on your body between your feet and the top of your head. Feet represent minimal power and top of head represents full power.

I ask Keri, one of the leadership students, where her power is. She places her hands at the level of her knees. She laughs slightly shamefully, judging herself. She senses how those administrators and doctors take her power away.

She takes a deep breath and imagines projecting her full power into the room. With each inhalation she pumps up her power until the room is full of it. She is amazed that just imagining can have such an effect.

Two weeks later in the leadership class, Keri shared an experience that involved attending another unit meeting. She used the technique. She positions her hand at hip level. 'It worked!' she exclaims, 'I still felt a sense of fear ripple through me but I took courage and found my voice. The projection was astonishing, I couldn't believe how it made me feel so different. I am now more mindful of my power.'

'Feel your power now.' Keri positions her hand on her waist. Just imagining her power empowers her, as if I am an energy catalyst. We explore a parallel technique of giving someone back their intimidation. 'I think this is your stuff not mine – have it back.'

Keri laughs: 'I can't do that!' I laugh in response: 'Oh yes you can! Just imagine that you hold the moral high ground and he is below you … and that he cannot touch you.'

Two weeks later Keri looks different, more self-assured, as if her power is radiant.

'I couldn't believe it … the medical director was sarcastic as usual. I asked him why he felt it necessary to put people down. The room went quiet. He was non-plussed. He apologised and said he hadn't realised he came across in that way. My power surged. I felt triumphant and thanked him. The meeting took a very different turn. It was so good. I think I can begin to put my hand on my shoulder at least … not the top of my head yet because I still felt fearful he could retaliate.'

'You are amazing. You helped him see another way, a more human way grounded in dialogue. We must celebrate with some tea.'

Perhaps this was the most significant part of Keri's leadership journey, plotting her personal power over many months, being mindful to remember her power especially when the going got tough. Slowly she inched towards the top of her head, where all great leaders must position her hands. Only then can she be truly dialogical with her colleagues.

Hank's complaint

Karen is an associate nurse working at a community hospital. In one supervision session she revealed her dejection about a recent event at the hospital.

Karen: One night last week Hank complained to me about the actions of one of the night staff. He was very angry about it, so I wrote about his complaint in the notes, really to cover my own back because if something had happened because of that … if he had got worked up and had a heart attack. I didn't state who was involved or the nature of the incident. Christine (a night associate nurse) picked up what I had written in the notes and said that she felt 'very sad I had to write that, that some things were better said, not written'. She didn't deny the incident but criticised my documenting it.

CJ: The way you handled it?

Karen: Right. I re-read my notes of the incident because I had written them in a hurry. I realised I had used a word that could have been replaced by a better one.

CJ: An antagonistic word?

Karen: Yes. I made a comment further on in the notes and replaced my initial note to make it clearer to people reading it.

CJ: Less volatile?

Karen: Yes, but what got me was Christine criticising me about my way of documenting it when *The Nursing Times* goes on about 'whistle blowing' and how complaints should be documented. I felt she was trying to cover for the person involved though she acknowledged that the event had happened.

CJ: And now?

Karen: I pointed it out to Leslie as he was the primary nurse. He commented – 'I'll have a word with the person involved'. I went home and worried about it all night, worried how she would take it, what she would say. So I need feedback.

CJ: What would you do differently if given the same situation again?

Karen: Only thing I could have done would be to ring her and ask her to explain from her point of view.

CJ: Think of the response you might have got from doing that?

Karen: From my perspective, if it was me … I would have appreciated it.

CJ: And knowing the person involved?

Karen: I can't say … she could nearly be my grandmother.

CJ: How do you normally get on with her?

Karen: I see her in the evenings and nights when she works … but I don't have much to do with her … I suppose my relationship with her is superficial.

CJ: Do you think this action against Hank was out of character for her?

Karen: I think it was an exaggeration of her normal character.

CJ: You think?

Karen: I don't work with her. It's difficult to know how she is with other patients. The event itself was quite trivial, it's Hank's anger that got to me.

CJ: Do you think Hank's anger was reasonable?

Karen: I felt at the time that if it had been me then I would have been upset and angry. She was inflicting her values on him, not respecting him.

CJ: Perhaps you didn't handle Hank's complaint in the best way, although writing a report in the notes is a proper way of reporting patient distress. Altering the notes was unprofessional, and perhaps should have been picked up by other staff, but it wasn't because it was righting a 'wrong' rather than being seen as 'wrong' in itself. You were making good your crime of 'reporting' her.

Karen: Discussing the situation at shift report would have been better but by then the night staff had departed. Reporting the incident to the primary nurse is good practice and it is not unreasonable to have expected Leslie to deal with it – but he is a coward and conveniently forgets about it – or put another way, he brushes it under the carpet. I could have reported it to the senior nurse but that would have made it worse … I can imagine that they would have said I went running to mother and got them into trouble …

CJ: So what could you do differently given the situation again?

We explored her options and agreed she should talk this through with the care assistant. This was not possible face to face but she could ring her at home. I asked Karen if she still wanted Leslie to deal with it. Karen felt she hadn't wanted him to do it in the first place, it was only because he had offered.

We rehearsed Karen's response in phoning the care assistant at home, reinforcing that Karen's response was morally correct. The key factor was to keep the situation grounded in the therapeutic situation rather than it becoming a secondary situation of interpersonal conflict (as it had already had become). I urged Karen to live the supervision maxim – tough on the issues, soft on the person – and take action because of her integrity even though she was fearful of this prospect.

In our next session 3 weeks later, Karen says 'I went home and phoned her!'.

CJ: How did you feel when you picked up the receiver?

Karen: Terrified! She was angry but she didn't get as angry as she possibly could have done.

CJ: Have you learnt that it pays to belong to the harmonious team? If so, if a similar situation occurs you will think twice before confronting it?

Karen: Remind me about the harmonious team?

CJ: The harmonious team is concerned with maintaining a facade of togetherness or teamwork. It does not talk openly about difficult feelings or issues between its members and seeks to protect itself from outside threat. Conflict is brushed under the carpet. As a consequence, conflict is inadequately resolved and continues to simmer under the harmonious surface (Johns 1992). It undermines the ability of practitioners to collaborate in resolving conflict. It nurtures a perverse culture of being loyal to staff rather than to patients as you have discovered. As a consequence people become inauthentic and lose their integrity. What can you do about it?

Karen: I don't know. I'm really dejected and yet I can sense it's vital that I am not intimidated. If we can't raise issues because of fear of conflict then we all go about as if wearing masks. I can't simply sweep this under the carpet.

CJ: Could you share this experience with your colleagues – to secure their support and to assert the therapeutic team to off-set this malignancy?

Karen: I felt like a chicken at the prospect of Leslie acting on my behalf. I'm now truly humbled. I didn't stop to think. I'm feeling very stupid. Why did Hank wait to see me!? He was probably just thinking about it when he saw me.

CJ: How do you think Mandy (the care assistant) might be feeling now?

Karen: I hope she thinks I had the courage to ring her.

CJ: Be positive about this – your phone call to Mandy was a cathartic intervention; you enabled her to vent her anger at you, yet she was also confronted with the fact that she did not act appropriately towards Hank; her angry reaction was to being exposed. You can rationalise her anger in this way. It's imperative that you do not see yourself as in the wrong.

Karen: I know … I hear what you say but it's not easy …

CJ: I know … I am frustrated listening to you … If I was still senior nurse here I would want to intercede and confront the staff myself but feel it would be better if you did this.

As the text reveals, Karen was bruised in retaliation for breaking the norms of the harmonious team. It was Karen who was in the wrong rather than Mandy. The issue had twisted from being a patient-related issue to an interpersonal one where loyalty to the 'team' took precedence over loyalty to the patient.

Karen's distress was the outcome of vilification – a reflection of the *force* of the harmonious team to regulate its members. Karen was motivated to limit the damage by accepting her villain role. As she noted, she was learning to play by the rules.

The dialogue reveals the way I urged Karen to take action – pushing her against a gradient that threatened her. To her great credit, she acted responsibly but was wounded in the process. My role was to help her lick her wounds and gather strength to tackle such issues more positively in the future. You can imagine what might happen on another occasion – once bitten twice shy or could she grasp the bull by the horns? Yet despite Karen's distress, she said that she enjoyed going through the situation in supervision. She hadn't wanted to come to the second supervision session because she thought it was going to be too hard. She had a slight residual fear about retribution from the night staff but at least the care assistant had gone on holiday for a month!

Horizontal violence

Karen's experience reveals the way staff can be violent to each other when threatened, in what is termed horizontal violence – a toxic form of dealing with stress. The idea of *horizontal* stems from bureaucratic-hierarchical systems, whereby the subordinate person (the nurse) is unable to project her anger or frustration at her more powerful oppressors. She can only fire at those on her own level. Yet, even on her own level, this violence is muted within the harmonious team, perhaps because people are motivated to be partially invisible, to keep their heads down to avoid criticism (Street 1992). Hence, being *harmonious* is a collusive strategy to paper over the team's potential violence.

Support

'It doesn't pay to be assertive here' (Johns 1989). These memorable words were uttered by a staff nurse who feared voicing her criticism to a senior nurse. Her words suggest that becoming assertive is not simply an individual effort but requires an organisational effort to create a collaborative team who work together on the basis of shared vision and mutual support.

Caring is a reciprocal relationship. If nurses and other healthcare practitioners are expected to care, then they need to work in caring environments. If the practitioner is suffering it is likely that other colleagues are also suffering, sapping their energy and limiting their availability to be with patients. Or as Remen (1996:70) puts it:

> Whatever we have denied may stop us and dam the creative flow of our lives ... avoiding pain, we may linger in the vicinity of our wounds ... without reclaiming that which we have denied, we cannot know our wholeness or have our healing.

The subtitle of Rachel Remen's (1996) book *Kitchen table wisdom* is 'stories that heal', suggesting that in telling our stories, by reflecting on our experiences, we can connect to something vital within us, something healing. In sharing our stories with others, we realise we are connected to others and that we are not alone in the world. Connection is healing. And yet often, nurses seem to need to cope, to not expose their vulnerability as if it is a weakness not to cope or admit to strain. They would prefer a collusive silence. To care, we need ways to penetrate the silence to support each other and create a therapeutic team – a team whose members are actively and genuinely available to each other. As such, the reflective and holistic practitioner is mindful of her colleagues' well-being.

So, consider the following questions.

- Are adequate support systems in place?
- Are people stressed or, worse, burnt out?
- If so, why do you think that is?
- Do you see seeking help as a strength rather than weakness?
- Do you explore your anxiety as a learning opportunity?
- Are you truly available to support your colleagues?

Nicklin (1987) observed that 85% of managers considered stress to be only a moderate problem, which they had no specific policy to deal with. The Briggs Report (DHSS 1972) identified that services supporting nurses are rare, inadequate, fragmented and not targeted to those most in need. There is no evidence to suggest this situation has improved since 1972. In fact, the situation may have deteriorated due to the persistent stripping of nursing resources since the development of the business culture prompted by NHS trusts. To say the least, it is profoundly ironic that a caring service should care so little about those who care. The emergence of clinical supervision is an acknowledgement of the need for formal structures and the failure of informal support systems. The cynics amongst you might consider that support is not the real agenda of supervision but a means of surveillance, however it is wrapped up. Whatever the truth of that, clinical supervision is no substitute for the therapeutic team.

Debriefing

At a recent clinical audit meeting at the hospice, it was felt that staff needed to be mindful of debriefing as a group at the end of each shift, in recognition of the emotional impact of caring for some patients and issues of misunderstanding. Staff had occasionally debriefed following particular incidents, but debriefing as a daily ritual acknowledges that work can be stressful and that staff have a responsibility to be mutually supportive. Debriefing has a number of obvious benefits.

- It acknowledges that sometimes, for whatever reasons, practice can be tough. It provides a space where practitioners can safely reveal their feelings, where it is OK to be distressed, angry. It cuts across a culture where practitioners have hidden their feelings in the (misguided) belief that 'good' nurses 'cope' or do not burden their colleagues.
- It allows practitioners to be heard above the din, to be recognised and valued as persons with human needs and human frailties.
- It helps with constructing the therapeutic team by bringing staff together to create a new culture of mutual support in their caring quest, bringing vision into clear view.
- It promotes the understanding of the nature of conflict.
- It encourages confrontation of inappropriate attitudes, behaviours, assumptions and defence mechanisms that disrupt therapeutic ways of working with patients and colleagues.

- It provides opportunities for leaders to role model the disclosure of feelings, and to encourage and facilitate reflection with colleagues.
- It promotes the morale, self-esteem and motivation of colleagues, with organisational consequences of retaining staff, enhancing quality of care and reducing staff sickness.
- It encourages the realisation of the learning organisation.

Therapeutic benefits of disclosure

An important dimension to coping with stressors concerns the degree to which people discuss or confront traumas after their occurrence. Jourard (1971), for example, argued that self-disclosure of upsetting experiences serves as a basic human motive. As such, people naturally discuss significant experiences with others. Talking about a trauma with others can strengthen social bonds, provide coping information and emotional support, and hasten an understanding of the event, while the inability to talk with others can be unhealthy.

Pennebaker (1989:213) noted:

> When given the opportunity, people readily divulge their deepest and darkest secrets. Even though people report they have lived with these thoughts and feelings virtually every day, most note that they have actively held back from telling others about these fundamental parts of themselves ... Over the past several years, my colleagues and I have learned that confronting traumatic experiences can have meaningful physiological and psychological benefits. Conversely, not confiding significant experiences is associated with increased disease rates, ruminations and other difficulties.

Pennebaker and his various colleagues have demonstrated the benefit of therapeutic journalling in well-being, notably the benefit of connecting strong feelings to past traumatic events. Smyth *et al* (1999) have developed this work to show the physical benefits of journalling on reducing symptoms in asthma and rheumatoid arthritis. Smyth's (1998) review of the literature suggested that emotional expression has a salutary health effect, whereas emotional inhibition has a detrimental health effect. Emotional expression may take the form of writing or telling another person your story. Smyth cites Pennebaker *et al*'s (1997:175) claim that:

> Written emotional expression leads to a transduction of the traumatic experience into a linguistic structure that promotes assimilation and understanding of the event, and reduces negative affect associated with thoughts of the event.

Smyth highlighted that the review studies demonstrated significant superior health outcomes in participants – psychological well-being, physiological functioning, general functioning, reported health outcomes, but not for health behaviours. Smyth noted that these studies demonstrated that short-term distress was increased but is thought to be related to long-term improvement.

Pennebaker *et al* (1990:536) note:

> The present experiment, as well as others that we have conducted, found that writing about transition to college resulted in more negative moods and poorer psychological adjustment by the end of the first semester. Our experiment may have effectively stripped the normal defences

away from the experimental subjects. With lowered defences, our subjects were forced to deal with many of their basic conflicts and fears about leaving home, changing roles, entering college.

All indications from this study suggest that the power of confronting upsetting experiences reflects insight rather than cathartic processes. In follow-up questionnaires, for example, the overwhelming majority of the subjects spontaneously wrote that the value of the experimental condition derived from their achieving a better understanding of their own thoughts, behaviours and moods. The stripping away of defence mechanisms means that practitioners and patients may need guidance to support them through the consequences of the writing experience.

Conclusion

In this chapter I have explored issues around creating and sustaining an environment in which practitioners can be fully available to patients. I have revealed how the practice environment is governed by social norms embedded in power/force and tradition that are embodied and reinforced within normal patterns of relating and create dilemmas for practitioners such as Cathy and Karen. To be available, practitioners need to realise their power, reflected in assertive behaviour grounded in ethical knowing. To be assertive requires shedding the fear that others have power over you who are likely to resist the growth of assertive behaviour because it threatens the status quo even when patients' best interests are not being served.

In Chapter 8, I explore the therapeutic value of patients' stories, both written and spoken.

Chapter 8

Therapeutic journalling for patients

Therapeutic journalling is a powerful healing modality for people who suffer (DeSalvo 1999). Consider any patients you work with who have been through a difficult time or have difficulty in expressing their feelings. Ask yourself – would keeping a journal benefit them? Of course, they might be reluctant to write or if they did, to share their writing with you, but I suggest that such writing is therapeutic. It enables the person to tell their story and reveal their suffering.

Writing is cathartic and healing, enabling the person to make sense and reintegrate a self so often torn apart by suffering. It also helps carers to appreciate the person's life, even more so when the person is unable to speak coherently, as with Moira Vass who suffered with motor neurone disease.

Moira Vass – living with motor neurone disease

Moira wrote her story of living and dying with motor neurone disease because she wanted her carers to understand what she was experiencing. Writing gave her dying some purpose and enabled her to express the feelings of despair and anger that she struggled to say.

Moira wrote:

I have motor neurone disease (MND). This is a disease that relentlessly destroys the nerves that enable us to control all our movements, while leaving the intellect and senses unaffected. There is no cure for this disease. I was told the cause was unknown and it was terminal. However, there is a ray of hope – the drug Rilutek. This is not a cure, but has been shown in trials to extend survival in people with MND. Its cost is somewhere between £1000 and £2000 per patient per year, yet it gives the patient time and some hope. It slows down the paralysing effect. My attitude to Rilutek is if it does not cure then why take it? It only prolongs the agony and postpones the inevitable. The paralysis goes on unabated and death is by strangulation, a form of choking due to the fact that the intercostal muscles are affected and you cannot breathe or cough. From day one I became slowly and deliberately useless and within 6 months I could no longer speak, eat, drink or walk unaided. Artificial ventilation via an endotracheal tube merely prolongs the suffering. Patients remain alert to the end and many need treatment to relieve their distress, as well as oxygen to assist breathing.

Living with feeding at home

MND affects the nerve endings and consequently affects the muscles in most of my body, but particularly all the muscles in my throat which means I cannot speak, eat, drink or swallow. I was referred by my neurologist to a dietician as the time had come for me to be fed by tube. My reaction was disbelief, anger and a lot of tears. Then more tears.

By the time I came to see the nutritionist consultant, I had calmed down and accepted the fact that this was my only option if I wanted to go on living. The tube is attached to the gastrostomy. My reaction was despair. How can I live with this? The first thing that crossed my mind was no more baked or roast potatoes. No more predinner sherry, wine, all the joys of living. One of my favourite hobbies was cooking: adventurous cooking, dinner parties, BBQ with the family, like any normal person.

The first feed was only 200 ml. At 50 ml per hour. The feed type was 'Nutrison' and it was not a painful procedure. When the feed was finished this was followed by a 60 ml syringe of water to flush out the tube and give you extra fluid and thereafter a water flush every 4 hours, totalling 240 ml per day to prevent me from getting dehydrated – feed at night and water during the day.

However, it did little to calm my anger. I just wanted to stop the whole business and go to God. I could not see myself living with a 'Kangaroo' pump and a plastic bag full of 1000 ml of 'Nutrison Energy Plus' to be given overnight. The idea of the night feed was to enable me to be free during the day apart from the water flushes.

I laid awake for the first 3 nights in hospital, my anger only getting worse. Anger that felt like someone pouring boiling oil over my body. On the third night, I reached down and closed the roller clamp. I forgot about the bleep sound from the pump, which brought two nurses to the pump who duly restarted the feed. They sat with me for a while and we had a chat. I was finding it impossible to come to terms with my new way of life, but I decided to take a more positive look at my feelings and especially the word ANGER. It struck me the word 'anger' is almost a cocktail of emotions:

A   Aggressive, to myself and the staff – zero tolerance
N   Negative thinking
G   Grief, crying
E   Emotions out of control
R   Resentful –'why me' syndrome

So I decided, for the sake of my family, my husband but especially my three grandchildren, to make an effort because they all thought the feeding pump was a great idea. I made up my mind to come to terms with tube feeding at home although the sight of the tube at my stomach brought back the anger.

On Saturday morning, 14th February 1998, I was found unconscious by Gordon, who was unable to rouse me. It was decided to admit me to the hospice. I have no recollection of the tragedy. I came round with my grand-daughter Kerry, aged 16, crying, telling me to squeeze her hand if I could hear what she said: 'Please wake up Nan, we love you'. Twenty four hours later, I was awake to the reality of my condition. My living will meant they could not feed me if I went unconscious. As a result they were anxious to start the feed but I said 'No, no, leave me be'. By the fourth day I gave in and the 'Kangaroo' pump and plastic bag with the 1000ml of food was back. I was back to square one – I had to give in for the sake of my family.

Once I had come to terms with home feeding I found it extremely easy to live with and having the feed at night was more convenient. You are free during the day to do what you please and go where you like. It is very easy to take a water flush with you. It took about 6 weeks to establish a routine. I would set it up downstairs in the kitchen, sit back in my armchair and watch TV. The feed takes ten hours to go through. When I am in bed I make sure the tube is free and to do that I attach the tube from the pump by holding it in place with Sellotape on my thigh – so far it has never woken me up. If you can still eat anything that is a bonus.

The hospice

Following my admission to the hospice as an inpatient in February, I received wonderful care, especially as I spent 4 days on 'hunger strike'. To me, this was the only way out – to stop all treatments, drugs and feed. The staff respected my wishes and while I was unconscious my living will (advance directive) stated *no treatment*. When I regained consciousness I made the decision to continue cessation of all treatments. I found my family were devastated and my three grandchildren cried and pleaded with me. On day 5, I came back to earth to the delight of everyone. The nursing care in the hospice was a special kind of nursing but I would rather have had my rights and my way.

On discharge I was invited back one day a week as a day-care patient. On the first day this caused me unbelievable distress. They collected me in a hospice ambulance; there was the driver, a nurse and myself. As my husband waved goodbye I started to cry – another step down the MND road to death. Suddenly my anger exploded and I lost control, crying excessively and choking. The nurse told the driver to pull over to the side of the road until I had calmed down sufficiently. On arival at the hospice I was taken into the quiet room and there I remained for the rest of the day. With their special kind of care and continuous oxygen for 20 minutes, I calmed down enough and fell asleep again.

I have come to terms now with the hospice-type care for terminally ill patients. I am going into the hospice for a week of respite care – the last week of the World Cup!

Care in the community

Learning to live with a progressive neurological condition, and in my case the advance has been rapid, has not been easy. Since my collapse in February on St Valentine's Day, I am totally helpless and require 24-hour care. The equipment needed to assist in my care has built up gradually over a period of time. It takes one nurse to get me up in the morning, washed and dressed. I bring myself down on the chair lift. We found the easiest dress code for my needs consists of a silk top, slacks, knickers with pad, socks and sandals. What does break my heart is that I can no longer wear my size 12 outfits. Since the introduction of the tube feeding my waistline has increased to size 16. The position the night team leave me in bed has to be the right one for comfort as there I remain until morning. I can no longer move in bed or raise my head. I was provided with an air mattress to prevent pressure sores. My gratitude to the team.

They always chat to me about nursing, clothes and fashion. I feel guilty that I need so much of their time. My particular hate was losing my independence, and in particular my personal hygiene. This added to my despair and anger.

It is at times like this when I wish we had voluntary euthanasia. The patient should certainly have a say when and where to die. Life with MND is like a living hell on earth. Your whole body is dead. All I am left with is sight, smell, taste, hearing and sensation. Family gatherings and Sunday dinners have never been the same. I can take no part in family laughter and discussion. I take no part in the kitchen or food shopping. Anywhere I go I must take the suction machine, my talking machine, a large bunch of tissues and a carer familiar with my management. Controlling the saliva which flows from my mouth is not only depressing but also embarrassing. I fold the tissue into one inch widths, four-fold deep and roll the top end down into a narrow roll. I put about three rolls in the side of my mouth since I can no longer cough, but I have an occasional sneeze. This prevents me from biting my tongue and my lip which is very painful. If I sneeze again within 5–10 minutes I hit the same spot. The surgery lent me a nebuliser to help remove very thick mucus.

Through Social Services I have obtained a wheelchair. I cried my heart out when it first arrived. Life in a wheelchair is a very different world. You feel so vulnerable and at risk. As the disease progresses I find waking up in the morning a slow process. My friend, the practice nurse, suggested taking 10–20 minutes oxygen to help me. Someone has to open my eyelids for me – usually Gordon. The only way I can sum up the sad journey is with a poem I have written. What more can I say?

My living hell on earth

I walk alone
Along this path
Leaving life's hope,
Sorrow, love and pain
Standing at my gate.

I speak no more
I sing no more
I eat no more
IN MY LIVING HELL.

Sometimes I wish
I could swallow,
But there's always
Something at my throat.

I drink no more
I kiss no more
I smile no more
IN MY LIVING HELL.

I see and hear
My world go by,
But reach out
I cannot do.

My smiles have gone
I have no joy
I walk no more

To join my crowd
IN MY LIVING HELL.

I'm wheeled along
In my wheelchair
To a sea of knees
And a lot of pushchairs!

Some smiles I get
Some yawns and cries
Thank God they're not
IN MY LIVING HELL.

I tried to find
The peaceful way
But the road is closed
And I must stay.
IN MY LIVING HELL.

Animal rights have a say
They can die
When they say;
Please God why can't I?

Reflection

Moira was keen to publish her journal. Louise, the day-care senior nurse, discussed this with me and I agreed to meet with Moira and discuss possibilities.

I wrote in my reflective journal:

August 4th, I arrive ten minutes late. Moira is not there. Louise says she has been delayed because her catheter had blocked – will arrive in about 20 minutes. I am happy to sit with the group preparing for the day. Moira arrives. We move to a table. She is small and frail in her wheelchair. She has a piece of tissue coming out of her mouth that soaks up the excess secretions she can no longer control. She has her 'lite speaker' with her to communicate with me. I tell her who I am and clarify why we are meeting together – to consider her journal on living with motor neurone disease and ways it might be published. I had been strongly moved by her journal. I also felt strongly moved by Louise's experiences that she had shared in clinical supervision. As one of Moira's carers, Louise had become deeply involved with Moira.

Using her 'lite writer', Moira tells me about her experience this morning with her catheter being removed. The district nurse has asked Louise to replace it. Moira says it was awful. I sensed this and ask if it was embarrassing. Moira grimaces. She says she could write so much more. I say she has written enough, that her message is powerful and will enable others to understand and learn. I pause and wonder what it must be like to suffer from MND.

I say to Moira that I understand she wants to publish whilst she is still alive. I ask her 'How long do you expect to live?'. I feel my pulse quicken on asking this question yet Moira takes it in her stride. She says her GP refused to answer that question, but she expects to die soon. Of course, no one knows for certain but do we as practitioners avoid such difficult questions and conversations? Do Moira's despair and obsession with euthanasia encourage us into avoidance tactics?

I understood Moira's need to write as a testament that her life and death were not without meaning. She had been a health visitor and teacher. She said she loved nursing and wanted to give something if it would help others to understand. Keeping a journal was a therapeutic act for her. It was cathartic, enabling her to pour out her feelings and helping her make sense of her despair in the face of her relentless physical deterioration towards death.

The catheter was yet another marker along this trajectory. She had become incontinent and she is a proud woman. Another devastating blow as it took away what pride she had left. I asked her if there was anything that made her smile – the sun shining in the morning or a sparrow singing? In response she did smile … but she said she felt like the weather. It was raining hard outside. Indeed, she had shed many tears that morning. In her absence of words she drew the tear lines down her cheeks with her fingers. There was no way anybody could take away her despair. There was no way she could rationalise what was happening to her, yet focusing on something positive such as her journal and the possibility of publishing it did ameliorate her despair, as if the sun had come out for a moment. She was grateful to me … she joined her hands in thanks.

I felt touched by this woman in this moment, privileged to sit with her and experience her dying. I was conscious that she, like other patients I had met and written about, were teaching me something profound along my own journey to realise myself as caring. When I left her, I sensed a lightness, a soft spring in my feet. Why was this? Perhaps I should have felt burdened with her despair. But no, the contrary. I had been lifted by the experience, as if I had been touched by an angel. I felt such a calmness and sense of humility. I felt that I was an angel, that I had given Moira some warmth and light within her living hell, as indeed Louise gave her.

> Moira nourished others, comforted and cared for those who would care for her. She did not want to be a burden but sensed the struggle her carers must feel caring for her. She had shared her story with her carers when perhaps they had not realised how she felt and had been insensitive to her plight. They were touched and it changed their caring towards her. It had opened their eyes to what Moira was feeling inside. Moira died shortly afterwards.

Such journal accounts as Moira's offer deep insights into the way people respond to disability and terminal illness, and how they face death. Her writing became her sanctuary, her space where she could scream out loud and communicate to others, so they knew and could understand. That was so important to Moira. Perhaps she sensed it was only too easy to see the demanding, complaining, depressed and angry woman rather than the suffering woman who deeply loved her grandchildren. Her writing made it easier for her and family to dwell together.

How might you encourage and guide a patient to write? Well, most people will struggle with the idea because it is not something they usually do. Writing about feelings demands an acceptance of those feelings that the person may prefer to bottle up and defend against. So, I might sit with the person and help them talk about their experience and then suggest writing about the experience – perhaps as a letter to someone they love, to help them to understand. Perhaps start by writing down the strongest feeling, especially if they have been resisting it. As such, writing the word down is both cathartic and confronting. I would then suggest they write something positive about their life, either something happening now or from memory. The intention is to balance any negative thoughts or feelings with positive ones, to seek balance and harmony through writing. To help find a still place inside themselves where they can be reflective (bringing the mind home), I might suggest writing in the afternoon, play some music or have some complementary treatment beforehand. When they feel more at ease, I suggest they explore the feeling or thought they have written – why do I feel that way? And of course, to be available to the person to help them talk through the things they have written. In doing so, offer them guidance, courage, compassion and let them know they are not alone.

Listening to the patient's story

Liehr and Smith (2008) have developed 'story theory' to give structure to working with patients through their stories. They note:

> We describe story as a narrative happening of connecting-with-self-in-relation through intentional dialogue to create ease. Ease emerges in the midst of accepting the whole story as one's own … a process of attentively embracing. (p207)

The theory has three inter-related concepts. The first is listening attentively to the patient's story. By listening attentively, the practitioner opens a space for the patient to reveal his or her story. The patient senses the practitioner's interest and concern, and in doing so feels safe to reveal self. Only when we know the meanings the patient attributes to their health-illness experience are we in a position to nurse the person. Hence listening is vital. It is the empathic process to know the person.

The second concept is connecting-with-self-in-relation; the practitioner guides the person to reflect on and find meaning within their experience. The third concept is creating ease, whereby the practitioner works with the person through their story towards a more satisfactory health status.

Liehr and Smith (2008:212) note that 'creating ease is an energizing release experienced as the story comes together in a movement towards resolving'. This resonates with my own vision of clinical practice as the intention to ease the other's suffering and enabling the person to grow through their health-illness experience. In this way, the story is lived as a therapeutic journey unfolding whereby the practitioner tunes into and influences the person's health journey towards a more satisfactory way of being. In other words, practice is narrative unfolding towards finding ease (easing suffering/enabling growth).

Telling the story may be more significant than just writing it. Smith & Liehr (1999) note that when individuals tell their personal health story to one who truly listens, a change in perspective takes place. Citing Campbell (1988), they state:

> Self-discovery is embedded in story. Through story, persons search for clues or messages that potentiate understanding and the experience of being alive described as a 'resonance within one's innermost being and reality'. (p5)

Smith and Liehr (1999) demonstrated the therapeutic impact of enabling another person to tell their story in reducing blood pressure, suggesting that the therapeutic benefit of writing may be enhanced by sharing the stories with a person dedicated to listening and guiding learning through the particular experience. They give the example of a female attorney who experienced considerable stress in her work. In response to her story, the therapist helped her to pay attention to her bodily responses, teaching her to breathe deeply and focus on calming images. Over the sessions she noted an increasing sense of calm as she came to take control of her life. Smith and Liehr note:

> As the disjointed story moments come together as a whole, there is simultaneous anchoring and flow through recognition of meaning, which empowers release from the confines of the old story. This is ease. It is calmness and vision even for a moment. It is a powerful moment creating possibilities for human development. (p10)

Smith and Liehr did not ask their respondents to journal. However, as they note, the woman's story was disjointed, suggesting the difficulty many people may have in expressing their thoughts and feelings. Hence writing may have helped to shape her reflection.

Smyth *et al* (1999) sampled 112 patients with asthma or rheumatoid arthritis and assigned them in randomised controlled trial (RCT) groups to write about either the most stressful event of their lives or about emotionally neutral topics. Outcomes were evaluated at 2 weeks, 2 months and 4 months after writing. They reported that patients with mild to moderately severe asthma or rheumatoid arthritis who wrote about stressful life experiences had clinically relevant changes in health status at 4 months compared with those in the control group. These gains were beyond those attributable to the standard medical care that all participants were receiving. For the asthma patients, the primary outcome measure was forced expiratory volume in one second (FEV_1). An improvement is measured as 15% improvement in functioning. Evaluations of (Rheumatoid Arthritis RA) patients were made with a structured interview completed by the treating rheumatologist rating diagnostic symptoms, global assessment of disease activity, symptom severity, distribution of pain, tenderness and swelling throughout the affected joints, presence and severity of deformities, assessment of daily living capacity, and general psychosocial functioning.

This was based on a categorical scale (asymptomatic/mild/moderate/severe/very severe). There was a 47% improvement (shift in rating) in experimental groups compared with 24% in control groups. Improvement was maintained in asthma patients whereas the change for RA patients was not evidenced until the 4-month check, suggesting that underlying physiological processes differ in different chronic processes. This study was the first of this kind undertaken with groups of patients, in contrast with earlier studies using healthy respondents.

The study by Smyth *et al* indicates that writing about illness experience does reduce physical symptoms. Alexander (1998), in her role as writer-in-residence at a hospice, noted:

> Writing is no solution to pain or illness. It cannot cure or heal physical damage but it can help a person to feel whole again, a human being with a story to tell. (p178)

Alexander's role was to help others to express themselves in words. Whether words can heal is an interesting challenge and the focus for her present study. As Burkhardt and Nagai-Jacobson (2002:296) note:

> In the process of telling and hearing stories, persons often come to new insights and deeper understandings of themselves because stories include not only events in our lives, but also the meanings and interpretations that define the significance of events for particular lives.

Conclusion

Encouraging and listening to patient stories is a therapy in its own right, alongside other activities that enable self-expression and healing such as art and music therapy. From a research perspective such journals offer a privileged view into the life of others, enabling practitioners to really appreciate what it means to live with something like motor neurone disease. Only when we can appreciate this can we begin to respond as carers in meaningful ways.

In the next four chapters (9–12), I share four narratives written by practitioners seeking to realise desirable and effective practice. These four chapters reflect the power and diversity of reflective writing, following the format of the six dialogical movements (see Fig. 3.2). Apply the being available template to see how these integrated dimensions of being holistic are woven within the narrative. Remember, narrative helps you to dialogue, to draw your own insights and to reflect on your own practice.

All four narratives were written as academic assignments at undergraduate level. All achieved an A grade.

Part 2

Narratives of being available

Chapter 9

Jill Jarvis: reflection on touch and the environment

Jill undertook the BSc Palliative Care programme at the University of Bedfordshire. The assignment for the holistic practice module asked her to reflect on the development of three aspects of her practice. She chose touch, spirituality and the environment. Only touch and environment are included in this chapter. Jill's narrative is a story of great beauty that raises significant issues for those who claim to care and offers an exemplar of reflective writing for academic purposes at postregistration undergraduate degree level.

Introduction

> Give the gift of touch. Touch understands and is understood. Touch is the harmonic healing the grieving spirit craves. A gentle touch on the back, the shoulder, the head, the hand tells the receiver more than what can be expressed. Hands held can quickly heal and bind together more than months of psychotherapy. Touch is the great gift of self that offers immediate renewal and certain connection for both the receiver and giver. Allow yourself to heal, to touch. Simple. Momentary. Revealing. Touch brings a unity of spirit to ease the pain … Give or receive the gift of massage. The painful memories are stored in your muscles. Touch them. Honor them. Release them. Heal them. Honor your body. It is as important a part of who you are as is your spirit. Remember, we live in two worlds. Then experience the peace that follows. It will close the circle. (Blackwolf and Jones 1996:184–5)

The use of touch is fundamental to nursing practice and yet how mindful and skilled are nurses at using touch? Every practitioner should be mindful of touch as an expression of caring presence and relaxation, whether bathing, comforting, massaging or whatever.

Jill Jarvis works as a night staff nurse in a hospice. She chose to write three exemplars around one patient, Sally, concerning touch, the environment and spirituality, all concerned with a broader question – how can we create places of healing?

Of course, creating a healing environment should be deep within the mind of every practitioner. Yet, as Jill's reflection reveals, practitioners are not so mindful of the therapeutic impact of environment. I sense they become almost oblivious to the environment, as if it isn't their business.

After *Touch* I enter into a dialogue with Jill's story as I begin to explore its significance. In doing so I draw on a further literature to heighten the story's significance. After *Environment* I am silent, leaving the reader to enter into a dialogue with the story.

Touch (Jill Jarvis)

This narrative focuses on my experience with Sally who struggled to accept her horrific circumstances as life slipped away. Sally was diagnosed with acute lymphoblastic leukaemia 2 years ago. She underwent a bone marrow transplant, which completely cured her illness. Eighteen months later she developed cutaneous T-cell lymphoma caused by graft versus host disease. There has only been one other case like this reported in the world! Filled with astounded disbelief, Sally is left to suffer the consequences of this devastating condition with the knowledge that no curative treatment is available. On admission to the hospice, Sally is in the terminal phase of her illness.

Using selective literature, I enhance and substantiate my intuitive awareness that many skills used in palliative care are not formally taught in nursing school but acquired during life experience and personal study. I aim to explore the depths and meaning of touch to gain insight into its therapeutic value. By reflecting on my thoughts, feelings and reactions of the care I administer, I aim to reveal ways in which I can improve my nursing.

My evening report states: 'Her skin is burnt all over, each movement causes pain creating many difficulties with her care. She is having trouble coming to terms with her condition.'

Leaving the office, I wander along the corridor, greeting patients and informing them that I will be here tonight. A penetrating nauseous vapour fills the air leading towards an open door. Standing at the doorway my eyes transfix onto the small wispy figure covered only by a thin linen sheet. Her face, peaceful in sleep, disfigured by ferocious, sore red patches which connect and weave their way into every crease and feature of beauty. The main attack centres on her eyes, producing a monstrous appearance of two cracked shivering starfish oozing from tentacles. Small mounds of decaying skin cling desperately all around her head, reluctant to completely give up and let go. Goose pimples emerge on my arms; my body shudders coldly, ending the momentary glance. On autopilot, I continue to the next room. Disgust and horror overwhelm my mind as I smile at the clean-shaven unblemished tanned face of the gentleman sitting comfortably reading. Conversation readily flows, we discuss the beautiful view from the window but my brain struggles to dismiss the suffering in the previous room.

Sally has called for assistance; she requests that I cream a very sensitive sore area on her back. As my hand approaches, an invisible layer of heat 3 inches from her body penetrates my skin. Like entering a hot oven, I carefully make contact with her slippery flesh. The cream has dissolved into oil and trickled onto the sheets. With gentle circular movements my fingers attempted to coat the raw burning tissues of Sally's back, lubricating the rippled surfaces. Feelings of sadness and hesitance are replaced by pleasurable sensations. The moist warmth infuses through the dryness of my hands, creating suppleness and ease. In silence I continue covering any area of need, enjoying the experience of Sally's relaxation radiating through my fingertips. 'That's wonderful,' she whispers, 'You're not wearing gloves.' Startled I question, 'Should I be?'. 'Well, I'm not contagious but everyone wears them because it's so revolting.' Sally's reply is nonchalant. Checking for approval, I ask, 'Would you prefer that I wear gloves?'. With eyes closed, Sally relaxes, smiles and mouths, 'No, no, it's lovely'. Continuing our intimate interaction until the peacefulness of sleep encompasses Sally, I leave feeling enriched by this encounter.

Returning to the office, thoughts of gratitude swell my mind. How privileged I am to work in an environment that values and prioritises time with patients. Gone are the days when I was considered a time-waster! (De Hennezel 1996: 61).

As morning slowly emerges I draw back the curtains, enabling Sally to witness the beauty of the sunrise over the lake. She smiles whilst beckoning me to her; taking my arm, she thanks me for last night. Our eyes meet as I reassure her that I also benefited by creaming my neglected hands.

Sally rushes into conversation about her history and prognosis, as if frightened that I might leave her; she holds my hand tight. With resentment she recounts her story, bewildered as to how or why she has to suffer such torment. Restrained by her grasp, I can only listen, no words are available to explain or bring comfort. Normal responses of stroking the hair or hugging are inappropriate due to causing excruciating pain. Motionless, I stand as the painful darts of information enter my heart and compassion is portrayed through facial expression and contact. Consumed into the depths of reality and truth, I feel Sally's pain opening disturbing craters in my soul. My mind wanders to things I should put right and others that I want to do before I die (Autton 1996: 123). Slowly an awareness of death is expressed, as De Hennezel (1996) has observed may times. Like panning for gold, I sieve through each word. Trickling down the mountains of despair is a tiny but clear meandering stream of hope and desire. The simplicity of Sally's needs bring tears to my eyes. Lowering my head, a spontaneous kiss reaches her erupting cheek; fragments of her scabby skin cohere to my lips but I only feel love. Sally mouths a return gesture; smiling, we squeeze hands and disengage. 'See you later', I whisper, leaving her space. Sally nods, closing her eyes.

On reflection, Sally's history left me dumb struck. What could I say to her that would make a difference, alleviate anguish and help her find peace? As Autton (1996) agrees, 'In some circumstances words can be more of a hindrance than a help' (p121).

By using touch as the first form of communication, I relayed my feelings to Sally (Talton 1995). I had the intention of achieving connection with Sally through physical contact. Sympathy and empathy can be exchanged by touch as Edwards (1998) explains, using a quote from Wyshcogrod (p801): 'fellow feelings that you and I are one'. I wanted Sally to know I cared, to break down the barriers of being strangers and facilitate her journey of acceptance. Estabrooks and Morse (1992) use the beautiful phrase 'bumping souls', which sums up what I wanted to achieve (Fredriksson 1999:7). Sally and I 'tuned in' to each other through the caring touch as Fredriksson (1999) has noted. I find amazing peace inside me that so much can be gained without the use of words!

Touch has been categorised as task oriented, caring and protective (Fredriksson 1999, Talton 1995). Task touch is the most commonly used by nurses and does not always have the intent to communicate in a positive manner. It can be defined by 'hurried, rough, jarred movements' relaying 'frustration, anger or impatience' (Fredriksson 1999:2). I find this very disturbing and not true in the hospice where I work. Because of the horrific condition of Sally's skin I was very wary of how I should commence the application of cream. Taking time to register Sally's reaction to my contact and constantly reassessing our intention, I was able to ensure that we understood each other (Davidhizar and Giger 1997). To make the mistake of hurting Sally would create fear of me administering treatment and in turn cause anxiety instead of ease (Davidhizar and Giger 1997).

The disgust I felt on first seeing Sally produced intense guilt. The T-cell lymphoma had totally consumed her skin into a revolting, stinking mess. On reflection, I suppose as a nurse, it would have been normal to reach for gloves. However, I feel they create a barrier within the touching process, preventing skin-to-skin contact. I wanted to communicate my acceptance of Sally despite her disfigured body. Autton (1996) describes how reassuring physical contact can be by transferring a healing message (p123). If I had created a barrier within the touching process, by wearing gloves, would Sally have received my message? No, I would have intensified her feelings of self-repulsion and ugliness. Sadly, when I tried to discuss this with my colleagues, they dismissed the idea and requested that we should all wear aprons as well to protect our clothes! How useful tacit knowledge becomes with experience. I knew she wasn't infectious. I didn't even consider using gloves and that brought Sally such pleasure.

Transmissions of pain and touch have joint nerve pathways (Talton 1995). The gentle movements of my fingers on Sally's back initiated relaxation and eventually sleep. What better way, during the night, can there be of dealing with personal mental trauma? So often, as hospice nurses, we turn to sedatives to induce sleep but through experience I am learning that giving time to patients is much more effective and rewarding. This can be demonstrated clearly in the way that Sally acted in the morning.

To conclude, Davidhizar and Giger (1997) state that 'touch has been described as the most important of all the senses' (p203). However, it does not follow that touch is used more often than sight, hearing, smell or taste, all of which I observe to be in almost constant function. Chang Ok Sung (2001) observe that 'touching is an integral part of human life' (p2). Within the nursing environment using touch is a normal, frequent method of administering care both physically and psychologically (Chang and Sung 2001). Nurses are also allowed to enter the private zones of the individual through intimate touch due to societal agreement (Hickman and Holmes 1994). Surprisingly, Estabrooks and Morse (1992) note: 'One of the most neglected areas of touch in nursing research is the investigation of the touching behaviours of nurses'. These authors suggest that nurses develop their own touching style through individual life experience and training. It is a comfort to know that touching can be a learned behaviour, especially when observing those who appear to have a comfortable natural ability for its proper use (Estabrooks and Morse 1992). Unfortunately self-evaluation and reflection is not a spontaneous process and therefore, some nurses do not learn to express positive feelings through touch. This research has heightened my awareness of the physical and therapeutic areas of touch.

Consideration must always be given to ethnic background, personal history and social connotations to ensure that touch is appropriate and authentic (Talton 1995). Ochs (2001) suggests that we should always ask permission before touching patients or family. I find it more agreeable to continually assess the person's reactions (Talton 1995). The meaning of touch is personal and can only be translated by the recipient (Chang and Sung 2001). To assist my own interpretation of touch, I indulged in a full body massage. This opened my eyes to the further pleasure of body therapies that complement nursing such as reflexology and aromatherapy.

Commentary

Through Jill's words, I experience the exquisite beauty and significance of caring. It is beautiful because Jill's action makes such a difference to Sally's care. I feel Sally's plight.

I ache for her. Sally feels cared for. Jill's care is the essence of palliative care perhaps more than anything. Jill's disgust at Sally's blistered and festering skin is a powerful confession, yet she saw the deeper beauty. Sally had learnt that her skin was disgusting for the nurses to treat. She had embodied that knowing. Hence she expected Jill to wear gloves whilst applying cream. Jill was ambivalent; part of her wanted to wear gloves because the skin was disgusting. But another, deeper and more powerful part of her rejected the gloves because she knew tacitly that she was rejecting Sally and this engendered guilt. She could not easily live with herself if she chose to wear gloves. As practitioners go about their practice, they touch people in different ways. I shall assume that touch is a vital part of healing, not just physical touch but also the sense of touching someone in an emotional way. As Turton (1989) says:

> To put our hand on someone's shoulder or take someone's arm are such apparently simple and commonplace acts that we can easily forget that touch is the most important sense in human growth and development. (p42)

Turton reminds practitioners to be mindful of their use of touch and its therapeutic impact. As a therapist, I ask myself – what messages do I give patients? Do I convey disgust in my posture? If I am mindful enough, then I would not but am I mindful enough? I recognise how easy it is to slip into habitual patterns of taken-for-grantedness, of complacency, as if we think we know what is going on. Arthur Frank (2002), who was being treated for cancer, describes his experience with a blood technician.

> As this technician went about her work I remarked how skilful she was compared to some other technicians. She then said something to me that had a direct reference to my complaint but also elevated the occasion to a wholly different plane – 'Remember', she said slowly, 'everyone who touches you affects your healing'. (p18)
>
> That technician [amongst many] is the one who drew me into a relation of care, in the full sense of *remoralisation*. She recognised, and she found a way to express that recognition, that she was not just extracting blood as a part of a diagnostic procedure, but was also affecting a change in who I was as a result of touching me. (p18)

Frank makes the point that caring 'is not a substance or thing … not merely the taking of blood but is possible only within relations of caring … not as a puzzle to be solved but as a mystery' (p13). Frank asked what the technician meant by using the words 'touch' and 'healing'. The words capture the sense of caring: the mutual exchange as something in Frank touched the technician, that she was open to and could listen to his suffering. From this perspective, for touch to be recognised as caring, it needs to be more than a technical thing. Indeed, being touched without a sense of being cared for, without a sense of intimacy is demoralising, the sense of being treated as an object. It is the antithesis of caring.

Frank says his experience with the technician was remoralising – she placed him firmly on his healing journey. In other words, the role of any care-giver is to remoralise the patient, to help him or her grow through the illness experience, to emerge as more whole having been cut to pieces by the cancer experience, even for patients who are dying, who feel torn apart. Touch is then healing.

I am always inspired by the stories of Marie De Hennezel, a psychologist working at the Paris hospice, from her book *Intimate death* (1996). Her words powerfully resonate with Jill's story and illustrate the way reflective texts are both evocative and provocative.

Patricia

Creating this atmosphere of warmth and calm around a sick person who is in torment is unquestionably the most beneficial thing one can do for him or her. Chantal has known this for a long time. The doctors have always been astonished to note so few tranquillisers or anxiety-reducing drugs are given on nights when she's on duty. She just prefers to give them a massage or tell them a story, or simply let them talk while she sits quietly at their bedside. (p46)

Charlotte

'I've become so hideous', she goes on. Last night, she dreamed about a crow. 'Crows reek of death, just like me.'

When I leave, I'll tell the nurses that she needs to feel recognised and loved. She's just given me the key to her agitation. When children are playing in the park and go to pick up a dead bird, you say, 'Don't touch. That's dirty'. She believes she smells of death; she's afraid of being rejected, pushed away like some dirty thing. We have to be able to help her to see herself differently, to feel accepted as she is. (p64)

Environment (Jill Jarvis)

What impact does the environment have on the physical, emotional and spiritual well-being of patients and their families? I aim to explore the patient environment within my workplace. Are any changes required? If so, how can change be implemented?

Slowly washing my hands in the cream enamel basin, my eyes wander around Sally's room through the mirror above the sink. Wilting, shrivelled stems interspersed by youthful blooms hang from vases. Stagnating in discoloured water, they silently scream for attention. Twisted chocolate wrappers hide between magazines haphazardly balanced on the bedside table. Walkman cables, compact discs and tubes of cream create a 'modern' work of art. 'Get well' cards lie abandoned, children's drawings huddle in a corner and photos of loved ones face the window.

An unintentional arena of chaos faces me as I turn around, feelings of claustrophobia creep inside my body. I need some space. Each item of furniture is overburdened with unnecessary clutter. The floor extends storage pads and dressings, red 'infected' linen bags openly display their contents.

Reaching for a paper towel, I dry my hands carefully, ensuring that nothing is knocked from the nearby shelf. Gadgets of hygiene engulf the small wash area whilst the sad magnolia walls absorb the atmosphere of dull isolation and neglect. Sally is asleep so I tiptoe away.

Standing outside the hospice, a refreshing night breeze hits my skin. A stabbing tightness tightens my chest. Sally finds even ripples of air painful on her burning flesh. She is cocooned in the moist 'foul-smelling' warmth of her room. Aromas of freshly mown grass fill my nostrils but Sally's sense of smell has become numbed by continuous stench. Confined to her bed through weakness but craving independence, Sally is rendered helpless in personally changing her surroundings. I wonder how she would arrange things if able.

Entering the main entrance, a beautiful arrangement of fresh flowers adorns the foyer. 'Welcome' signs invite my arrival and homely décor instils comfort. Windows proudly display wonderful views of nature, a lake, gardens, wildlife and an abundance of glorious, towering protective trees. the corridor turns revealing a quiet area of cosiness to relax, chat with family or befriend other patients. Visually nothing to fear is apparent except the word 'hospice' all around the building!

An intoxicating fetid odour invisibly digests the air, as I get closer to Sally's room. 'Can't sleep,' she whispers as I move blankets and clothes by her bedside. 'Can I tidy your room?' slips from my mouth. Smiling, Sally giggles: 'Where will you start?'.

Mesmerized by activity, Sally remains quiet. Within half an hour her environment evokes order, cleanliness and thoughtful comfort. Nursing supplies are secretly hidden in cupboards. Smeared surfaces now shine with approval. Photos smile at Sally from wardrobe doors and cards hang overhead, displaying their messages of comfort. Wiping tears of joy from Sally's eyes, I ask if the room is to her liking. Nodding contentedly, Sally pours into conversation centred on memorabilia. Time rushes by, twilight creeps across the sky bringing a new day. Exhausted, Sally drifts leisurely into the land of dreams.

Reflection

How many times do I ignore the irritating untidiness of a patient's room? Actually, the answer is never. Mess constantly annoys me but I don't always clean it up! Neither do I consistently take time to consider how the patient feels about their surroundings. Literature relating to patients' or nurses' thoughts on their environment can be picked from a variety of sources, as I have done.

Morse and Dobernect (1995, cited by Summer 2001:4) mention the determination of the patient to endure the unpleasant 'side effects' of illness. Sally appeared to have lost interest in her surroundings, she was forced to endure the clutter. In an investigation by Rogers *et al* (2000) on the sources of dissatisfaction with hospital care, the environment comes right at the bottom of the list! This research included 229 people but only 26 complained about untidiness or dirty bathrooms. Am I to believe that hospitals and hospices are very tidy, clean places? Unfortunately, we nearly all have personal stories to tell or have heard disturbing reports to the contrary. Is it good that people are so grateful for our care that they feel unable to express their concerns?

The intrasubjective world of the patient is discussed by Summer (2001), who claims that the patient becomes vulnerable, in need of help due to illness. Summer states: 'the patient comes to the illness-induced interaction hopeful that this exquisite vulnerability will be acknowledged' (p4). Hope that this will happen comes from 'a yearning for a recognition or consideration by others of unmet needs' (p4). Although Summer's work is focused on the interpretation of nurse–patient relationships, I feel it can be applied to environmental issues.

Loss is described by Robinson & McKenna (1998) as having three attributes:

- that someone or something one has had or ought to have had in the future, has been taken away
- that which is taken away must have been valued by the person experiencing the loss
- the meaning of loss is determined individually, subjectively and contextually by the person experiencing it. (p7)

Sally craved her independence but it had been snatched from her. She would have loved to keep her room tidy, bright and cheerful. The glow on her face when seeing her family photos answers my questions: 'Is Sally vulnerable?', 'Does Sally endure her surroundings?', 'Is Sally grieving due to loss?'. The daily nursing ritual of ward rounds, checking that everything is 'ship-shape', has long gone (Biley and Wright 1997). Sometimes I feel that in nursing we have gone from one extreme to another. For example, delegating the task of cleaning to a particular person usually, in my opinion, gets the job done, whereas relying on individual commitment unfortunately often doesn't! This is a good example of why the stench from Sally's room has not been dealt with. Everyone has to be aware of its existence, with the exception of Sally, but nobody took responsibility to act.

The sense of smell is the most immediate of our senses due to the olfactory nerve being directly connected to the brain (Davis 2000:278). Smell is also the most fleeting of the senses; fading occurs when one is exposed to a smell for a long time (Davis 2000:279). Sally sadly had become a victim of this. Bergamot is one of the most effective deodorising oils (Davis 2000:283). Why didn't I take the time to discover this oil and use it? Davis also informs that bergamot is an 'uplifting' oil, producing a relaxing atmosphere for the anxious, depressed person (p57). Although Sally had lost her sense of smell she still could have absorbed the oil into her bloodstream through inhalation via the lungs (Davis 2000:281).

Music can be used to improve the nursing environment and has been demonstrated to decrease pain, reduce anxiety and promote relaxation (McCaffrey 2002). Sally obviously appreciated music – a Walkman and compact discs were in her room. Given the potential effectiveness of this non-invasive pleasure, 'it should be offered to all hospital patients in all situations that are known to be stressful' (Evans 2002:9). Music improves the mood of patients and may reduce the need for sedatives (Evans 2002:9). My mind fills with a picture of Sally's room. The light is dimmed, bergamot penetrates the air and soft sounds ripple in the background. Serenity. How easy it is to produce a peaceful haven. Why didn't I achieve this for Sally?

On reflection, I can think of many other ways of improving the boring surroundings for patients. Empirical evidence is very limited but reactions of individual patients plentiful. Art can bring such pleasure, Videos, especially those of family, distract patients from circumstance and create opportunity to express feelings. Creative hobbies, jigsaw puzzles, nail-care, facials and massage all give a short welcome break to discomfort and despair. Alternative approaches such as reflexology and aromatherapy concentrate on the mind, body and spirit. Shouldn't they therefore be given more recognition within palliative care?

Summary

I feel the environment has an enormous impact on both patients and their families despite the lack of research to prove this. Street (1995) encourages nurses to notice the unnoticed through journalling. By concentrating on the setting, Street (1995:149) advises that we should consider the following questions:

- Where was I?
- What could I see, smell, hear and feel?

Self-inquiry data can therefore be a source of information on which I can improve and initiate change within my workplace. Caring ideals are described by Wuest (1997) as images of how things should be and these ideals shape the way in which we respond to caring demands. Wuest illuminates environmental influences of woman's caring and areas in need of nursing action on a social level. She argues that a broader conceptualisation of environment needs to become a focus for nursing action.

At present we are reviewing the name for my place of work. It has been noted that the word 'hospice' means 'a place to die' for many people. Improved symptom control and respite care allow a lot of patients to go home and continue living. With this in mind, we feel a less disturbing title would be more appropriate.

Conclusion

Jill's narratives of touch and environment written at an academic undergraduate level give vivid insights into her practice whilst achieving a good academic standard. Jill has the gift of drawing the reader deep into her story through her rich engaging description. Her story is more engaging because she doesn't interrupt the story with interpretation – keeping story telling apart from story analysis. Then she stands back from her art to reflect and consider the significance of these stories, illuminating the impact of reflection on shifting her practice and her challenge to others. Without doubt, she becomes more available to Sally, illuminating how each element of the being available template is an indirect focus for reflection – her intent to ease Sally's suffering, her compassion, knowing Sally, responding with skilful action, knowing and managing herself and, perhaps most significantly, creating an environment where she can be available to Sally.

Through her writing, Jill lifts the mundane into significance and in doing so, lifts herself to a higher level of mindfulness. These issues are no longer mundane. Indeed, she is resolved to act on her insights to change hospice practice. These stories are transgressive in confronting normal individual and collective practice.

At work tomorrow, just pause and consider some of the issues that Jill raises in her narrative. Ask yourself – is the environment therapeutic? How could it be more therapeutic?

Chapter 10

Simon Lee: reflection on caring

Introduction

Without doubt, 'who I am' is my major therapeutic tool and needs to be kept sharp enough to cut the cloth in skilful action. In the following example, consider Simon's existential struggle in the face of Bill's and his wife's suffering. Simon is a charge nurse on a medical ward. His story is a search for meaning in the suffering and joy he experienced, reflecting the deeply emotional aspect of holistic practice and the fundamental need to know and manage self within relationship.

Simon wrote this as his final reflective account whilst a student on the Becoming a reflective and effective practitioner programme.

Simon writes

Nursing is a demanding profession. The commitment we invest in our roles provides us with our greatest source of reward – the ability to use our position to aid others. This interpersonal aspect of nursing when encountering people at their most vulnerable is the foundation of our practice and its fulfilment the foundation of our satisfaction even though the price of constant exposure to emotionally challenging situations can be very high. Can we avoid this expense? Or can we grow as nurses through it? Can we become overexposed to death and dying, resulting in emotional detachment that undermines holistic care and prevents us from using ourselves in therapeutic way or learning from the experience?

By reflecting on my involvement with Bill, a 40-year-old man who died of cancer, I am attempting to discover the factors that influenced my feelings and actions.

Standing at a shade over six feet tall, weighing a muscular 14 stone, the smiling face on the photograph provided a shocking contrast to the image of its owner sleeping in the bed. I use the word 'shocking' in response to how cancer specialises in the distortion of features and expressions more rapidly than a cosmetic surgeon's knife and in a fashion that only first-hand witnesses could believe. When the bones, normally concealed beneath a physique developed through good living and exercise, become not only visible but the dominating feature in Bill's experience, it becomes a cruel irony of nature that many years of development can be so undone at a rate that growth can never equal.

We described Bill as cachexic, a single word to describe so much. As professionals, we are very comfortable and familiar with our terminology. It becomes very easy to use and the words can soften their meaning. This is a user-friendly language that cannot portray what it describes. Cachexia is defined as abnormally low weight, weakness and general bodily decline associated with chronic disease, most notably cancer.

In reality, however, it is the image that Jane [Bill's wife] tries to spare her sons – Joe and Tim – from seeing, fearing nightmares and difficult 'why?' questions. It is the sight of a loving son, a devoted husband and doting father reduced to a living skeleton barely able to acknowledge everything in life that is dear to him and those who love him struggling with their pain.

Bill was admitted to our ward when symptoms of his lung cancer began to overwhelm him and his family. It had been a short disease process typical in its presentation and diagnosis. The dry cough that had failed to respond to linctus annoyed Jane so much that she wore down Bill's reluctance and persuaded him to go to the GP who sent Bill for a chest X-ray. The film showed a shadow that in turn resulted in bronchoscopic biopsy and diagnosis. Simple, systematic and effective intervention. It is the impact that has the medical profession floundering like a bully having its bluff called: 'So what are you going to do now?'. You can almost sense the taunt.

Radiotherapy was marginally successful in reducing the size of the shadow. Isn't *shadow* an easy word to use, avoiding the dreaded 'C' word but managing to remain mysterious, sinister and often, for the patient, ambiguous? But tragically, postponement of the inevitable was its only consequence. Subsequent community management with the input of Macmillan nurses had kept Bill at home until uncontrollable pain and nausea necessitated admission to hospital. The original plan was to achieve symptom control to facilitate discharge as soon as possible. However, the best laid plans of mice and men …

Bill could feel the pain through his chest wall. A subcutaneous syringe driver containing diamorphine and cyclizine was used to manage his pain and nausea. These drugs were initially effective but the diamorphine needed to be increased within hours to achieve adequate pain control.

Bill had lost his appetite and was unable to keep fluids down long enough for them to be of any value. He looked dry and blood tests confirmed this impression. An intravenous infusion was commenced to correct his dehydration. Secondary to his reduced fluid intake, Bill experienced oral candida and some painful oral ulcers. Antifungal and ulcer medications were prescribed and regular mouthcare provided. Bill was nursed on a pressure-reducing mattress.

Over the next couple of days Bill's condition stabilised and improved enough for him to have visits from his sons. They were aged 8 and 12 years old. Jane had protected them as much as possible by shielding them from seeing their father when he had looked so unwell. During this period, over 3–4 shifts, I got to know Bill quite well. He was intelligent, articulate and we shared mutual interests in sport and music. We shared a similar sense of humour and managed to make each other laugh frequently. I wished I had the opportunity to know Bill for longer. Bill and I were disagreeing about England's World Cup chances as I left the ward for 2 days off. Bill invited me to call round and see him when he was at home as we were aiming for discharge in the next 2 days. I replied that I would try but I knew deep down that I wouldn't. Not because I doubted that Bill would get home, but once a patient goes home we prepare for the next one. Our busy schedules are exactly that and how much time and involvement should one invest?

On one occasion, whilst completing some paperwork, I found myself watching Bill as his family visited. The indelible image was that of seeing the boys at the foot of his bed and simultaneously touching their dad's feet as their mum hugged him. The boys so needed the physical contact but seemed reserved and hesitant until Bill held out his arms and the boys rushed to him and held him tightly. They seemed scared to let go and Bill, eyes closed, tried to absorb and retain every precious moment, knowing how valuable time was.

Later that evening, I checked on my sleeping son and cried as I recalled what I had seen earlier. My emotions were a combination of anger at how people's lives are so sense-lessly destroyed and fear generated where the fine line between life and death is made so visible and where our own mortality is questioned.

Returning from my days off, I noted that Bill had been transferred into the side-room. I immediately asked the nurse looking after Bill what had happened. She informed me that Bill was close to death. He had become increasingly dyspnoeic due to the development of an extensive pleural infusion. A pleural aspiration had been performed which had alleviated some of his breathlessness. However, the effusion was a sign of general deterioration that warranted increased analgesia and a sedative to control his developing agitation. Bill's deterioration was rapid, the disease's only concession to Jane's feelings – 'he's not in pain, is he?' Jane urgently inquired. Before I could respond, Jane continued 'I wish we could have him home'. I responded by saying that Bill was asleep and peaceful, indicating that the medication was effective and that we were continually assessing his condition. Jane was obviously distressed that Bill had not got home as she repeated her statement to herself shaking her head and crying. 'I think Bill's main concern was to have you all here,' I responded, looking towards the sons, trying to highlight to them how important their presence was to their dad. I continued: 'Holding his hand and talking to him is the most you can do regardless of where you are'. Jane forced a smile in my direction and nodded in agreement. She turned her attention to Bill and her sons. Feeling somewhat uncomfortable with the ensuing silence, I asked a typically English question: 'Can I get you a cup of tea or anything?'.

Bill's family visited at regular intervals as he slipped into unconsciousness. I continued to let the family know that I was there for them should they need anything. Within an hour Bill died. I stood silently, deprived of the sanctuary of offering tea. I withdrew to allow the family privacy. Jane was very protective of her sons and through her grief she remained strong for them. They were distraught and through their tears betrayed a vacant, disbelieving look; in this instant they were experiencing emotions with demands beyond their tender years. Their sobbing provided a heart-breaking image and I was revisited by the twin impostors of anger and fear and a feeling of frustration at my helplessness.

I offered my condolence simply by expressing how sorry I was and instinctively touched Tim's arm as he stood next to me. Jane took my hand and thanked me for all I had done. I repeated how sorry I was and said how I liked Bill a lot. She seemed to appreciate this and smiled. I was glad that I told Jane this. I felt for some reason that this was important to say as I knew that I would not get another chance to hint at the impact that looking after Bill was having on me. The practical aspects were discussed with Bill's brother-in-law and provided a sense of relief that comes with taking refuge in practices over which we have some control.

Bill required a subtle balance of physical and psychological care typical in palliative nursing. But its influence on me as a person, and subsequently as a nurse, was atypical.

I found myself experiencing fear, helplessness, inadequacy, anger and levels of distress that I had not felt since my earliest nursing exposure to death and dying. Farrar (1992) recognised these emotions in novices. However, my experience is far beyond novice so why do I seem to be regressing? I initially perceived these feelings to be barriers to effective care as they can elevate stress levels and compromise my ability to carry out clinical care objectively. In providing psychological support, I have always felt it prudent to keep some distance between my empathy and my personal feelings, a kind of conditional empathy whose extent is determined by my feelings of discomfort and my emotional self-defence. In short, the experience has exposed barriers in my attitudes that, unless resolved, will impact negatively on my practice.

My reflection illuminates the darkest areas of my practice and reveals the source of my fear, anger and frustration, and guides me in my attempts to learn from them and apply my understandings in practice. Bill and I had much in common that stimulated me to empathise to the extent that I was forced to confront my own personal experience of loss and my own mortality. I felt helpless at not being able to alter the course of Bill's prognosis or lessen the impact on his wife and sons. These are perfectly normal human responses but need to be fully understood to turn them into positive emotions, rather than areas for personal conflict and distress. The majority of my nursing practice has been in care of the elderly environments and my dealings with palliative care in my own age group have been limited. In managing the needs of the older patient, I can see that I could have more easily employed my coping mechanisms that dilute the personal impact and subsequently lessen the felt distress.

This is not to say that terminal disease is any less tragic for the people involved or that it requires any less skill or commitment on the nurse's behalf. But I am able to rationalise the event and see it more objectively. In examining my thoughts related to my own mortality, it is clear to me that it is a subject that I have actively avoided. McSherry (1996) details the importance of discovering our attitudes to mortality in order to resolve our barriers to death and dying. The experience of observing the trauma of Bill's sons brings back memories of my own father's death that I have not allowed to impact on my nursing due to the upset that they still evoke. Reissetter and Thomas (1986) state that these are the very emotions that we need to expose and incorporate into our practice. In avoiding applying my own experience into my practice, I am denying a major source of personal knowing. Utilising this knowing would enhance my care as I could use my subsequent increased capacity for empathy to understand my patients' needs more acutely and view this closeness as a bridge rather than as a barrier.

Applying my own anxiety and fear of death and dying to provide a door to another's actions and thoughts rather than a subject to be dispelled immediately on appearance gives me the opportunity to provide true holistic care. The question 'How would I feel if that were me?' should not only be accepted but encouraged if holism is our objective. In revisiting my father's illness, I am reminded of the doctors, nurses and therapists that we came into contact with and the way they made me feel. Whispering at the foot of the bed, head shaking when reading the notes and being stared at by curious student nurses are memories that I seldom, if ever, relate to my own ideas of nursing. Do I whisper over my patients, leave patients perplexed and terrified with the shake of my head or the raising of an eyebrow, or forget the individual's right not to be a source of medical curiosity? I wish that I could cast the first stone at these sins but in reality I fear that I cannot. I worry that a lack of true empathy that can prevail when we lessen our humanness leads to a provision of care guided by a form of nursing 'autopilot' that demands little from us. I am equally reminded of the staff who respected my father and our family with their time, skills and most of all their understanding that meant so much to us so much of the time.

I want to leave a positive impression of my caring on those with whom I come into contact and recognise the factors that reduce this possibility. I hope that Jane's memories of Bill's hospital care are reassuring. I will then have achieved something. At times I feel like a voyeur, impotent, unable to achieve practical goals that would make myself or Bill's family feel better. The danger of containing these feelings is that I carry them around with me into the next similar scenario, immediately creating a barrier.

Through reflection, I am now in better shape to use my frustration and anger to enhance my care. Being able to value the care I give reduces my frustration and allows me to accept my limitations, whilst my anger can be channelled into striving to improve in all areas of practice. Anger experienced by patients is often part of the grieving process (Kübler-Ross 1969), but its impact can be damaging if there is no justifiable recipient to direct it at. In harnessing memories of my own anger when experiencing my father's illness, I can detect this in difficult and aggressive people and avoid dismissing them as irritating or their behaviour as meaningless.

The anger I felt at seeing a man deprived of the opportunity to love his sons, enjoy and nurture their growth has to be managed and resolved to avoid extreme levels of stress and potential burnout. In response to this, I am committed to working with our palliative care team to establish a support network for ward nurses to explore, share and hopefully resolve emotional fall-out from our work. I am now a more complete nurse through knowing Bill. Reflection has been enlightening, supportive and rewarding.

Commentary

Simon reflects on his involvement with this family. Part of him is drawn into the family's suffering and as a consequence, he suffers himself. Through reflection, he strives to make sense of his feelings as he positions himself alongside this family. Part of him is also distant, staying on the edge, uncertain of the extent to which he should become involved. Simon illuminates that becoming involved is not a rational thing or a technique to apply but heartfelt soul bumping. Involvement is giving the self to the other. Or, put another way, the practitioner's depth of involvement, or intimacy with the patient, is a reflection of compassion – for compassion is only possible to the extent that the practitioner can loosen herself from her concerns. If the practitioner is wrapped up in her own stuff how can she be available to another? If my gaze is upon myself how can I gaze at the other?

For many nurses working on busy medical wards, Simon's story will be well known. I know from teaching such nurses on palliative care modules at the university that there is always a deep tension between the prevailing dominant medical model and a palliative care attitude. The frustration of not realising ideal care is strongly felt, especially when associated with patients who are dying.

Simon articulates the way reflection helped him to understand his feelings, linking back to his identification with Bill in terms of similar age and interests, having young children and the impact of Bill's death on the children, and his unresolved anger about his father's care and subsequent death. The idea that we can separate the personal self from the professional self is challenged by Simon's story.

The X-ray film showed a shadow, the shadow of death that hovered over Bill and his family. How do we learn to live in the shadow of death with its suffering? Simon felt this suffering and suffered himself. As Rinpoche (1992) notes:

Suffering … gives you such an opportunity of working through and transforming it. The times you are suffering can be those where your greatest strength really lies. Say to yourself then – 'I am not going to run away from this suffering. I want to use it in the best and richest way I can, so that I can become more compassionate and more helpful to others.' So, whatever you do, don't shut off your pain; accept your pain and remain vulnerable. And don't we know only too well, that protection from pain doesn't work, and that when we try and defend ourselves from suffering, we only suffer more and don't learn what we can from the experience. (p316)

Such powerful words. Simon lives these words through his narrative. He reveals and transforms his own suffering in response to Bill and his family.

Benner and Wrubel (1989) argue that burnout is the loss of caring and that the remedy is to reconnect to caring. It is the loss of caring that is truly harmful. And on medical wards such as Simon's, caring can be submerged in the pressure of time and cure priorities. Reissetter and Thomas (1986) showed a significant relationship between high-quality palliative care, reduced stress levels and the individual nurse's ability to draw on personal experience of death and dying. This would seem to suggest that practitioners who have the motivation and ability to reflect on their experience as a method of development are better equipped to respond effectively to the needs of their patients. In contrast, Atkinson *et al* (1990) detail the way people deal with personal loss by viewing it in abstract terms that 'prevent us from internalising and personalising questions surrounding our mortality and death'. Atkinson *et al*'s research indicates that nurses who are able to utilise their own experience to enhance their personal knowing are in a better position to respond to the needs of their patients and the impact upon themselves, and understand the feelings, attitudes and prejudices that influence behaviour.

Involvement

Morse (1991) identifies the risk of 'overinvolvement' whereby the therapeutic gaze becomes blurred through entanglement with the other. This is always a risk when the practitioner does not know herself well enough. Becoming overinvolved may be a necessary learning journey, for how else can the person come to know herself? Simon noted his fear of 'getting in too deep'. The metaphor suggests drowning, of becoming submerged in another's suffering. Yet, as Simon's reflection illustrates, his willingness to 'go there' and dwell with Bill and his family opened up possibilities for his own learning. In dwelling with the family and letting go of the urge to 'fix it' for them, he could explore the depths of their suffering with them. That he absorbed their suffering and suffered himself is human nature. None of us is immune from that but through reflection and guidance, he could make sense of his feelings and grow through the experience. He emerges from the chaos of his feelings wiser, more caring, more able to manage himself in similar situations. If Simon had resisted these feelings then he could only have fled from the situation to save himself. As it was, he tuned into the suffering on the different levels of Bill, Bill's wife and children, and flowed with it in its unpredictability.

Most relationships fall within a person's 'normal' intimacy boundaries and are not problematic. But as Simon's experience suggests, experience sometimes falls outside normal boundaries, resulting in anxiety. Because of this, practitioners are urged to balance engagement and detachment in care giving (Carmack 1997). As Menzies-Lyth (1988) notes:

> The core of the anxiety situation for the nurse lies in her relationship with the patient. The closer and more concentrated this relationship, the more the nurse is likely to experience this anxiety … a necessary psychological task for the entrant into any profession that works with people is the development of adequate professional detachment. (p51-4)

The alternative to professional detachment is to know and manage self within involvement. To avoid the situation is a response whereby everyone loses. A more positive response is to 'go there' better equipped because, as Benner and Wrubel (1989) assert, the risk of detachment is a loss of intimacy and a denial of self as caring. Yet, as Simon suggests, this is not easy work. We must learn to become confident with who we are if we are to help patients like Bill and his family.

As so often, the wise and compassionate words of Blackwolf and Jones (1996:183-4) put things into the right perspective. They say:

> Uncomfortable with the griever's uncertainty about life, deep sadness, encounter with death, and changed self, we turn away when we are needed most. Look at times when, perhaps, you have turned away … what were you avoiding? Most likely it was your own uncertainty, your own sadness, your own changes, your own mortality. In order to be comfortable with the uncomfortable, you need to confront your life issues. take this time to look at your life. How do you view death? How do you view life? Take the time to answer these two questions. They are the most important questions you will ever have to face … your physical presence reassures the griever that life is still a familiar scene. The griever needs your presence more than words. Your presence gives a sense of order in the world that has been turned upside down. Your presence offers peace and comfort. Your presence connects the griever to the world. Connection is needed more than ever.

Through reflection we develop presence and poise to be present when shaken by the experience. Through reflection we learn to tune into and flow with the other along often tempestuous wavelengths, with the appropriate level of involvement within the moment even when the patient or family rejects involvement or demands an inappropriate level of involvement. We learn to appreciate the person's pattern. Resistance may also be felt within the practitioner – that something about this person or family brings a negative attitude or prejudice to the surface and triggers rejection. The mindful practitioner senses and reflects on the rejection and responds appropriately.

The practitioner does not set out to 'fix it' for the other person, but to work with the person to help them find meaning in the experience. As many of the stories illustrate, flowing with another in their suffering is not easy work, it is not comfortable. Yet within a caring relationship caring is reciprocated where the practitioner can express her own humanness. Where caring is reciprocated, the patient or family can care for the nurse – it is a dwelling together along an uncertain path. This reciprocation is inevitable and must be expected and welcomed because in being cared for, the other person has a need to give something back.

And this practice can only be learnt through experience and sustained guided reflection.

Simon shared his story in a small guided reflection group consisting of six other practitioners and a guide. The group had been together for several weeks and had developed a strong bond of trust that made it safe for Simon to reveal such deep aspects of self. Simon had not met any of the other practitioners in the group prior to its commencement and the guide was not from his organisation. It is the positive aspect of the 'confessional' – an opportunity to unburden and cleanse self. Sharing his story enabled others in the group to relate with similar stories. As you might imagine, it was very cathartic yet through the suffering caring was valued. The whole group felt reconnected to caring. Simon had shifted his energy from dwelling on his suffering to celebrating his caring. Profound energy work. He made the point that he had never been 'taught' how to use himself in a therapeutic way or to deal with feelings that such work evoked. Such revelation gives support to James's (1989) observation that *emotional labour* is generally unrecognised, viewed as unskilled and as such, not taught. Yet Simon's narrative reveals that such work is the he(art) of holistic practice.

The narrative itself is beautifully crafted. It blends emotions and reasoning. I image that few practitioners will not feel the emotion and transformation within and between the words. They will inevitably reflect on their own feelings and practice with dying patients and their families when next at work. The narrative is a powerful 'call to action' when caring on medical wards is threatened by diminishing resources. Initiatives such as the Liverpool Care Pathway are helpful to draw attention to dying patients but I suspect that they become little more than checklists. On the palliative care degree, we read and explore how such stories as Simon's can impact on our practice and require the practitioners to write their own reflective accounts. Powerful medicine.

Chapter 11

Clare Coward: life begins at 40

It was Pitkin (1932) who coined the phrase 'life begins at 40' and how right he was. On Thursday 2 October 2003 I attended the first session of the Becoming a reflective and effective practitioner course. It also happened to be my 40th birthday and when my life as a reflective practitioner was to begin although at that point in time I could not have envisaged the significant impact and influence the course would have on me.

What follows is the story of my journey of endeavouring to become a reflective and effective practitioner, how my practice has developed as a result and what factors have constrained this process. This will be illustrated through a series of unfolding experiences using entries from my reflective journal which, when viewed alone, are perhaps not of great significance or worth. However, like a children's dot-to-dot picture, it is only when the dots are joined together that a tangible picture becomes clear.

At the beginning of the course I recorded my feelings and thoughts at the end of the day on a separate piece of paper in my journal. I felt I was reflecting. This made me question why I needed to be on an 8-month course to do this. It was only when I began to share my experiences within the group that I realised that all I was doing was stating what had happened and how I had felt. It was when I was challenged and *forced* to examine my feelings and view the situation from different perspectives that I started to learn from my experiences. However, it still took some weeks and a comment from Chris, the course tutor, who informed me that 'an effective practitioner is an informed practitioner', for me to ashamedly acknowledge to my self that knowledge acquisition does not happen magically but does in fact require a degree of effort on my part.

ECGs

Within my current practice, one of my clinical responsibilities is to perform electrocardiographs (ECG) for all the inpatient units of the hospital. Initially I found this interesting. However, once the novelty had worn off I viewed it as a task that had to be done. My lack of enthusiasm was quite evident in my journal entries until one day following an attempt to perform an ECG, my journal entry was very different:

When I arrived on the ward I was shown in to the lady's bedroom. I introduced myself and started to explain the procedure; the nurse interrupted me; stating that I was wasting my time: 'she doesn't understand a word you are saying, she has dementia'. My anger levels rose but I carried on, trying not to let my feelings show. The lady looked at me with watery pale blue eyes and, speaking in a language of her own, was trying to tell me something but I was unable to understand her; she kept tugging at my arm, getting more frustrated with tears falling down her cheeks. I reassured her that I would not be performing the ECG and left the ward. The image of her eyes stayed with me; had they once been sparkling deep blue, full of life, and what had those eyes seen in their 82 years of existence? I felt disgust with the nurse for treating her with disparagement and disrespect but I also had to acknowledge the uncomfortable feelings within myself about my view of performing an ECG as a tedious task and had appreciated the privilege of entering into this intimate relationship ...

The impact this experience had on me was immense; it forced me to examine my attitudes, beliefs and focus my thoughts upon the nurse–patient relationship, especially the challenges faced when the patients' ability to communicate is compromised.

What sense do I make of this? Morse (1991) states that the nurse–patient relationship is established as 'the result of interplay or covert negotiations until a mutually satisfying relationship is reached'. She discusses the types of relationships that exist and divides them into two categories: mutual or unilateral. The latter she describes as being asynchronous, with one person unwilling or unable to develop the relationship to the desired level of the other. Morse (1991) provides an example of why mutual involvement is not possible, that is when a patient is unconscious or in a psychotic state. The fact that the lady with blue eyes was suffering from dementia automatically forced her into a unilateral relationship.

Rao (1993) believes the act of communication comprises all of the ways that people send and receive messages. However, Miller (2002) draws to our attention that most people do not think about the way they communicate on a day-to-day basis and are often unaware of how they relate to others yet communication is essential to our development as social beings and it is the ability to communicate that enables the development of short- and long-term relationships. What happens then if the ability to communicate becomes impaired? Bush (2003) suggests that people who cannot communicate or who communicate inappropriately are often marginalized by society and run the risk of social alienation and diminished function and that as a result of the frustration of being unable to make needs and feelings understood by others, challenging behaviour and behavioural disturbances can occur. It has been proposed by Lliffe and Drennan (2001) that communication with the patient suffering from dementia may be the key to understanding and resolving behaviour disturbances. One method of communicating with people with dementia is validation therapy. This was developed by Feil (1993) and attempts to help the person deal with their feelings by validating them, subsequently helping them to move from their inner world to the shared reality of the present. It is claimed that validation therapy promotes communication with the severely confused older person on their own terms, on subjects and issues that are chosen by and are important to them. In validation therapy it is assumed that all the words and actions of a person with dementia have a real sense of purpose and value.

Picking up the story, as a consequence of confronting and examining my feelings, my attitude towards performing ECGs altered. I no longer viewed it just a task that had to be done as quickly as possible but recognised that although only brief, I was engaging in a relationship with another person which should be given time and respect. Having shifted my viewpoint, I found that once again I found performing ECGs a positive experience. I was mindful of this when I received an ECG request from one of the wards that specialises in treating elderly people who are more severely confused, suffering from dementia or other organic brain disorders. The name on the ECG request seemed vaguely familiar; however, I was not prepared for the shock when I was introduced to the lady. Sitting slumped to one side with saliva dribbling out of the corner of her mouth was a lady with whom I had contact about a year ago when she received a course of electroconvulsive therapy (ECT) to which she responded well. My last memory of her was of a bright, smiling, physically fit lady in her 50s who was able to return to her work, which incidentally was as a healthcare assistant on one of the other elderly wards. This is an extract from my journal entry for that day.

> When I first saw her the shock was immense, like a jolt of electricity had surged through my body, causing my skin to prickle and take a sharp intake of breath. It took me a moment to recover. What message had my face portrayed and had she seen it? How lonely must it be to be trapped inside a body unable to communicate verbally and how must it feel to be reliant upon nurses, with whom you had once worked, to feed, wash and dress you … what is it about this situation that I find so uncomfortable? I perform ECGs on other patients who are unable to communicate verbally and do not feel the same. Perhaps the sadness I feel is that she is too young to be treated on an elderly mental health ward and that her own profession has in some way let her down …

I remembered Chris had recommended an article about silent advocacy (Gadow 1980) and I set about finding it. However, it was then that I started to question my motives for doing this. Was it that being more informed about a situation helps me to become a more effective practitioner or was it to help me resolve my uncomfortable feelings and feel better in myself?

It was this conflict that I shared with the group at the next session. I began by sharing the experience and discussing the conflicts I faced, which was helpful. The focus of the discussion wandered slightly with issues around communicating with patients with communication difficulties examined. One of the group members made a comment about how some nurses, without realising it, treated people as an object and lost sight of the person and challenged me on one aspect of my practice ECT. I was defensive and categorically stated that within the ECT department people were treated with respect, dignity and as individuals.

This comment niggled away at me. During the next two ECT sessions I metaphorically took a step back and observed with more critical eyes how we regarded and treated the patients receiving ECT. I was reassured that the mental health nursing team did show respect for the patient, taking time to explain procedures and provide reassurance, although once the patient was asleep the focus of them as a person was lost. One thing that struck me was the amount of people that are present during treatment; on that day seven people, including the patient, were present in the treatment room (Fig. 11.1). Conversations took place that excluded the patient.

In the next team meeting I shared this experience and my observations and in order to generate discussion. I posed some questions. How would you like to be treated if you were to receive ECT, what aspects of our practice are positive and what areas could we improve upon?

In order to gain a better understanding, I suggested we recreated the scenario as fully as possible to experience first hand being on the trolley with people attaching various

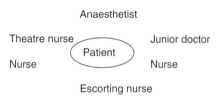

Figure 11.1 People in the treatment room.

monitoring equipment to you. Benner (2003) highlights that good nursing practice requires ongoing clinical knowledge development through experiential learning. However, it is not automatic and requires openness, attentiveness and responsible engaged learning on the part of the practitioner. One of the team members was not a willing participant at first but did join in and at the end of the session commented that she had never thought about it from the patient's point of view.

We discussed this exercise within the next team meeting. We all felt it was worthwhile and that it gave us a better understanding of how the patient feels before they are anaesthetised. What struck us all was how vulnerable and intimidating it felt lying on the trolley with so many people surrounding you. From this we considered ways we could improve our practice, limiting the amount of people surrounding the patient until they are asleep, encouraging the doctors to have discussions about treatment regimes out of earshot of the patients and instead of having the radio on play more soothing and relaxing music. This exercise was only carried out with the mental health nursing staff, who felt it would be beneficial for the whole treatment team to undergo this, particularly with the theatre nurse and the anaesthetist who by the nature of their work spend the majority of the time with unconscious patients. As Morse (1991) highlights, nurses working in operating rooms use a strategy of depersonalisation which includes transforming not only the person into a patient but also the patient into a case.

According to Sisson (1990), hearing is the last sense to go when a person becomes unconscious. Studies of patients' memories of their unconscious state indicate that they heard and understood various conversations that took place while they were unconscious (Lawrence 1995, Podurgiel, 1990 Tosch, 1988). It is imperative, as Leigh (2001) points out, that health professionals evaluate the way in which they communicate with unconscious patients. Russell's (1999) study concludes that hospitals are often noisy, which can make the patient anxious, whereas reassurance and explanations by nurses help them to feel safe, secure and feel less vulnerable. This study also found that where nurses became overinvolved with technical equipment and the physical aspects of care, this reduced the level of communication with the patient. While Podurgiel (1990) and Green (1996) both recommend that personalised care should be given through the use of effective communication strategies such as speaking directly to the patient and using touch to enhance communication and express emotional support, Dyer (1995) cautions that touch is a two-way process and permission should be sought before a nurse invades a patient's personal space.

At the end of an ECT session I shared our experiential experience with the theatre nurse, hoping that she would be receptive to the idea of participating in a similar exercise with the anaesthetist. 'Whatever did you want to do a thing like that for?' was her reply. I attempted to explain that I felt it was important to view the care we gave from the patients' perspective. 'What a load of poppycock, how do they know what they need,

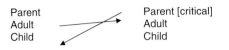

Figure 11.2 Transactional analysis: crossed transaction.

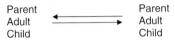

Figure 11.3 Parallel transaction.

we are the anaesthesiology specialists not them, so how can they possibly know what they need and I certainly do not need to lay on a theatre trolley to know how to do my job.' She left the department with very ruffled feathers and I felt irritated and disappointed as this extract from my journal entry shows.

> My emotions are all in a muddle like a big ball of spaghetti lying heavy and uncomfortably in the pit of my stomach. I have experienced these feelings before; when I was a child in primary school there was one particular teacher who no matter how hard I tried to please and gain her approval she always knocked me back, leaving me feeling angry and frustrated and confused. Only now I am not a schoolgirl, I am a professional practitioner and believe in what I am trying to achieve. Why do I always let her get to me? Why do I feel intimidated by her and unable to assert myself with her when I can with other people?

I connected this experience to another that I had shared with the group about the difficulties I had experienced with a junior doctor who was constantly late and on one occasion did not show up at all. Chris, in his ubiquitous coaxing manner, asked how I felt about the doctor and how I had asserted myself, which at the time I had felt no hesitation in letting the doctor know my feelings. Chris then introduced me to the idea of collaboratively working with the doctor to improve things. Using transactional analysis (TA) (Berne 1961) to examine the pattern of communication between myself and the theatre nurse, I discovered where the breakdown of communication lay. The response from the theatre nurse was not the adult response I had invited; instead she moved into a critical parent state and her response invited me to move out of my adult and into my child (Fig. 11.2).

Stewart and Joines (1987) describe this as a crossed transaction, so called because the vectors of the diagram usually cross. Also *cross* is an apt description of how I felt in this exchange. For a transaction to be complementary, the vectors of the diagram have to be parallel, what is often described as a parallel transaction.

Looking again at how I communicate with the theatre nurse, it became evident that I often revert into 'child mode' in response to her 'critical parent mode'.

Examining the communication patterns between the theatre nurse and myself was illuminating and challenging. That encouraged me to examine my patterns of communication with other members of the team and establish if they are parallel or crossed. By having a heightened awareness of these communication processes, hopefully this will empower me to shift the pattern to become more effective and promote collaborative working.

Vision, what vision?

One of the workshops on the reflective practice course was about being reflective in everyday practice, in which Chris provided an example of a philosophy that had been constructed through reflection. This was a sharp wake-up call. I recalled that the department had its own philosophy but if I was challenged as to its contents I would have failed miserably. Once back in the department I eventually found the operational policy buried away in a filing cabinet. Included in its contents is the department's philosophy of care; however, it did not state who had devised it and when. I asked one of my colleagues who had worked in the department for many years as to the origin and author of the philosophy; she looked at me blankly and said 'I am sorry, I did not know we had one, duck'.

In my next management supervision I raised this issue with my manager who also was ignorant of these facts but thought it might have been based upon the acute services philosophy. I compared the department's philosophy with one of the acute inpatient wards, only to discover that it was exactly the same. Johns (2000) draws attention to the difficulties caused by having an imported philosophy imposed on a practice; it denies articulation of the practitioner's own beliefs and values and is easily forgotten. What then is the point in having a generic philosophy devised by someone else, locked away in a filing cabinet? None whatsoever.

Reflecting upon this, I established that the team believes that we provide a high standard of individualised care for patients within the department. However, we lack evidence to validate this. By not having a philosophy of care that had been constructed on our collective beliefs and objectives of our practice, how do we know where we are going and the rationale for the journey?

> One day Alice came to a fork in the road and saw a Cheshire cat in a tree. 'Which road do I take?' She asked. 'Where do you want to go?' was his response. 'I don't know,' Alice answered. 'Then,' said the cat, 'it doesn't matter.' (Carroll 1988:26)

This is my journey so far as a reflective practitioner, and like many journeys obstacles have had to be negotiated and choices to be made, which have been tested and disputed. Although my voyage is still within its formative years I realise that having embarked upon it changes have occurred within me and even if I could return back to the beginning I could not disengage with these changes.

One of the biggest factors that hindered my development of becoming an effective practitioner was myself. At the beginning of my journey my attitude was arrogant and the reasons for attending the course were influenced by the 60 level 3 credits that could be obtained. Although I consistently kept a reflective journal my entries were descriptive, inexpressive and once written were not returned to. I am not sure when exactly my transformation happened as it was a gradual process. However, I remember feeling uncomfortable when other members of the group shared their journal entries. The words of a teacher who taught spelling came back to me; he said 'If you cheat you are only deceiving yourself and it will be you who has to face the consequences'. I felt like an impostor and my atheism would be exposed at any minute.

One of the ways I overcame this was by reading some of the recommended literature, which up until that point had sat unopened on my desk. I found Johns' (2000, 2002) work inspired and motivated me. Reading narratives from everyday clinical practice helped me to develop and learn through my own reflections. This development of self-awareness was a key issue in me advancing as a reflective practitioner. Self-awareness, as identified by Atkins and Murphy (1995), is an essential activity in reflection. It not only enables a person to recognise their beliefs and values but facilitates analysis of feelings and behaviour and how these can affect the behaviour of others.

My journey has also been lonely at times, having undergone a complete transformation of my attitude and realised the power that reflection has to change and improve practice. I wanted to share this enlightenment and sought after converting my colleagues to my newfound faith. However, in my passionate and overzealous approach what I in fact achieved was to alienate my colleagues, not bring them on board. I realised that in order for me to have any influence then a drastic modification of my approach was needed.

There were times on this journey that I became exhausted and on occasions I wished that I could remove my reflective lenses and view things with my old eyes. Reflecting daily on my practice was constantly highlighting areas that need modification or change. I could see my focus was on problems and that I was ignoring the positive aspects of my practice. Perhaps that is inevitable.

Has attending this course helped me to become an effective practitioner? The answer is unequivocally yes. Although I am a novice in the world of reflection, I realise the potential reflective practice has on shaping the future of our profession. Reflection on action can provide us with a route whereby we can begin to value our practical expertise as a profession (Bulman 2004). In a relatively short period of time I have undergone a revolution of myself as a practitioner. For me one of the immense values of this course was that the process of reflection was guided. Being in reflective group help me to remain focused and motivated me to continue on my journey. If my reflective journey had not been guided, then I feel it may well have been more of a magical mystery tour.

Commentary

Many practitioners, like Clare, are initially resistant to the idea of reflective practice. She had the idea that reflection was just writing things on a bit of paper. I am sure many practitioners feel this way, especially if they are just asked to write and do not have the opportunity to share their writings in expertly guided sessions. The insight is that reflection needs to be dedicated and guided. When Clare broke through her resistance to experience the transformational potential of reflection, it was a revelation.

Chapter 12

Jim Jones: balancing the wind or a lot of hot air

Jim writes

> If you take the Christian bible and put it in the wind and rain, soon the paper on which the words are printed will disintegrate and the words are gone. Our bible is the wind. (Anon, Native American)

I intend for you to join me on my journey towards becoming a reflective practitioner. The journey has been exciting, challenging and cathartic, as I have travelled, nomadically through theory and practice in an attempt to regain the vision I once had as a fresh-faced nursing student. My ideals and visions clouded over by the bureaucracy and politics which is mental health nursing.

Sharing of my experiences in guided reflection group sessions has enabled me to accept the challenge of the first few steps of my journey. Have I achieved the outcomes that will allow me to wear a hat with tassels? The proof is in the reading.

First I must ask myself – What is reflection? How does it fit within modern nursing practice? Indeed, does it have a place at all? Johns (2004a) states:

> Reflection is being mindful of self, either within or after an experience, as if a window through which the practitioner can view and focus self within the context of a particular experience, in order to confront, understand and move towards resolving contradiction between one's vision and actual practice. Through the conflict of contradiction, the commitment to realise one's vision, and understanding why things are as they are, the practitioner can gain insight into self and be empowered to respond more congruently in future situations within a reflexive spiral towards realising one's vision as a lived reality.

If so, then reflection is looking, but not at what you see, more at what you do not see, that which is not obvious, that which lies within.

Reflection has its critics. Mackintosh (1998) argues it is flawed and a passing fad which will be replaced by another. However, I come to praise Caesar not to bury him. I will attempt to show the reader how reflection has enabled me to develop my practice. I understand and fully acknowledge that had I been studying advanced needle-point there is a possibility that I would now be advocating its usage within nursing as a comple-mentary therapy. I can only let you know what is true for me. I do know that without guidance I would still be sinking in Schön's (1987) metaphoric swampy lowlands. I have become a more effective nurse, a positive practitioner, a more caring person and, to cap it all, a jasmine tea drinker!

My patient, Mary, has given me permission to talk about her in this narrative. There is no happy or sad conclusion for her. This narrative is merely my quest to find some answers to life's complicated questions for the sake of Mary and all the Marys I have yet to meet. As Mary says, 'Life is not like the movies … maybe there will be a sequel'.

Names have been changed to protect the innocent or guilty.

Mary

The sun filters through the patio windows. Wogan in the background prattling on about this and that (have I really become a tog?). Strange! Radio 2: who would ever have that on at 07.30 in the morning? Wogan plays 'White man in Hammersmith Palais' by The Clash. As Joe Strummer sings, my mind wanders back to the late 70s when, as a pimply faced youth with freshly bleached spiky hair, I wandered down the King's Road in London, deaf, hoarse and exhilarated having just seen The Clash perform at the Hammersmith Palais.

Inspired, Terry Wogan turned off, I place my 'Best of the Clash' record on the turntable, pump up the volume as much as acceptable. A 'fluffy moment', the iron in front of me, I set it on 'linen' and prepare to press my suit – Matalan, £40, navy blue, wash 'n' wear. I bought it when I commenced as acting ward manager on an older person's ward for mental health. I am due to take the lead in a multidisciplinary team meeting later this morning. I feel I need to make a good impression. My insecurity bites.

Twenty-five years from the release of The Clash; from safety pins in ears, bondage trousers and leather jacket to a £40 Matalan suit. Have I really become the establishment? A different uniform for a different time, but what of the uniform of the mind? Have I changed that much inside and if so, how did it sneak up on me without me even knowing? Can I find me again within a job I love yet still be accepted by my peers and fight for the right of patients?

Mary has been known to the mental health services for about 5 years. She saw her nephew who she raised murdered by another member of the family. Her own mother had died when Mary was with relatives in New York. During her time there she had been trapped on a burning train whilst riding the subway. The clinical diagnosis – post-traumatic stress and psychotic depression. Physically this manifests as chronic facial pain. Many treatments had been tried: dentist, analgesia, X-rays, referrals to pain clinic, ECT, none of which has had a satisfactory outcome for Mary. On two of her many admissions, whilst on leave, Mary had succumbed in desperation to overdosing her prescribed medication. As a consequence she was placed under Section 3 of the Mental Health Act that allows the authorities to detain her in hospital for 6 months.

This resulted in her being nursed on a high level of observation, granting me the opportunity as her key worker to engage with Mary in plenty of conversation. I knew her and she trusted me. Therefore, negative comments such as 'She's putting it on', 'It's all in her mind', 'She's not helping herself' and 'She's attention seeking' that are flippantly bandied around by my fellow professionals give offence (the right hump!). As Mary's key worker, I could argue that I knew more about what makes her tick than other members of the multidisciplinary team (MDT). At the meeting today I need to get 'our' point of view across and advocate her needs.

My trusty suit may just assist in this process; I would be in a room full of 'suits', being 'one of them'. Playing the game – the game identified by Stein (1978). The object of the game is for the nurse to be bold, intuitive, and be responsible for making significant recommendations whilst, at the same time, appearing passive so that it appears that the doctor made the decision. The game is designed to preserve the doctor's authority. The reward for the nurse is the doctor's patronage. Failure to play is 'hell to pay'. Through reflection, I have become more mindful of this game and my part within it, becoming better able to express my opinions without being passive or subordinate. The game sucks. It insults my self-respect to play it. Yet I play it ... I play it because I fear the consequences of not playing it, not so much for myself, as I admire my freshly ironed suit, but for the Marys.

The referral to the pain clinic by the SHO (senior house officer) has been overlooked. Everyone had assumed this had been done. Frustration went from simmer to boiling, anger vented at the nursing team. Hackles on the back of my neck start to rise. It was the doctor's responsibility, why should we have to chase after them? The doctors close ranks – the finger of blame pointed towards myself. They are trying to put me in my place.

I feel the tension as I struggle to stay in the right place to advocate for Mary and for myself. My collar is too tight. My integrity hung out to dry! Dear reader – you may think that as an old punk rocker I would relish 'hell to pay' but there is something very sinister about the way nurses are oppressed. Maybe if I was wearing bondage trousers I could have overthrown the establishment. Perhaps it is 'the suit' that keeps me in place.

Benner (1984) argues that in the initial stages of learning we are acutely aware of what we are doing and our failings. I would liken this to being consciously incompetent, knowing that you are struggling with something, and the frustrations that ensue. In not knowing how to deal with something it is always best having one's arsenal, somebody or something to aid me. My arsenal was a battery of reflective tools and guidance within the guided reflection sessions. But most of all was being open and honest with myself – as I have always endeavoured to be with patients like Mary. No longer hiding behind my 'funny man' posture and cropped shock of bleached hair. No longer trivialising academic effort. I had to grow up and take responsibility for myself, supported by a cup of jasmine tea at the ceremonious tea party that infuses each guided reflection session and a glass or two of beloved Stella Artois to shift the blockages when reflection becomes stuck.

Mary's family mysteriously appear for 15 minutes on pension day. They had agreed at an early family meeting to pay Mary's bills whilst she was undergoing her healing process. Several months later Mary was £750 in arrears with her rent and utility bills – yet more stressors adding to her distress and depressive state. She was unwilling or unable to challenge her family. Should I intervene on her behalf? If so how?

Using 'ethical mapping' (Johns 2004a) to weigh up where everybody involved in this situation is coming from and ethical principles, I conclude I should act but not directly. I contacted Age Concern who offer an advocacy service. This action was paternalistic – acting on behalf of Mary when she was being harmed and was unable to act for herself. Benjamin and Curtis (1986) set out three factors that must be justified to warrant therapeutic parentalism.

- Harm – Mary was being harmed.
- Autonomy – Mary was unable to make decisions or act on her own behalf.
- Ratification – my judgement that Mary would thank me for my actions when she was able to.

My decision to contact Age Concern further met my agenda of avoiding coming into the muddy waters of conflict with Mary's family. Was I too close to the situation, emotionally entangled and losing my objectivity? It's tough to sit by and watch helpless people be abused.

Writing in my journal as this situation played itself out enabled me to freeze the moment and view it more objectively from different angles, digesting and dissecting it, bringing the experience back into focus, surfacing and working through my mixed emotions of anger towards the family, sadness and pity towards Mary, and residual feelings of anger at my colleagues. All stuff bubbling away inside my body cauldron. It's hot in there ... what was that about getting out of the kitchen if you can't stand the heat?

This is not the language I would use when at work. It (the journal) does not judge, criticise or threaten to use my words against me at a later date. Holly (1989) believes keeping a journal enables development of an educational archive, to aid insight and enrichment in future practice. Ferruci (1982) argues that journal writing stimulates the 'interchange between the conscious and the unconscious' – how true I have found that to be. Burrows (1995) thinks journals are too time consuming. Burnard (1995) thinks that they are too superficial. I wonder if they keep journals. My journal allows me to express my anger, thereby diffusing it, allowing me space to deal with events in a more reasonable and professional way. Do I mean professional? Let it go. Johny Rotten once sang about anger being an energy ... I channel my energy, using it as momentum to press forward to finding a positive outcome for Mary. I don't like feeling angry – for others would then perceive me as unprofessional (buying into an idea that professionals are impassive or are good at wearing masks to deceive). Buddha states that anger will never disappear so long as there are thoughts of resentment. I sense my residual resentment at the consultant for not hearing me and at the relatives for abusing Mary and ... and the list goes on. Anger and resentment are self-harming. As one American chat show host said, 'Remember, when you point the finger at another in anger, you have three fingers pointing back at you'. Wish I could remember his name.

I write in my journal: 'They [the family] don't give a damn about Mary, they are fleec-ing her blind. I need to be more assertive and shed my fear of conflict'. Reading this out in the guided reflection session, I feel embarrassed as if I am some kind of failure. The punk rocker brought to his knees. Exposed as a fraud. Yet the group are amazingly sup-portive. They all recognise the conflict avoider in themselves, giving credence to research (Cavanagh 1991) that conflict avoidance was the primary mode of being for nurses and nurse managers. What are we frightened of? Why are we so willing to ditch the patient to ensure peace with the relatives and patronage of doctors? Surely dialogue is a better way, being open and honest or, as Chris says, being tough on the issues and soft on the people.

Chris talks me through the assertive action ladder to see at what level my blocks are (see Fig. 7.8). I can see I am blocked at rungs 3 and 4 – lacking confidence in my author-ity vís a vís others, and with making a good argument, at least in language that is heard. I can see my weaknesses at each rung. It's not easy being assertive in a power-driven hierarchy.

I digress. Getting back to the meeting. During a break for coffee and a smoke, as these meetings last several hours, my mobile phone rings. Elvis Costello ring tone, 'Every day I write the book' seems a fitting tune ... it's my Mum. 'Dad has been to see the urologist, it's his prostate ... they want him to have more tests.' Sensing her concerns, I say 'Sorry mum, I'm at a meeting, ring you later'.

CANCER – the very thought burns into my being. I need time to take stock. Ethical dilemma – my father's medical records are confidential yet I can gain access. He will have to wait a fortnight for his results but, at the push of a few buttons on the computer, I can get them tomorrow. I contact Dawn, the specialist urology nurse. She has assisted me in the past with clients on my ward. She listens, explains possible treatments, gives me statistics: 60% plus of all men in my father's age range – 70 plus – have prostate cancer and are blissfully unaware of the situation. It's slow growing. Reassuringly she says, 'He will probably die of something else before the cancer gets him'. Dawn never pulls her punches – again honesty. Maybe the moral or insight of this story. We arrange to meet later in the week.

The urology team are now aware that the man under their care is my dad, not just another patient. At least I feel I have done something for now. I also share this dilemma at the guided reflection session. Waterworth (1995) argues that such workshops allow nothing more than a forum for expressing negativity. In my experience this is not so. The session supports and guides and nurtures creativity. So stick that in your pipe! Of course, Chris would argue 'Where is Waterworth coming from, what is the basis for her claim?'. And it's true, I partially read stuff and draw hasty conclusions. Stick that in my pipe!

Back at the meeting, the consultant is advocating further use of ECT to raise Mary's mood. He argues that the Mary's (psychosomatic) facial pain will be addressed. I chirp up: 'What about stronger pain killers?'. 'I'm not prescribing anything else until the consultant pain specialist has seen her.' I tap my fingers in frustration. More delay. My eyes burn into the SHO. He avoids my gaze – I smell his guilt.

Cut to several weeks later. Mary has been having two ECT sessions per week. No change in her facial pain, little positive change in affect. Still no word from the consultant in pain. The wheels of the NHS turn so slowly. My frustration increases. The ends of my fingers will soon be worn thin.

Friday I set up the ECT on my ward. The anaesthetists are on rotation. I check the list. Dr Zaphon. Something jolts my attention. A 5-minute check on the computer. Yes! Yes! Dr Zaphon is the consultant in pain specialist, the one and only Scarlet Pimpernel (they seek him here, etc.) and he is walking right into my sticky web! By pure chance, destiny, good luck, say what you will, I have the opportunity to affect change and move Mary up his waiting list. Imagine the scenario: 'Good morning Dr Zaphon, would you like a cup of tea?'. Learnt behaviour. Hitler is raining bombs around my patient's head yet still the English make a cup of tea.

I sensed the challenge that awaited me as he came with a formidable reputation – 'I am the Boss and what I say goes'. Be careful, Jim, he is a right one for putting people down and making complaint if you cross him – so say my pals from theatres. Little room for manoeuvre. I imagine the scenario: 'Dr Zaphon, while you are here can I please draw your attention to a referral we made some months ago (suitable fawning posture)? His face like thunder, assuming the stance of the critical parent. I do not wish to be perceived as pushy, must remember the game. I can't simply change the rules and expect him to be different. It would only lead to conflict as we cross vectors of communication.

Through the thick veil of self-concern I see Mary and remind myself – what do we do our jobs for? So sorry if my patient gets in the way of a smooth day at the office.

I mentioned Mary and got short change. A curt response: 'I'm not wearing my pain hat, here to do ECT ... focus on the task ahead'. He is giving me the right hump, again trying to put the little nurse in his place. But the old Jim is still there – a voice in my head says 'focus the anger', reflecting in the moment, drawing upon the assertive action ladder, playing the game, acknowledge the doctor's position, back to the job in hand.

Part of the ECT procedure is to give the doctor a brief history of the patient prior to treatment. Adjust the tie, make good eye contact, positive stance (show your professionalism, Jim, blind him with your personality). Back and forward from controlled self, pushy and yielding, finding the balance, being adult, not being put into child mode. Anticipating the situation gave me the chance for my scheming self to come to the fore. What better optimum conditions to maximise my effectiveness would I ever get? My vision was focused. I understood intuitively the boundaries and my authority within the game. I had the right to assert myself on behalf of Mary. I felt empowered and by being coercive, maybe I could just make him listen. So much for my ruminations – what about the real event?

The procedure went smoothly. I like to create a positive atmosphere for clients and staff alike but this morning I had to use more coercive tactics or, in other words, to be sneaky. Dr Zaphon likes traditional jazz music. I had found this out earlier from Geoff from the anaesthetic team when jazz pianist legend Oscar Peterson was on the stereo.

Whilst Mary was being recovered and I was thanking the team, I turned the conversation to the choice of music. I mentioned that my father had once met Oscar Peterson at a showcase in the mid 1970s. Dr Zaphon's eyes lit up. I spoke about this experience and mentioned that my dad had recently been seen by the urologist, casually mentioning the urologist by his first name, and saying how delighted my father was with the care he was receiving. Using the first name term of reference, I was aligning myself on first name terms with Dr Zaphon's peers. Levelling the playing field. Light banter and a second apology for confusing Dr Zaphon's remit this morning. The previous tense atmosphere is diffused.

Dr Zaphon had been on call the previous night; three emergency caesareans and a road traffic accident had contributed to his tetchiness. He said he would look into Mary's referral but made no promises, stating that he was a busy man and my client was just one of many. He would ask his secretary to arrange something.

Buddha's teachings come to mind: 'to utter pretty words without acting on them is like a fine flower without a fragrance'.

I felt better. I felt cleansed. I had used a newly acquired skill, an art form, and understood it. I had played the game skilfully and yet I had still played the game. Patterns of relating are deeply embodied and not easily shifted. But I feel stronger, the balance has shifted.

'Ring, ring' … 'Hello, older adults mental health, Jim here, how can I help you?' 'I am Dr Zaphon's secretary. I have an appointment for next Tuesday for Mary. Do you think you can make it also? You must have left an impression, he never changes his mind.' Will wonders never cease? Excuse me if I feel slightly smug.

Blackwolf and Jones (1996) say that 'Before we can help another we must first address our own bruises and in doing so become real, really become who they must be'. The truth of these words floods through me … as if for the first time. I cannot help Mary until I had helped myself. That is why we fail patients because we fail ourselves. Reflection is enlightening, empowering and ultimately transforming. If we remain stuck in oppressive patterns of relationship we simply cannot grow. Instead we fester and rot, stewing in our oppression and misery. I climb out of the box I was put in.

The suit has now been consigned to the charity shop. The bondage trousers, although not suitable for work, still make the odd week-end appearance, much to the annoyance of my partner. But without her support this journey would not have been possible. Better than safety pins to hold my trousers together. I have forgotten now who said that we are the sum of many parts, possibly something I read many moons ago whilst training to be a nurse. Bit like this narrative really, more than the sum of its parts when taken as a whole. At least I think so. I'm still learning, not just to play the game but to shape the game towards a better state of affairs for myself and my patients. A game that has its basis in values and integrity. I'm not always agreeing with points of views and climbing the ladder to work on that assertiveness thing. Demanding in dulcet tones my right to have a voice and be heard. Voltaire said: 'I may not like what you say but will defend to the death your right to say it'. Again I can't finger the source. Sorry Chris.

I still listen to The Clash but have to sit in the conservatory, but at least my partner now appreciates the lyrical delights of Elvis Costello. Her son is upstairs with a friend. 'Aaron, will you turn that bloody rubbish down!' Hip hop, what's that ball about then? Time to reflect. Intolerance to other views and arrogance that I am right are such destructive negative events. As I read back through this work I acknowledge all the assumptions I have made. I first wrote pseudo-assumptions but that is daft. Assumptions are assumptions although their basis may be questionable. But that's the point of reflection, to reveal assumptions and ask that question – what is their basis? And is that basis right?

Schön and his ilk came from disciplines outside my field of practice. Just because punk music and Native American ideology is not nursing, is it less relevant to inform our values and practice? Indeed I would argue that it adds flavour and new perspectives. So when Chris enthusiastically says 'look what I've found in Native American dancing philosophies' why should I doubt? Get out of the box for it is a coffin.

As I sit in my self-built Japanese tea house (roof structure ongoing … you can't rush these things), sipping jasmine tea (thanks Chris), I see baby blackbirds follow their mother, eager for the worms and insects – learning, growing, waiting for the chance to break free and fly from the nest. I too (when my belly is full of worms and juicy bugs) will find the right time and strength to make my own way in the nursing world, not held back by politics or traditions. I am getting there. Reflection has expanded my view of the world. My horizons are infinitely broader. I can breathe more fully. I am enriched through this process. Less bondage.

So back to Mary and my journey to ease her suffering.
'What about acupuncture? Is there a policy? How much would it cost? Would she (the object, not patient), who is taking up valuable time in the MDT meeting, accept it?'
'She has said to me on many occasions, she would try anything. She even stated to me that she regrets the offer from her parents to have all her teeth out for her 21st birthday – apparently that was commonplace for Scottish working class of her generation.'
'They will bring back foot binding next,' says some unhelpful wag.
I could not help but see the humour. To find humour in a negative situation has for me always been beneficial. It relieves tension, creates bonding and does not show up on the monthly fiscal deficit.

Commentary

Chapters 9–12 are all examples of reflective writing that reflect the practitioners' efforts to be more available to their patients. Reflective writing is a moral endeavour to that end that nurtures vision and commitment. As you compare these narratives, what comes to mind about the nature of reflection and narrative? Which do you prefer and why? Which ones are most convincing and reflexive?

In Part 3 I move into exploring the creative environment.

Part 3

Creating the reflective environment

Chapter 13

Reflective communication

Communication is vital. It is the collagen that holds practice together to ensure the patient and family receive consistent, continuous, congruous, compassionate and collaborative care within and across practice settings.

Using reflective techniques, the reflective practitioner communicates to ensure:

- continuity of care over time despite changes in personnel
- consistency of care between different care workers
- congruence of care between care workers in tune with shared vision and best practice
- that talk should always be compassionate, positive and affirming
- collaboration between care workers to ensure the above points.

Communication is both verbal, through language, and non-verbal, through body posture, senses and intonation. Communication is both formal and informal: formal verbal communication takes place through writing notes and reports, through shift reports, ward rounds and various care meetings that may include patients and families. Informal verbal communication takes place in the way practitioners relate to each other and with patients and families throughout the day: corridor conversations, passing remarks, the sluice room conference, coffee chat, etc. I am sure the reader can provide many euphemisms for such informal verbal meetings, all accompanied by a vast range of non-verbal communication that conveys positive and negative power messages.

Dialogue is the core of reflective communication. To reiterate, the significance of dialogue is opening a space in which we can listen to each other and work collaboratively towards realising a common vision without our own agendas and egos closing down the space, resolving conflicts and problems in its wake. Indeed, conflict, from a reflective perspective, is a learning opportunity. To dialogue effectively, the practitioner must first be mindful of self and her own mental models and assumptions and hold these in check in order to listen to the other's perspective and be open to what others have to say, loosening attachment to her own ideas so as to be open to possibility. Easier said than done but if we shared a vision to dialogue and developed dialogical skills then it is possible. Imagine the positive energy that would become available as a consequence! What a difference that might make to caring and the working environment.

Talk

The way practitioners talk with patients, families and with each other is a caring act. What we say is a reflection of our values. Therefore if I intend to be caring and compassionate and work in collaborative ways with my colleagues, you might expect my speech to reflect those values. Anything less would be a contradiction that the mindful practitioner would acknowledge and work towards resolving. Talk is both a process – an act in itself – and an outcome – it aims to achieve something. Hopefully it is both of these, but talk can also be uncaring; tongues can be sharp and venomous.

Reflective handover

Consider the way nurses talk to each other at shift reports. Just sit and listen – what messages do you get?

Traditionally, nursing has been communicated through an oral culture typified by the shift report. The function of the shift report is to communicate relevant information to ensure the smooth transition of care and responsibility to the next shift.

How is this done most effectively? The practitioner might say 'read the patient's notes' but would these be an adequate account? In my experience, notes rarely adequately reflect the patient's care or treatment patterns simply because of the shifting nature of treatment and care. If this was true then what is the purpose of written notes? Given the general inadequacy of written notes, the verbal report is probably the most significant form of communication to ensure continuity of care because it is traditional and more accurately captures the current patient status.

At the hospice, the new shift nurses gather in a room for the 'report' by nurses from the current shift. Conscious of confidentiality, the door is most often closed to prevent others overhearing what is disclosed. The nurse reports on the patients, with the patient notes in front of her to refer to if necessary, although this happens rarely. The emphasis is on the nurse reporting – the new shift nurses write notes of what is said on scraps of paper. Some exchange of views takes place but this is usually in the form of opinions rather than dialogue around decision making or care dilemmas. Nurses rarely express their personal feelings, especially if these feelings are problematic in some way. The report usually lasts for about 30–40 minutes, which for 10 patients is longer than most units give to this activity. Often the difficult patient is singled out as a health warning.

I have often discussed this format with the nurses involved, suggesting we might move to a more reflective format with a greater emphasis on dialogue, creating the opportunity for people to reflect on the way we think, feel and are responding to care issues around the patients and their families. Most practitioners agree this would be helpful but practice does not change, as if we are locked into a habit. Why do nurses write notes on scraps of paper when the patients' notes are available? In response I am told that 'it's handy' to have a list in the pocket rather than keep referring to the notes.

Writing such notes is a distraction from dialogue; indeed, it is a means of avoiding dialogue. I have challenged the senior nurses to role model dialogue by revealing their own thoughts and feelings and to challenge others to respond. A dialogical approach shifts the culture of the report from essentially information giving to reflection. This does not mean information will not be given – but the emphasis has changed. The notes can be read either before or after the report, and considered in light of the shift report dialogue. But old traditions die hard.

Bedside handover

Sitting around in a room discussing patient care can be challenged from a holistic perspective of involving the person and their family in their care (Ward 1988). Yet do patients want to be involved in decision making and taking responsibility for their health? A considerable literature emerged in the 1990s that explores the idea of patent participation in decision making (Ashworth *et al* 1992, Biley 1992, Jewell 1994, Trnobanski 1994, Waterworth and Luker 1990). Yet like many innovations in practice, the topic has seemingly faded from professional interest. Perhaps, like the hospice in which I work, they tried it and it didn't work. The idea was resisted, and ultimately rejected, because nurses did not feel comfortable with this shift in the pattern of communication and the constant threat to patient confidentiality by disclosing information in public areas or such was the excuse.

Working with and negotiating decision making is fundamentally an 'attitude' – whether patients are able to or want to be involved is another issue. For many reasons patients may resist taking responsibility for their own lives. The mindful practitioner appreciates this dynamic and judges whether to accept the other's dependency or confront it. However, if practitioners do value patient involvement in decision making, then it is incumbent on them to create space where this can happen. What better opportunity than the shift report rather than sitting in a closed room?

The approach to implementing bedside handover at Burford Hospital in 1990 was written as a protocol that involved visiting each patient before moving into 'the office' to complete the report. We anticipated that this approach would enable:

- the nurse to say hello and greet the patient (and family)
- the nurse to invite patients to reflect on their care and care decisions
- the patient to give their perspective first
- the nurses to make care values and processes more transparent
- the nurse to make better sense of information having seen and spoken with the patient beforehand.

The protocol emphasises the primacy of written notes as the means for continuing care, written as narratives (see below) rather than in nursing process format. We decided to store these notes with each patient simply because we viewed them as patient notes. The idea of patient-held records is well known in community settings, again reflecting the philosophy of working with the patient in terms of their health. This practice really challenged practitioners to become mindful of what they wrote, knowing that it might be read by the patient or the patient's family.

Confidentiality

The crux of appreciating confidentiality was to determine the meaning of 'public space' as set out in the UKCC Code of Professional Conduct on confidentiality (UKCC 1987). Shared ward areas are public spaces and hence the nurse could not say things about the patient or family without the patient's permission if others might overhear (Johns 1989). As such, any patients unwilling or unable to engage in the report were not talked about at the bedside. The nurse would cue the patient to self-disclose, for example 'how are

Standard statement – Patients do not have confidential information disclosed accidentally

Date .... Handover observed by ....

1	Patients are involved in the handover of their care	Yes So-so No
2	Patients control the disclosure of information concerning themselves	Yes So-so No
3	The nurses do not talk about the patient outside the patient's hearing	Yes So-so No
4	No accidental breach of confidentiality takes place	Yes So-so No
5	Patients' notes are not left open in a public space	Yes No
6	Ask each patient: 'Do you think your nurses have always treated what they know about your health/illness in a confidential manner?' (Sinha and Scherera 1987)	Yes So-so No

Score 3 for yes, 2 for so-so, 1 for no

Figure 13.1 Confidentiality scan sheet.

things this morning?', encouraging participation. In this way it was the patient who would disclose information about themselves. At least in principle.

One morning I observed the night associate nurse and primary nurse communicate at the bedside of one lady in the three-bed ward. They stood at the foot of the bed as the night nurse informed the primary nurse. The primary nurse was a little deaf and so the night associate nurse spoke loudly – loud enough for me to hear at the end of the ward and loud enough for the other two patients to hear what was being said. The woman in the bed was also deaf. She was sitting up trying to listen. However, she was not involved in the discussion. Clearly the protocol had failed and confidentiality had been breached.

We had a teaching session in which each nurse was talked about in public as per the observed incident. The staff's reaction was a revelation – they felt very uncomfortable. As a consequence we wrote a standard of care – 'Patients do not have confidential information disclosed about them accidentally'. (Constructing standards of care is explored in Chapter 14.)

We invited students to shadow the walkround handover and feed back their observation using the scan sheet in Figure 13.1 to ensure we both involved patients in the handover as appropriate and did not breach confidentiality. As you might expect, such scrutiny of practice helped staff to become more mindful of patient involvement and confidentiality. It was also an excellent learning experience for students.

From a holistic perspective, not to involve patients in the handover of their care was a contradiction that reduced them to objects of care rather than active participants in their own healthcare. Involvement may take more time and may create some risk of public disclosure, but it does lead to greater trust that more than offsets bureaucratic concern of risk: the constant tension between managing risk and being therapeutic. Unfortunately, organisations, wary of litigation, tend to lean heavily towards risk management even when risk is minimal.

Patient notes

In the first edition of this book I gave this section the heading 'The nursing process'. I like to think the nursing world has moved on just a little beyond the nursing process to more creative and reflective ways of thinking about and writing patient notes. For most practitioners since the late 1970s, the nursing process has dominated the approach to thinking and writing about patient care. Essentially the nursing process is a linear problem-solving approach that structures thinking through four stages.

- Goal setting – an interpretation of assessment in terms of identifying specific actual or potential problems/patient needs and goals to be achieved in responding to the problem/need.
- Planning – establishing the best response to solve the problem/need.
- Intervention – carrying out the planned care.
- Evaluation – determining whether the set goal has been met, including redefining the problem or goal as necessary in light of events.

The care plan is designed as a table consisting of these four columns. In theory, a practitioner should be able to pick up the care plan and continue the patient's care as a seamless activity. However, most aspects of care cannot be prescribed in advance, at least not without reducing the patient to an object to be manipulated. Some aspects of care may be more amenable to prescription, for example technical solutions to medical problems such as wound dressings and responses to pain and nausea. Yet these responses are better framed within a protocol based on evidence of best practice as guidelines to inform the mindful practitioner. Aspects of care concerned with the human–human encounter are almost impossible to prescribe given the uniqueness of each individual and each caring encounter.

The nursing process has attracted much adverse criticism (Howse and Bailey 1992, Latimer 1995, McElroy *et al* 1995, White 1993). Although the nursing process was intended to promote a culture of individualised and negotiated care (De La Cuesta 1983), ironically the opposite tended to happen when it was amalgamated with the prevailing nursing culture in the UK characterised by allegiance to the reductionist medical model. Rather than changing practice, the nursing process was accommodated to fit within this existing culture, resulting in a minimal or lip-service response to the ideology of individualised care (Latimer 1995). It is easy to see why, because the splitting up of the patient into problems mirrored the medical model. The nurse was now able to diagnose problems. The patient became a set of problems or needs (problems being viewed as too mechanistic) based on complex systems advocated within an accompanying array of nursing models. These models were almost exclusively from the USA. These models were theory driven and, as in the nature of any model, sought to find a comprehensive representation or conceptualisation of nursing.

The nursing diagnosis movement (NANDA) has been a natural development from the nursing process within the USA, yet in my view, it is a process fraught with difficulty because it imposes abstract meanings on 'nursing' concepts in the futile attempt to ensure consistency of diagnosis. In this respect this movement mirrors medicine's approach to diagnosis. Practitioners might find some common understanding of what a grade 4 glioma is, but can they find common meaning in using the words suffering, spirituality or agitation? Of course not. It is a positivist illusion to think otherwise.

So pause for a moment and ask yourself what individualised care means to you. Do patients' notes reflect the wholeness of care?

These are profound questions. Yet is it necessary to put the adjective 'individual' in front of care? How could care be anything other than individual? The opposite might be termed institutionalised care. Ray (1989) coined the expression 'bureaucratic caring' as a reflection of the way the individual might become obscured within the layers of bureaucracy. The human within the machine becomes a contradiction. As Wilber (1998) puts it, systems are the language of 'it' and 'it' is a stark colourless landscape of labels. The individual's cry can be difficult to hear amidst the din. To compensate, we need to say 'individualised' to remind ourselves that we care for unique human beings and that we carers too are unique human beings. We can only find meaning in the unfolding moment and respond with our humanness … humanness which is at risk of being buried beneath an avalanche of concepts and prescriptions. The nurse becomes a technician.

As practitioners begin to respond within a holistic perspective, they realise the nursing process is a contradiction, making little allowance for holistic and intuitive processes that are acknowledged as significant in the way experts make decisions about complex caring situations (Cioffi 1997). The Dreyfus and Dreyfus (1986) model of skill acquisition indicates that the expert practitioner intuitively makes clinical judgements based on grasping the whole situation. The model sets out five characteristics of intuitive judgement.

- Pattern recognition – perceptual ability to recognise relationships without pre-specifying the components of the situation.
- Similarity recognition – an amazing human ability to recognise 'fuzzy' resemblance despite marked differences.
- Common sense – a deep grasp of the language culture so that flexible understanding in diverse situations is possible.
- Skilled 'know how' – the practitioner can respond without resorting to rule-governed behaviours.
- Deliberate rationality – the expert practitioner has a web of different perspectives that causes them to view a situation in terms of past situations.

The inadequacy of the nursing process to guide patient care means that practitioners do not use it, or at least not in any meaningful way. Clearly communication systems need to be based on the way the expert practitioner thinks. Anything less will be absurd. Does a skilled carpenter choose a blunt spoon to chisel wood? Of course he doesn't – he chooses a sharpened chisel of the right width.

In an observational study of the impact of primary nursing on the culture of a community hospital (Johns 1989), one practitioner commented: 'Much of it is just nursing, you don't have to write that down'. This comment reflects the pattern recognition and common-sense knowing that this practitioner and her colleagues possessed, and their struggle to write down what was so obvious to them. Another practitioner commented: 'Patients we know well don't need care planning' – a comment that again reflects all elements of intuitive knowing.

I asked one staff nurse on her return from holiday if she had read her patients' care plans. She commented: 'I haven't had time because it's so busy'. This reinforces the comments above, symbolising the way the nurses on the unit did not use care plans as part of their daily planning. However, I sensed that this apparent intuitive knowing was not based on appreciating the patient's life pattern, but from knowing the patient in terms of the report given to the nurse at the shift report and normal routines. In other words, patients do not need care planning because we know them as a group of similar patients. This was reflected in the notes, that had a strong emphasis on medical and physical care issues with very little focus on emotional, psychological and spiritual aspects of care.

As one of the primary nurses said, 'When I deliberately change something on the care plan, I come back from my days off and it hasn't been carried out … is it because they disagree with what's been said or are they too busy to read the care plans?'. Other nurses countered this comment by saying they resented less experienced nurses telling them what to do or that they disagreed with what was written and therefore disregarded it, that is, if they had read it in the first place.

Completing patients' notes is often seen as a task to be done at the end of the shift. Practitioners recognise this task as generally meaningless and yet feel anxious about writing something, possibly motivated by an internal censor that if nothing is written, then care has not been carried out. The fear becomes reinforced when audit systems are constructed around the completion of patient notes. Hence, what is written tends to be descriptive rather than evaluative, and meaningless in terms of communicating the essential nature of continuing care. If the nursing process is meaningless then, as Batehup and Evans (1992) have challenged, 'Why do we keep this sacred cow?'.

The nursing process is an inadequate form of communication for the reflective practitioner because it does not represent how she views and responds to situations. It constrains thinking simply because practitioners no longer think that way. Most practitioners know this, yet have been unable to move beyond this deeply embodied worldview because the nursing process dominates the way nurses conceptualise their practice. Even when practitioners acknowledge the absurdity of the nursing process, they seem powerless to move to more meaningful and practical ways of communicating care.

So, what alternatives are there given that a holistic approach eschews any reductionist and deterministic approach to nursing practice, yet values the idea of best practice?

Narrative

At Burford hospital, given the inadequacy of the nursing process, practitioners embraced the idea of narrative as a more adequate form of communication in tune with the vision of reflective and holistic practice (see accounts by practitioners in *The Burford NDU model: caring in practice* edited by Johns 1994).

Practice is a reflexive narrative unfolding, reflexive meaning that when one looks back over the narrative, a concise account of patient care unfolds. As I have emphasised, the reflective practitioner tunes into the patient's wavelength and pays attention to what is unfolding – a constant process of appreciating the shifting patterns of the patient's experience. In noting the shifting pattern, the practitioner compares what is unfolding with what has gone before. Has the analgesia made a difference? Is Mrs Jones more restful? Is the wound healing? Is Alison better able to breast feed? Has the new bed for Mr Smith been delivered to his home? As such, assessment and evaluation are two sides of the same coin – what is unfolding now and what has happened before.

In writing, the reflective practitioner is mindful of being meaningful and pragmatic. Therefore, narrative should always be concise, reflective and evaluative, and capture the drama of the unfolding story.

Narrative intends to capture the unfolding experience of working with or journeying alongside the patient through their health–illness experience, illuminating the way care issues emerge and are responded to, guided by the Burford reflective cues (see p36). Writing a brief background story of who the patient is really helps to see the person in their humanness and not just as a disease object. This makes such a difference to perception, especially in hospices with their primary focus on symptom management. Facing death is not a collection of symptoms but a human being and family experiencing the most dramatic point of their life.

Remember, reflective cues are not concrete questions that require specific answers. They are merely prompts to guide the practitioner to tune into her thoughts and feelings. Hence if the patient makes me feel anxious I might acknowledge this: 'Sheila is very anxious. I acknowledged her anxiety and enabled her to surface and talk through her fears ...' My emotional reaction might be: Sheila's anxiety manifests itself as demanding and abusive. I may initially have felt abused and defensive as these darts of anxiety were fired at me but being mindful, I see my reaction is a defensive ego response. My skill is to see beyond my own concerns to tune into and appreciate the patient's perspective, as difficult as that might be sometimes. In other words, I write about what I have done with my concern rather than about the concern itself. I acknowledge the patient's feelings as valid and convert my anxiety into positive action, acknowledging that Sheila may be overwhelmed and bewildered by events and possibly angry at the way things have unfolded, especially when she faces a life-threatening illness and has experienced a lack of caring prior to transfer from another hospital.

Reg Simpson's narrative

In Reg Simpson's narrative, note the presence of each of the Burford reflective cues (see p36) and the way the cues (Fig. 13.2) have helped me weave the narrative. If you are used to filling in boxes (for example, as per the Roper *et al* model) then your natural inclination might be to respond to each reflective cue as a question to answer. That's fine as long as you are mindful of seeing the whole person. With time, as with all models of reflection, you internalise the cues and construct your own internal model that emerges as your narrative style.

Date	Narrative	Sig
6/11	Reg was admitted this morning for one week's respite care. He has been attending day care for the past 4 months (see attached notes). He is 93. He has cancer of the prostate gland with bony spread. He lives alone although his daughters live close by and provide support for him on an ongoing basis. However, as Reg says, he is not managing so well. He feels very tired and unco-ordinated. Pain well controlled – on MST 20 mg bd (see pain chart). This morning he got himself into a real mess getting dressed. He feels he will need more support. His daughter needs a break from caring – hence this admission.	
	Reg wears a hearing aid and requires people to speak loudly to hear. He is very philosophical about this admission and indeed about his eventual death. He was tearful when talking about his wife who died 27 years ago. I asked him if he anticipated being reunited with her. He laughed and said 'no'! He has no strong faith – he thinks he will simply return to the earth from whence he came. He still enjoys the *Guardian* newspaper, doing crosswords and watching TV. He has been a very keen angler but fears he may now lose this – so dependent on help to continue fishing. He enjoys company, chatting – was appreciative of my chat with him, especially talking about philosophical issues. Worked in a bank for all his working life.	
	Reg presents with a number of issues: difficulty with sleep, has a catheter which he dislikes, poor appetite, fatigue, fragile skin – small break, loss of mobility and dependence, anxiety about future support. No pain. He is on a wide range of medication for his heart (see list) – he has some lower oedema for which he wears Tubigrip. He also takes an antidepressant.	

Figure 13.2 Reg Simpson.

How can we help this man?

Symptom management – stable but observe.

Difficulty and anxiety with sleep. He commenced sleeping tablets 6 weeks ago. These have been helping. He was waking up at 04.00 and becoming distressed as he lay awake for the remaining 5 hours before he got up. He goes to bed around 22.00–22.30.

Action – monitor sleep on visual analogue scale (Fig. 13.3).

Poor appetite and loss of taste. He enjoys soups. He says he has lost a lot of weight over the past months. However, he takes this in his stride.

Increasing loss of mobility. He has stopped using his electric scooter a home – because he was getting his feet mixed up! He walks with a zimmer frame – in fact, walked with one nurse to eat lunch at the table. Lacks confidence.

Action – refer to physiotherapist.

Fragile skin – he has a small break on left hand after an accident with his grandson. No other breaks. Will need pressure-relieving equipment (see Waterlow score/lifting-handling assessment).

Action – monitor pressure areas. Wound is 2 cm x 1 cm. Stage 2 (see wound care protocol).

Catheter in situ – he doesn't like it but it is working OK (protocol care). Reg says he is prone to constipation – bowels last opened 2 days ago. No discomfort – that's not unusual for him. He usually takes lactulose when it becomes a problem.

Action – monitor using bowel chart (Fig. 13.4).

Support for the future

Action – to discuss with daughters the current situation/to support his daughters.

Assistance with personal hygiene

Action – negotiate best way with him on a daily basis (see standard of care).

Consider self-medication – to ensure he maintains his competence with drug taking. He enjoyed his soup for lunch and managed some pudding!

Arrange delivery of *Guardian* newspaper.

7/11	New wound noted on outer side of right leg (size 1 cm x 4 cm. Stage 2). He knocked his leg on the side of the bed (see wound care plan). Seen by physiotherapist – he can walk with one person safely – need to encourage mobility but remember he is also fatigued! He really enjoyed 'jacuzzi' bath this morning. Sleep: Reg woke as usual at 04.00 and lay restless until breakfast. Medication is currently temazepam 10 mg. Sleep assessment (using VAS) did not reveal any particular factors that disturbed his sleep. Action: can we review our approach as it distresses him? This afternoon he was dozing in his chair as he does at home. He asked me the time. I said 4 pm – he groaned 'Oh no – when is dinner time?'. He is clearly bored, he structures his day through meal events (even though his appetite is poor). I asked him how the crossword went yesterday – he said he hadn't been in the mood. I found him the *Telegraph* for today. (We need to order the *Guardian* for him!) Hazel will help him later with it as he enjoys company. Seen by Dr Webb – he is booked for thyroid function test on Monday. Also to review use of sertaline- antidepressant. Does he need this? (depression assessment) Action: Offer Reg day care to engage him?
8/11	

Figure 13.2 *Continued*

Bowel chart

While it seems almost heretical to contemplate a return to the bowel chart, mapping or charting is a practical and meaningful approach to monitoring patterns for most aspects of care. At a glance the pattern over time is revealed alongside the response to shifting patterns and the efficacy of the response in bringing care back into a desired pattern.

Sleep VAS	Reg Simpson	6/11/02
Complete satisfaction with sleep	◄————————————► *	No satisfaction with sleep

Mark perception on scale
What factors influence this mark?
NB: pain, position, hunger, drink, temperature
   of room, environment, noise, bed, bedclothes,
   anxiety, emotion, usual sleep pattern, sleeping
   tablets, full bladder, other?
	Reg says he sleeps worse than he does at home despite
	   maintaining fairly normal sleep pattern. He feels
	   being in the hospice was OK, although it is strange
	   being in another bed – not so comfortable as his bed
	   at home. Comforted by nurse spending time with him
	   in the 'early hours'. No pain.
	Written up for night sedation if necessary.	

Sleep VAS	Reg Simpson	7/11/02
Complete satisfaction with sleep	◄————————————► *	No satisfaction with sleep

Mark perception on scale
What factors influence this mark?
NB: pain, position, hunger, drink, temperature
   of room, environment, noise, bed, bedclothes,
   anxiety, emotion, usual sleep pattern, sleeping
   tablets, full bladder, other?
	Reg is more dissatisfied with his sleep than last night.
	I sat with him and he talked about his wife and the
	   prospect of not being able to manage at home
	   anymore. Even had half cup of tea. He seemed more
	   settled afterwards.
	I offered night sedation but he refused this.	

Sleep VAS	Reg Simpson	8/11/02
Complete satisfaction with sleep	◄————————————► *	No satisfaction with sleep

Mark perception on scale
What factors influence this mark?
NB: pain, position, hunger, drink, temperature
   of room, environment, noise, bed, bedclothes,
   anxiety, emotion, usual sleep pattern, sleeping
   tablets, full bladder, other?
	Reg is more satisfied with sleep although he was awake
	   again – he said he enjoyed day care, that it took his
	   mind off things. I gave him hand massage with some
	   lavender and he managed to doze for another hour.	

[1] See Chapter 14 for information on constructing reflective standards of care.

Figure 13.3 Monitoring sleep. The sleep visual analogue scale (VAS) was originally developed at Burford Hospital as one of its standards of care: 'The patient is satisfied with their sleep'.[1] If appropriate, the patient is asked about their usual sleep patterns and marks their normal satisfaction with their sleep.

The chart in Figure 13.4 was designed at the hospice where constipation is a particular and often difficult symptom for many people – patients, families and nurses! Before the bowel chart was used, the hospice used a standard care plan with the ubiquitous goal that 'the patient should have their bowels opened every 1–3 days (depending on what is normal for that person)'. The care plan also stated the (almost) universal first line of action – 'if patient uncomfortable suggest one bisacodyl and one glycerine suppository'. Whilst this may, for many people, be the best response, it may not be. The risk with standard care plans and protocols is that they impose a 'best' response rather than being perceived as a guideline to inform the response. This is more so when best practice is prescribed through research such as National Institute for Clinical Excellence (NICE) guidelines. Protocols help to ensure consistency of response by practitioners based on best practice and therefore there must be good reason for deviating from the guideline.

Assessment of bowel habit Reg Simpson 6/11	Prone to constipation. Last went 2 days ago. Reg is not uncomfortable
Threats to bowel habit?	Morphine – would he be better on fentanyl patch? Poor mobility and fatigue, poor diet and fluid intake
Plan	Monitor

Date	Shift am/pm/ night	Open? y/n	Assessment/description	Response/evaluation
7/11	am	n	Doesn't take any laxatives and eats a low-fibre diet	Encourage Reg to drink more
	pm	n		
	night	n		
8/11	am	n	Again he says it isn't a problem	Reg declined bowel massage – he is reluctant to drink
				Prescribe Movacol
	pm	n	He says he feels uncomfortable (maybe movacol?)	
	night	n		
9/11	am	n/y	Reg accepted offer of suppositories (see protocol)	Small hard stools passed. He felt better.
	pm	n		
	night	y +	Diarrhoea ++ Probably overflow??	

Figure 13.4 Reg's bowel chart.

Using the bowel chart (as with the sleep VAS) enables the standard of care for bowel care to be monitored.

My narrative of working with Gerard

I visited Gerard at home to appreciate whether he would benefit from complementary therapy. My appreciation is written as an unfolding based on the Burford cues. Unlike Reg Simpson's narrative, I have boxed the Burford cues in order to guide other practitioners unused to working with them, despite my reservation that the cues might be viewed in a reductionist way.

I have incorporated two visual analogue scales into the narrative: 'relaxed – tense' and 'positive – gloomy' to appreciate Gerard's emotional and pyschological being. His scores suggest he is not as relaxed as he makes out.

In scoring Gerard, I am mindful that it may be perceived as insensitive and that I am concerned in the outcome rather than the process. Gerard was in free-fall towards his inevitable death. He clung to hope and exploring his feelings and thoughts would have been too painful. As it was, when I sat on his bed waiting for the doctor, his fears spilled out. There was no longer any point in evaluating whether reflexology or any other therapy was enhancing his sense of well-being. The scales also enable an evaluation and audit of treatment.

Name – Gerard Hanwell	Address 9 The Havens, Ludborough		
Age 43	GP Dr Candice Main		
Meaningful others: Lisa – wife, Jessie aged 7, Greta aged 3 Both sets of parents	District nurse/Macmillan nurse Amy – district nurse Esme – Macmillan nurse		
Diagnosis/synopsis of illness	Cancer tip of penis surgically removed 1year ago Lymph node involvement in his left groin – lymph node excised but the cancer has invaded the left leg and groin areas – poor response to chemotherapy.		
Wednesday October 16th	Wound now extensive and spreading rapidly through the leg and pelvic areas. Very offensive smell – being treated daily by district nursing and pads changed about every 2 hours by Gerard or Lisa due to heavy exudate. Charcoal being used to combat the smell although Gerard finds the edge of the dressing pressing on the wound causes discomfort.		
Who is this person? What meaning do they give to this health–illness experience? How do I feel about this person?	Gerard is pale and apprehensive. He is pleased to see me – and quickly tells me his history and the way he and Lisa are exploring alternative treatments – currently taking an exotic bark diet. Gerard knows he has cancer spread. His openness and Lisa's despair, seeing the pictures of his children on the window sill, I feel a strong connection with him and his family – I want to help them if that's possible.		
How is this person feeling? (mood/stress/anxiety/fears/ body image)	Relaxed ⟷ 2 Tense 3 Positive ⟷ Gloomy 5 4 3 2 1 On the surface Gerard seems relaxed and philosophical. Lisa is more anxious – a point Gerard picks up – that it is harder for the onlooker. They are both positive and expectant about my involvement – that it fits in with their chosen alternative approach at this time.		
How has this event affected their usual life pattern and roles? Sleep Eating/drinking Mobility Pain Elimination Work/play Relationships Energy/fatigue	Gerard finds difficulty getting comfortable at night with the movement and pain in his left leg – need to review his analgesic pattern? Lisa is not sleeping and still working. Diet – Gerard on his special diet – needs to drink 5 litres water each day – the diet is very challenging but he is determined. Gerard can just get about up/down stairs – pain increases significantly with movement. No comment on bowels at this time. Gerard was working up to a week ago. He worked as a computer software engineer in a small firm – his work very supportive, but Gerard anxious about this as his work is crucial to firm's success. Gerard was a very keen footballer – supports Charlton – fanzine on floor. Enjoys music very much – Queen – had to cancel concert at weekend to see tribute band due to leg.		
What is important for this person to feel comfortable?	Pain control and position for leg. Hope!! Support for Lisa.		

Figure 13.5 Gerard and Lisa's narrative notes.

What support does this person have in life?	Lisa – although her work have given as much time as she needs to be at home. Both sets of parents live nearby and support Lisa with the children. District nursing and Macmillan support.
How does this person view the future for themselves and others?	Gerard understands he has the option of further chemotherapy if the alternative approach fails to respond. Both he and Lisa are positive that he will beat the cancer.
Contraindications	None
How can I help this person?	Offer reflexology weekly using essential oils (patchouli for positive thinking/frankincese as blend to calm emotions/one drop of juniper berry – help with odour and rid toxins. Suggest lavender on wound gauze as deodorant and analgesic. Suggest lavender and bergamot in aroma-stone to fragrance room Possibility of therapeutic touch – ?? teach Lisa to give this
Evaluation	Gerard very relaxed and enthusiastic following reflexology – he would like me to visit again. They are going on week's holiday for half-term so make appointment for two weeks (30/10)
Wednesday October 30th	Amy, district nursing is leaving as I arrive. She reports the wound has worsened. Jessie, the 7 year old opens the door – she's off school with a cold. Gerard cheerful. Good break. He feels the wound is stable and the smell less offensive. Lisa allergic to lavender and bergamot! (she has asthma). They have stopped using charcoal because too painful cutting into his wound! Gerard's legs have swollen – tumour must be constricting blood and lymph flow. Reflexology treatment – Gerard asleep – says it was 'fantastic' afterwards. Suggest seeing lymphoedema nurse at hospital – but can he get there? Gerard's legs very dry – I leave some grapeseed oil for Lisa to apply. Gerard and Lisa are going to Lourdes tomorrow with his parents. As Gerard says, 'Who knows what might happen? I'm not particularly religious but maybe a miracle?' I wonder if that comment reveals how darkly Gerard and Lisa are thinking as they try and maintain a surface sense of hope.
Monday November 4th	The first thing I notice is the smell – not as bad as my first visit but still hangs like a cloud. I ask 'How was Lourdes?' They did not go as Lisa's passport had expired! His father had brought some holy water back and poured it on Gerard's leg. He says 'It felt warm'. Hope high. Gerard describes the way his wound continues to spread. Leg remains swollen although had gone down after my last treatment – now swollen again. He continues with alternative approach. I ask 'Do you ever contemplate that you won't beat this thing?' He responds 'I'm hopeful it will get better but sometimes it does cross my mind that I won't.' Lisa says Gerard had 'disturbed' weekend –not sleeping, confused, restless. Lisa is exhausted. Reflexology – Gerard quickly asleep. Again, he says the treatment was fantastic. I finish with therapeutic touch. Lisa asks if this was what I was going to teach her. I wonder if reflexology may help twice weekly. Appointment for Friday.

Figure 13.5 *Continued*

Friday November 8th	Speak with Esme before visit – she is on phone to Lisa. Things have deteriorated ++. Esme saying to Lisa that Gerard will die – need to tell the children. The wound nw solid black necrosis, infected and had haemorrhaged. I feel as if I am walking into a cauldron. Blood transfusion arranged for hospice next Monday.
	Arrive at house – children blank faces, shocked. Lisa brave. Gerard in bed – he is shocked, devastated with the news. I sit with him – helping him to talk through his tears and fears. Waiting for GP – 'any moment' – so he declines a treatment.
	Downstairs I comfort Lisa – and break the children's despair by doing Greta's feet – Jessie joins in. Children bounce easily.
Wednesday November 13th	Big mix-up. District nurse comes at 11am – give Lisa and Gerard more time in the mornings. Gerard in bath – he shouts his greeting down the stairs. Children back to school after 'colds'.
	Gerard's pain control improved, especially at nights, enabling everyone to sleep better!! Still some pain on movement.
	Arrange visit for Friday 15/10
Friday November 15th	Gerard back downstairs in his 'usual' chair. More colour in his face after the blood transfusion. He is cheerful and looking forward to his reflexology. Continuing with his alternative diet.
	Reflexology uneventful yet Gerard says it was relaxing and that he was transported to another place beyond fear. He can't explain it but it was profound. Lisa comforted listening to him say this – I give her a reflexology to relax her – she is very stressed although tries to be calm on the surface. It works well – 'at one point I was conscious that I did not have one thought in my head'.
	Appointment made for 25/11.
Monday November 25th	Gerard admitted to hospice – deteriorated last week. Children also sick – Lisa's mother at house with them.
	At hospice, Gerard not conscious. His sister, Leanne, has arrived from NZ. I stay with family.
	I greet Gerard and he stirs. Lisa jumps in expectation. I sit with them as Lisa unfolds the story of Gerard's deterioration. His breathing is very erratic, it bothers her listening to it. It also reflects Gerard's distress underneath the midazolam.
	I use therapeutic touch for about 20 minutes – shifting his breathing pattern from Cheyne-Stokes to normal rhythm. I take the heat out of him – he is more settled, more relaxed. Lisa says his hands are warmer – she is so grateful. She can sit easier with him now.
	I also give Lisa reflexology as she holds Gerard's hand to help relax her. She actually falls asleep for a short time. She feels relaxed and energised afterwards.
Wednesday November 27	Gerard died yesterday in Lisa's arms with children present. Very emotional. The staff are deeply affected by his death.

Figure 13.5 *Continued*

Reflection

I realise how tentative my plans to help Gerard were on my fist visit. And yet I recognise how all such plans must be tentative in response to his and Lisa's changing condition. The core of my care was establishing a relationship with him around the idea of helping him and his family let go of fear. Put another way – the idea of holding his and Lisa's *hope*. Yet I was mindful not to foster false hope. Looking back, I see how profoundly difficult it was to hold their hope as he deteriorated rapidly towards death. It was as if a panic set in and they went into anxiety free-fall.

I also recognise my need for support, my need to liaise with the other care workers and how I absorbed the family's suffering. In the face of the cancer's remorseless onslaught I knew my therapy had no 'cure' value – it was simply a way of being with this family to ease their suffering as best I could right through to the end and eventually attending Gerard's funeral.

Writing 'his narrative' was in reality writing 'my narrative' – it was cathartic. I wonder if I had sat and written the narrative before I left the house and left it with him – how differently would I have written?

Conclusion

I have considered some ideas concerning reflective communication or dialogue with regard to oral and written traditions within nursing. I now view my clinical practice as a therapist as an unfolding narrative which means I naturally write in a reflective vein. Through writing I become more mindful and evaluative, always challenging myself on whether I am most available to Gerard and his family and how I could be more available. I am always challenging myself on whether I am reading the situation correctly and responding most appropriately with skilful moral action. In other words, I live the MSR cues through the narrative.

In Chapter 14 I consider 'ensuring quality' as reflection.

Chapter 14

Ensuring quality

Reflective practice is always concerned with the practitioner realising desirable and effective practice. As such, it is always concerned with ensuring quality.

In the following reflective account, Lazell, a community midwife, is struggling with an organisational initiative to cease postnatal home visits. She feels this will compromise her vision of being with the woman and diminishing the woman's experience. Or in other words, the quality of care will be diminished.

Lazell's reflection was written as an assignment during her second year of the Masters in Health Care Leadership programme.[1] She had no previous experience of reflection prior to undertaking this study.

A narrative of a quality initiative to improve midwifery care to postnatal women in the community

All of the major religions of the world, being patriarchal, have, for thousands of years, suppressed the female aspect of God. This denial of the Goddess Mother has led to a major imbalance within the spiritual life of all of us. This spiritual imbalance, deeply imbedded within our culture, manifests into the mental, emotional and physical levels as dysfunctional energies. This essence is to assist in the healing of this deep-seated disharmony.

Seeking inspiration for the words I wish to write in this assignment, catching sight of my two sons together in a photograph on the wall aged 8 months and 4 years rewards me. After the birth of my first child, I was transferred to a cottage hospital on the edge of Dartmoor run by community midwives and ancillary staff. It was a warm spring. I sat for many hours recuperating in the sloping, scented gardens, staring at my first child in awe. The chaplain came and blessed his funny bald head, prayed for him and for days I imagined a golden spiritual haze around him! I was in love! I ate well in a communal dining room with other mothers. Auxiliary nurses held our babies if they cried during mealtimes, mothers were given milk twice a day, and rested in the afternoon. It was didactic care, but I was thoroughly well cared for.

After my second child, an elegant and gentle-natured midwife who was passionate about breastfeeding and motherhood visited me at home. She would arrange pillows and

[1]See Chapter 18.

adjust the baby's position until feeding felt comfortable. She would bring me a drink, and then for a few moments watch us both. I remember her saying how rewarding it was to watch a mother and baby relaxed and happy. I remember feeling very happy and beautiful at that time. We were both, I think, basking in something quite luxurious.

These experiences and memories of being 'mothered' after birth by midwives, and becoming a mother have considerably shaped my values as a practitioner and contributed to my vision as a leader of best midwifery practice.

This account explores how my vision of desirable and best midwifery practice after birth has been challenged by a quality initiative, which radically altered the place of postnatal care in the community.

By considering the National Service Framework for Children, Young People and Maternity Services (DoH 2004: 38–40), guidelines from the National Institute of Health and Clinical Excellence (NICE 2006), research and a local organisational benchmarking measure to assess quality, I consider whether managers and midwives have assured quality in line with recommendations. I also explore the problems of interpreting quality. I used a model of structured reflection to explore the discordant feelings this initiative provoked and to surface emerging insights as a leader (Johns 2004: 18).

From the reflective cue 'Have I been able to realise desirable practice', I used framing perspectives to help me explore the learning potential emerging from this initiative. I have tentatively looked to the future as to how opportunities might be seized from this initiative and the ways in which quality practice might be best measured and integrated into midwifery work in order to remain true to my vision, and the essence of midwives being 'with women'.

A quality initiative

Postnatal care in the community is going to be changed. This will, according to the head of midwifery, bring it in line with other maternity units under the new guidelines for postnatal care (NICE 2006), and we are reminded that in other European countries, there is little postnatal visiting. There is also word that money is tight and savings need to be made on travel and midwife time. I am unclear and suspicious as to the real motive for the initiative.

I work remotely from the hospital, so I call into the office one weekend when I am on duty and speak to Carol.
'Who knows what is happening? I hear it's starting next weekend. As from next weekend there will be no home postnatal visiting.'
'None?'
'There's going to be some sort of drop-in clinic. No arguments, it's drop-in or nothing.'
I am bewildered and angry that I do not know more. My 'patch' is rural, 15–20 miles from the hospital. I feel ashamed and embarrassed to imagine myself telling a woman after birth, tired and overwhelmed, that she has to travel back to the hospital to be checked and that my visits will be minimal. It seems almost a betrayal of a trusted relationship, an undervaluing of her achievement, a trivialisation of the enormity of the act of giving birth and becoming a mother.

Reflecting back on my early description of my vision as a leader, I write:

To offer a high-quality level of safe creative practice to my clients and their families. I aim to help women to have the chance to know the positive illuminating power of normal birth as a life experience, which contributes to happy parenthood and happy children. I believe that women who feel they have been strengthened by birth because they have experienced and enjoyed what their body can do might be termed as empowered through empowering midwifery practice.

My vision of practice, of helping women to know the 'illuminating power of birth as a life experience' extends into the postnatal period. I share so much of this enormous and amazing life-changing experience with clients. My work is as varied and changing as the skies. I remember kind words written in accolades reflecting the value they placed on seeing me, feeling reassured during their dark and doubtful days, moments of anxiety or just sharing something of those special early days of motherhood with me. My philosophy has little to do with checking and ticking boxes on the postnatal care book and it seems unbelievable that it can suddenly be so easily diminished.

I discover that minimal postnatal home visits will continue during the week. Any other visits required must be accounted for in the care plan. There will be a postnatal drop-in clinic on the weekends run by the community midwives, when the mother may or may not see her known midwife. The plan is to ultimately extend the clinics to weekdays too. The breastfeeding clinics will continue to run at both hospital sites in the week.

Checking a woman I don't know on a couch in a hospital drop-in clinic seems more like a check-up at the dentist. I muse that perhaps that's what we are becoming as we shed more and more of our role to maternity care assistants, and evolve into extraction technicians, functioning to survey and monitor the development of the child and deliver the woman. Obstetric work and dominance increasingly overshadow the essence of our role and further remove us from being 'with women'. Standardisation of pregnancy, birth and postnatal care through hospital protocol and policy means midwifery care increasingly regards women as baby-making machines and undermines the intuitive, nurturing role of midwives to be 'with women' and celebrate motherhood (Walsh 2006).

I feel like a puppet, manipulated by the organisation, my script written for me. Doctors get the leading role in the performance, with costly technology, which, for example, allows surveillance of labour without entering the room or speaking to a woman! There is a palpable sense of uncertainty about what this means for community midwives. Some midwives seem to disconnect from discussion in the office and bow their heads to whatever they are doing, seemingly in resignation to the change. Maybe they don't care, maybe it's too hard to think or be angry any more. Others are angry and rebellious, yet seemingly a weak, powerless group, behaving like children saying they will get women to write in and complain, a behaviour characteristic of individuals when authorities are parental. Transactional analysis is described in Johns (2004:142) and demonstrates this as a non-reciprocal pattern of dealing with conflict or anxiety. This behaviour reflected the powerlessness and rebelliousness of the midwives, a subordinate group or 'docile bodies' as termed by Foucault cited in Gillespie (2000), and the sense of authority and decision making coming from an unreachable parental height. Some midwives agree changes are needed, they think postnatal care is a waste of time.

A letter is going to be written by our acting manager to give to the women. Our usual manager is on sick leave. Another manager says she cannot have community midwives doing 'reassuring' visits to women at home when she has so few midwives staffing delivery suites. I read the minutes of a meeting about the alteration to postnatal visiting. 'No more T.L.C. (tender loving care) visits.'

Just the wording makes me feel volcanic. TLC is what caring is about sometimes, ensuring rest and food, infant feeding support, encouragement, sometimes just a hug for an overwhelmed, tired, anxious mother. It is intangible care at times. Being a mother to a mother. Or am I already feeling uncomfortable about the inference of the powerlessness that 'TLC' conveys?

However, I don't go to the head of midwifery and shout, or voice my concern or say how angry I felt. I don't write a letter of protest. I spend some time grieving and feeling a bit of me depressed and dying inside. Lindberg *et al* (2005) explored midwives' expressions of loss and grief during organisational changes although being ahead in ideas about caring, yet caught up in the past. I fear something important and valuable to me in my work is being cut away, I'm angry, and it hurts. Despite my anger, I can't express it to the managers, because what I have to say doesn't seem important against big financial decisions, evidence-based care and the hospital machine. Perhaps I fear the judgement described by Gilligan (1982) as 'the very traits that have traditionally defined the goodness of women, their care for and sensitivity to the needs of others, are those that mark them as deficient in moral development' (p18). Belenky *et al* (1986:106) speaks of the loss of voice when separate knowing has been the only voice allowed and voice is suppressed when faced with perceived displays of brilliance or superior intellect. I have always felt my emotional nature, 'my internal boil' and voice, should be controlled and suppressed, my mother making sure I stayed inside the box of respectability and attractiveness for a woman and my father speaking *at* me. If I do get angry, the organisation will consider me emotive, girly and stupid. So I'm wary of being associated with being 'for' something with a 'soft tag' because that epitomises everything I want to scream about, being a girl, powerless and not having a voice. I have spent my whole life feeling trapped in a box of different-ness, like a pressure cooker, wanting to break out and scream at the seemingly immovable walls and feeling powerless (Dickson 1982:72). When I do break out, privately, it is volcanic and fearsome and usually at things or people who reflect my feelings of powerlessness.

I have this sense of something coming in backstage undetected. A nasty big threat. I want to shout out to every midwife 'look behind you. ... BEHIND YOU'. Yet I am silenced, and I know part of that performance is that the players will not turn round.

The 'letter' appears for us to give to the mothers. 'We are always looking at ways that we can deliver a better service to the families we care for. We continually look at the different ways we work and the needs of the mother and baby to give tailored care to individual families ... community midwives will plan the timing and content of your postnatal visits with yourselves at first contact.'

The wording in the letter seems to shroud an unpalatable truth and is an effective stage illusion.

Ensuring quality

Our head of midwifery emails me. She knows I am looking at this initiative in my assignment.

She says: 'Midwives' time could be spent on doing better things if they are freed from routine postnatal visiting by reducing home visits, use of the drop-in clinic, and utilisation of maternity healthcare assistants'.

For many years postnatal care has been the poor relation in midwifery. It is undoubtedly the area that women are least satisfied with in their journey through maternity services (DoH 2004). Wray (2006) observes postnatal care is an area where there is minimal professional 'competition' and where midwives *could* reign and showcase successes. Yet the paradox seems that where doctors do not 'compete' with us, we have failed to embrace and value those areas of practice.

Postnatal care is the first victim when staffing is low, and in our unit tends to suffer low status in terms of valuable work. Perhaps, as described by Cattrell *et al* (2005), this is in part due to the sense that the organisation does not appreciate the stressful ward environment where too much time is spent on clerical duties, answering the door to visitors, staff often deployed to work on delivery suite, and not enough time with the mothers. There is an undercurrent that community midwifery and postnatal care are 'having cups of tea with women'. Perhaps we attach importance to midwifery business where doctors have greatest interest. On the one hand technology in childbirth has altered the craft base of midwifery and arguably 'deskilled' the role by undermining normal birth, and on the other, it has enabled midwifery to claim an occupational space in the professions. Therefore, 'skill' might be a work category disguising the power-based hierarchy of obstetrics (Hunt and Symonds 1995: 142). Midwives perhaps would rather be associated with 'skill' than 'craft' associated with untechnological postnatal care.

Statutory provision of postnatal care originates from 1905 when mortality rates were high and care was prescriptive and routine. Little has changed in routine practice and Wray (2006) argues we now need a clear purpose to our care giving. Cattrell *et al* (2005) support this idea that we remain attached to certain activities that are of arguable value, although most midwives valued the physical and emotional support of women in the postnatal period.

Considering the alteration to our postnatal services, I examined the national agendas for quality improvements in maternity. The Department of Health Framework (DoH 2004) challenges maternity services to review the routine discharge of mothers at 10–14 days and indeed suggests maternal health problems often extend beyond this period. This requires that services need to be flexible to extend into these wider time frames of up to 8 weeks after birth. A National Childbirth Trust survey, described in the document, found that women described help as lacking between 11–30 days after birth compared to the first 10 days. Concentrated visiting within the first 10 days and discharge shortly after this time is historical. The document states maternity care providers must be innovative in delivering ongoing maternity services. This indicates maternity care assistants to address aspects of postnatal services receiving negative comments, such as hygiene, food and breastfeeding support. Our maternity managers have not yet implemented the use of maternity care assistants in the community yet they have reduced our visiting.

Theoretical framing[2] helps me synthesise my knowledge about this quality initiative, I considered some literature on effectiveness of postpartum interventions. A systematic review of randomised controlled trials (RCT) found there was no evidence to endorse universal postpartum care (Shaw *et al* 2006). This research reflects findings that many long-term postnatal health problems have remained unidentified before postnatal discharge (DoH 2004). However, the research also recognised that these studies focus on predetermined measurable outcomes and that qualitative literature and non-randomised studies may add 'significant insights' into the benefits of postpartum support. Women still valued a healthcare professional visiting them at home in these studies but the nature of this value was not measured. As this review reveals, studies considered could not endorse postnatal interventions as effective. The view, however, is the empirical objective eye of a RCT. The study acknowledges that some outcomes *can* be measured but the patient experience is not easily measured in objective research.

---

[2]See Figure 3.7.

Clinical governance is: 'a framework through which Health Service organisations are accountable for continuously improving the *quality* of their services and safeguarding high standards of care by creating an environment in which clinical excellence will flourish' (DoH 1996). Improving the clients' *experience* of healthcare is seen as the central purpose of clinical governance (Halligan and Donaldson 2001). NICE has been integral to clinical governance setting quality standards for clinical care towards which trusts work by approving treatments, equipment, interventions and procedures based on current best evidence. It would seem that by adopting such an evidence base, effective and consistent transfer of the lessons of research should be integrated into routine practice, rather than traditional and historical practice that do not improve patient outcome. However, as expressed previously, much research and evidence base stems from a purely empirical scientific eye and the quality of the patient experience is often invisible.

Our maternity unit routine postnatal care has been benchmarked against the NICE guidelines. Benchmarking and auditing support clinical governance activities by providing a measure of current practice against a standard. Considering the audit trail as a measure to confirm a standard or a piece of information, Cutliffe and McKenna (2004) argue that 'confirmability' is driven by a positivistic stance to knowing, and perpetuates the empirical scientific need for objective reality and truism. Indeed, our benchmarking process asks whether specific postnatal practices are routinely performed, and demonstrates whether boxes have been ticked on the postnatal notes to indicate care and information giving. For example, NICE stipulates that women are to receive information on life-threatening conditions at specific 'contacts' with the woman. This governance activity demonstrates that at our unit we complied with many of the standards in accordance with NICE guidelines although there are some areas where information is not routinely given to women. I reflect on benchmarking, the doing of care to define quality, and the invisibility of aspects of quality not in the doing, but perhaps best illustrated as poor quality when it is not done. This was most clearly described when reading a reflective account of fieldwork carried out on a busy postnatal ward by Wray (2006). This revealed many of the frustrations and failings in the present system of hospital care. Amongst many observations, acquiring help, support and advice and interacting with staff on the ward had to be instigated by the women by ringing the bell. Redeploying staff to the labour ward frequently depleted numbers. Women seemed inhibited and deliberated as to whether to ask for help from busy midwives, and seemed to be unsure as to whether their request for support would be deemed worthy by the midwife. This piece of work scrutinised the *quality of experience* for the women on the ward and would not be revealed within our benchmarking process. Scrivens, cited in Bartlett (2000), states that models of quality assurance such as benchmarking and audit, relating process to outcome, are not readily transferable to the outcome of quality in healthcare.

The 'doing' parts of midwifery and 'being' a midwife are crucially different, taking my thoughts back to memories of motherhood, and later, some of the professional, yet hugely sensitive and intangible acts of caring I have shared with mothers I have worked with. The state of what it is 'to be a midwife' is the ontological enquiry of 'harnessing midwifery skills to assist a woman to fulfil her potential to do physiological birth and be alongside her in that'. Traditional empirical research renders invisible much of what midwives see and know (Walsh 2006.) Surfacing this knowledge would help us move away from the checking mentality that describes much postnatal care. Therefore, in the light of governmental and organisational party line implying quality improvements to patient outcome and experience, effective care should be based on a collaborative approach implementing qualitative and qualitative research findings into practice.

Running concurrently with evidence-based practice, and arguably the raison d'etre for NICE, at the top of all government agendas is the need for tight financial control and 'value for money' as the health service is utilising public money and the public increasingly demand evidence that the money is spent prudently to deliver high-quality care. Many treatments and interventions have been placed under scrutiny as to their effectiveness to decide where scarce resources should be spent. Nyberg (1990) and Fox (1995) cited in Timpson (1996) state that 'current financial management of healthcare appears to dismiss professional affiliations and challenge the humanistic and holistic framework in which ethical ethos of caring has been nurtured'. Deciding what quality *is*, therefore, from the financial director's perspective, the midwifery view, the doctors' opinion and the patients' experience could reveal many different stories.

Managers and clinicians have a duty to challenge the norms and work with best evidence. I am beginning to understand their perspective. I *have* begun to make sense of the need for change. I am internalising and understanding the concept of reshaping the terrain and perspectives I have been familiar with, and having a new fresh lens on my practice environment (Cope 2001: 93). Under clinical governance I have responsibility to challenge my entrenched and somewhat nostalgic beliefs about care. This is indicated within the leadership and lifelong learning elements of clinical governance and has emerged through these reflections. I remain sceptical, however, as to what 'best evidence base' is and how we measure what midwives do. I also remain unclear as to the long-term plan for the place of community midwives and postnatal care. The managers seem to have rationalised the existing postnatal support structure without introduction of maternity care assistants as recommended by the government framework.

The initiative has been running 5–6 months. The managers report few complaints! There has been minimal impact for the patients or me in my geographical area, as women are reluctant to travel to the drop-in clinic and prefer to wait until they can see a midwife in the week at home. I hear at a recent meeting that we will be provided with a couch at our outlying base and the drop-in clinic will be extended to the week and in all areas. This may, however, have an impact on breastfeeding rates in the long term and is a quality issue for audit in the near future. Tired women struggling with a feeding challenge may be more likely to give up without easily accessible weekend support. There have been financial savings effected from the reduced travel costs and midwife time as a result of this initiative, although it has remained unclear as to where midwives might be redeployed eventually, or whether there will be the introduction of maternity care assistants.

An audit is being carried out to determine how the clinic is being utilised, whether functions of midwifery have been carried out, and if there is continuity of carer. I am critical of asking a woman a question such as 'Were you happy with the care and advice received?'. There is nothing to explore the concept of 'what happiness is' and exactly what care/advice was given, and is an example of the dangers of a tick box culture, that a job has been done, to satisfy a quality standard. Midwives tell me there is reduced continuity of carer for many women now the drop-in clinic is routine on weekends.

Visions, maps and leadership

Throughout my reflections, I have struggled with my feelings of anger and negativity towards an initiative which I have perceived as eroding my values of what quality care means. I questioned the concept of a personal vision and have wondered if it is possible to hold onto this while all around me is shifting sand and an ever-changing horizon. There is undoubtedly a risk in my work to allow vision to erode, to give up, to believe I have no power, sink into the abyss of not caring and just do my job as I struggle to cope with the structural conflict. This erosion of vision might be applied to the fact we have redefined the 'bad news' of reduced visiting and glossed it up as something else, as described in the letter. I also fear the organisation redeploying us to work more medically within the hospital, which will eat up our 'freed up' time and not be the best use of midwifery, in turn contributing to a devaluing of our role and motherhood.

I was aware, during the writing process, of hesitation, picking my words guardedly about the things I wanted to say in case my manager reads this work. I am wary of confronting her with my views on the unpalatable nature of her decisions, and I am self-consciousness that she may think my views 'soft'. I try to offload this cumbersome baggage, as this is not congruent with an assertive leader's right to a view (Dickson 1982: 31). Neither should I allow myself to let others reflect a view to me of what makes me acceptable (p142). I am aware of a small voice telling me, this reflective writing *may* have skewed my vision and enabled me reach a comfortable place to *be* rather than *sit with* the perhaps unpalatable truth, that I do not really like any of this initiative. Have I allowed my desire for acceptability to echo back to me another voice? Have I conformed in some way? Have I compromised to the path of mediocrity (Senge 1990: 153)? I have wrestled with the idea that perhaps I am in danger of signing up to my managers' vision in order to comply (Senge 1990: 211).

I reflect upon the 'boiled frog parable', in which subtle and unnoticed alterations to our environment eventually threaten to weaken and destroy us (Senge 1990: 22). This was apparent in my moment of wanting to shout to my colleagues to watch what was coming up behind them. There is leadership weakness in merely having goals and objectives in our vision (Senge 1990: 164). Parallel process framing[3] has helped me see connections in my learning. My own obscured vision, focusing only on the *way* I want to practise, rather than keeping an eye on a meaningful vision, true to my purpose, the essence of what I am as a midwife, is similar to the 'visionary' problems of using benchmarks to measure postnatal care. It blurs the picture and does not give a clear image of what reality is, or purposeful direction. Perhaps the organisational obsession with measurable outcomes goes some way to explain why practitioners experience the ricochet effect of enduring one quality initiative after another, yet increasingly feeling they are losing sight of meaningful, quality patient care. Clarifying my vision exposes me to the gap, the creative tension between reality and where I want to be. It is the energy that can drive action.

'The ability to focus on ultimate intrinsic desires, not only on secondary goals, is a cornerstone of personal mastery' (Senge 1990: 148). As I have revealed, my vision has been easier to articulate, the challenge is confronting my current reality (p150).

Johns (2002) likens our process of learning and understanding through reflection to the sculptor chipping away at the constraining forces whilst keeping a strong vision of what he wants to achieve (p24). According to Cope (2001), confronting reality requires re-mapping of one's map. As I write using the reality framing perspective[4] upon this text I am reminded of map shifts, and shoots of understanding are beginning to sprout within me. I recognise a pattern of being which is obstructive to forward

---

[3] See Figure 3.7.
[4] See Figure 3.7.

thinking and action. I have been expecting my work environment to continue to appear according to my mental map, the way I see things, the roads and terrain I am familiar with. I am recognising a need to break with the past in order to begin to appreciate others' maps, and carve new paths and develop new ways of seeing and thinking for myself (p94).

I have steadily regarded my managers' decisions with less frustration and anger. To work within the framework of clinical governance, managers have responsibility and accountability to direct resources to make the clinical environment safe and that may indicate redeploying midwives to work where risk is greatest. They also have responsibility to work within the budgets. Mark (1995), cited in Timpson (1996), states 'to seek only bottom line financial solutions potentially affects the well being of both practitioners and clients alike, weakening relationships and damaging the very foundations of the system they are supposed to improve'. But 'seeking only human caring solutions could equally be detrimental to the well being of healthcare organisations' (Ray 1989). These are the challenges this assignment exposes.

The process of this initiative was not transparent and did not engender thick trust or contribute to creating a learning environment characteristic of a transformational organisation. The process engendered suspicion about power and indeed, camps became evident comprised of those 'for' or 'against' the initiative. Cope (2001) speaks of the hand dimension of behaviour and conduct in creating effective relationships to achieve outcomes: 'If people don't have to worry about making mistakes and protecting their turf, they're more willing to open up and share learning and knowledge' (p152).

Openness in organisations emerges when one group suspends certainty about the other and this creates free flow of meaning through *dialogue*. Bohm, cited in Senge (1990: 240), suggests that discussion alone creates a 'ping pong' effect with ultimately winners and losers. In this case there was some discussion, but the initiative was broadly considered by the midwives as a *fait accompli*, as illustrated in Carol's words 'no arguments, it's drop-in or nothing'. Midwives, and arguably the women, have lost.

I want to discuss with managers the way forward with postnatal care and to explore new ways of delivering care that I could be involved with. This might, for example, encompass a supporting and educative midwifery role aimed at new mothers beyond the 10–28 day discharge period, as midwives have been 'freed' from the constraints of a short and concentrated period of 'doing' care, which is not effective. The issue of introducing maternity care assistants needs to be addressed as currently we have reduced postnatal visiting without an adequate support structure for mothers and babies in place as described in the government framework. However, the current staffing and financial challenges may render this impossible or create further constraints.

Leadership is not moving the mountain, but presently for me picking a fairly difficult path through rocks towards the top, the goal of being and becoming a leader of best midwifery practice, not losing my footing, my vision, and persisting in hard times (Schuster 1994). Like a cartoon, I follow the sign toward doubt, thinking I am getting there.

Johns (2002) describes the process of transformation as climbing mountain paths, with each step an event in itself, and not just a means to get to the summit (p26). At this time I have no sense of anyone following me on this difficult path. I feel quite alone with the joy and tears described in this work. Perhaps that is what I am beginning to see along this path, that leadership *is* aloneness. I think I have always felt alone. I am quietly hearing an inner voice telling me to stop fighting against what I know and feel.

Conclusion

I have written a narrative about a quality initiative that I did not initiate; I was participant to the impact of a change to clinical practice. This initiative reflected the nature of the transactional organisation with authoritative power, tendency to be reactive to organisational objectives, and emphasis on outcomes.

The changes made in the name of improving quality did not sit comfortably alongside my vision or values. They were in response to the financial predicament the trust faced and to the government agenda and new NICE guidelines.

Delivering high quality of care to mothers and babies is undoubtedly a shared concept of government, organisation, managers and myself. I am unsure if *visions* are necessarily shared; the ever-shifting sands and various political strings that dictate our 'dance' suggest to me that we are goal and objective *driven*, rather than *led* towards an overall vision. The creativity must be in how we achieve what we want within the constraints and limitations we have.

I see opportunities for midwives to work within a quality framework in new and innovative ways, whilst still delivering intuitive and creative care that is 'with women' and in keeping with my values and vision. These opportunities presently do not appear to have been grasped or articulated by my midwife leaders. I am sceptical that quality has been assured in this instance as motives for the initiative have been blurred, and the organisational vision is not clear. The process of assurance as far as done has been of a quantitative nature, not addressing quality patient experience or acknowledging midwifery skill.

It remains to be seen in time, if the organisation and managers behave congruently with the spirit of clinical governance in embracing *my* potential leadership innovation and allowing 'clinical care to flourish'.

I hope this narrative conveys my growing awareness of 'coming through, and transformation' on a path of becoming a transformational leader of best practice in the hierarchical, chaotic and shifting environment I work in.

Reflection

As I read through Lazell's reflection I begin to absorb something of her restrained anger; the contradiction between the organisation's decision to curtail home postnatal visits and the value of *being with* woman. Now the woman can come to the clinic at certain times to sort any problems out. Breastfeeding a problem to solve. Yet women struggle with breastfeeding for complex reasons. Midwifery now reduced to a technology, the midwife becomes the technology rather than woman with woman. The sucking into the hospital of midwives to be the technology to produce a safe baby and mother. Lazell notes the tension between *doing things to* and *being with*. Neither the woman nor the midwife seen in their humanness. Is this midwifery?

Reflect on the Burford cues (p36) – who is this woman, what meanings does she give? How is she feeling? How do I feel about her? How can I help her? Opening space to be with woman.

Narrative seeks transgression. As Okri (1997: 63) says: 'In storytelling there is always transgression, and in all art. Without transgression, without the red boundary, there is no danger, no risk, no frisson, no experiment, no discovery, and no creativity'.

I feel Lazell's anxiety that someone might read this and punish her for the transgression in exposing such tensions, for having a voice, for daring to be loyal to her women before the organisation. The threat of sanction heavy in the air. She can feel her tension, needing to get her voice out there, but can she? Can she overthrow her oppression to be true to herself and to women? Powerful evocative writing that draws the reader into the drama, to enter into dialogue with the text. This is easier when the text provokes me in some way. Being provoked, I might defensively reject the text as nonsense. If I am a reflective practitioner I will always ask – what does this text have to say to me? If I take offence I must then ask 'Why do I take offence?'.

As a palliative care practitioner I am mindful of palliative clinics being set up, where people with 'problems' can attend at certain times, cutting back on visit time. I can sense the same sort of logic being applied by organisational leaders overly concerned with budget in contrast with service. Another reason not to audit caring is that it raises issues that might have to be dealt with. After 6 months few complaints. I almost feel Lazell's disappointment that women accept this situation so readily. Does that reflect a general passivity in women or simply that they don't know what they are missing?

Clinical governance

As Lazell noted, in the UK the quality agenda is centred in the development of clinical governance, defined as: 'A framework through which all NHS organisations are accountable for continuously improving the quality of their services and safeguarding an environment in which excellence can flourish' (DoH 1998).

Who takes responsibility for creating this *environment in which excellence can flourish?* To achieve this, practitioners must take ownership of quality and live it as part of their everyday practice and organisations must create the opportunities for practitioners to exercise this responsibility. If not, quality systems will be imposed determined by external criteria; for example, National Service Frameworks (NSFs) and the National Institute for Clinical Excellence (NICE) have begun to both indicate and dictate the quality agenda.

If so, then aspects of practice not acknowledged in these schemes, such as caring, become invisible. Being invisible, it is not valued and not seen as real work. If practitioners do not take control of the quality agenda then quality systems will impose conformity and compliance and the creative opportunity of quality will be lost.

Reflective approaches to quality include clinical supervision, standards of care and clinical audit that collectively provide a comprehensive response to realising an environment in which excellence can flourish. Each of these learning opportunities is grounded in reflection, highlighting the organisational value of reflection as a process of professional development and ensuring quality through double-loop feedback.

- Loop 1 Do practitioners' clinical judgement and skilled responses realise desirable practice? Do the conditions of practice hinder realising desirable practice?
- Loop 2 Is the understanding of desirable practice flawed? Are the indicators for realising desirable practice adequate?

Clinical audit

Lazell notes: 'An audit is being carried out to determine how the clinic is being utilised, whether functions of midwifery have been carried out, and if there is continuity of carer'. Clinical audit offers an opportunity for multiprofessional group reflection around specific patients with the primary purpose of answering two fundamental questions:

- Did the patient/family receive best care?
- Do we know what best care is?

Clinical audit in the NHS (DoH 1996) states that:

> Clinical audit is a clinically led initiative which seeks to improve the quality and outcome of patient care through structured peer review whereby clinicians examine their practices and results against agreed standards and modify their practice where indicated. The future development of audit would aim to achieve:

- a clear patient focus – by linking quality explicitly to patient experiences rather than abstract clinical outcomes
- greater multiprofessional working across the different clinical and managerial disciplines which contribute to the patient's episode of care
- an intersectoral approach where a patient's care is managed across primary, secondary and continuing care
- professional self-development
- better integration of effectiveness information. (p3–4)

While clinical audit has a powerful impact on those who take part in it, many practitioners remain uninvolved. Consider this question for yourself. If you are involved, what factors have influenced your involvement? If you are not involved then why not?

It is the same question as whether practitioners are involved in quality, although clinical audit is a very practical approach to assuring quality, more so than standards of care because the process is simply reflection on experience, keeping the two clinical audit questions in the foreground. Practitioners are only likely to become involved where they retain a clear sense of ownership of the process of audit and feel it is a safe environment for discussing sensitive details about their professional practice without the fear of provoking management sanction or civil litigation (NHS 1996: 4).

Project

At one hospice where I led a project to establish clinical audit and standards of care, a practitioner prepares and presents an overview of the patient and family's care and treatment at the clinical audit meeting. The patient/family is usually chosen because their care has challenged the caring team in some significant way and highlighted areas of practice that are problematic. Following dialogue, the practitioner then summarises recommendations for future practice which are subsequently audited and presented to the Clinical Governance Group.

Recent topics have included:

- appreciating the nature of agitation in terminal illness and knowing how best to respond
- patients who are off-hand and with whom it is difficult to create 'good' relationships
- conflict with aggressive and demanding relatives
- seemingly intractable pain
- patients who did not 'die well'
- very poignant or emotional deaths where staff have become (over-)involved or felt they have 'failed' in some way.

What has been most interesting to note is that these issues have no definite solutions. They are complex and indeterminate, what Schön (1987) described as the swampy low-lands of practice. It is only through reflection that the nature of these topics can be grasped and alternative ways of responding surfaced. Of course, each clinical situation is different and learning cannot simply be transferred from one situation to another. But through reflection a deepening of appreciation is becoming evident. Clinical audit, like standards of care, is a learning opportunity, as indeed are all reflexive quality systems.

Perhaps if Lazell could present a postnatal woman who clearly needed home visits at clinical audit, her voice of concern would be formally heard, challenging organisational decisions that have not been agreed with the professionals involved in the name of 'best care'.

Standards of care

The idea of 'best care' suggests there is some standard against which 'best care' might be measured.

Consider what it means to *be with woman* and how *being with woman* might be audited? Such ideas are reflected within the being available template – the idea of the midwife being available to the woman to help her find meaning, make best decisions and help her skilfully to meet her health needs (and those of the baby and family). As such, an audit would consider:

- the midwifery vision – is it valid? is it intended?
- the extent to which the midwife and others knew the woman as the basis for care
- the midwife and others' concern for the woman
- how the midwife and others responded with skilful action to help meet the woman's needs and judged the efficacy of her actions
- how the midwife managed herself within the therapeutic relationship
- whether the midwife and others created a therapeutic environment and what factors constrained this.

The most concrete of these criteria is skilful action and indeed, much of research is geared to providing technological answers to the problems of clinical practice, albeit in a limited way given the uniqueness and unpredictability of the human condition.

It is these more concrete aspects of care that are formulated as protocols, pathways and guidelines informed by 'evidence', as far as it exists. Often anecdote (practitioner experience) is discounted as valid 'evidence' even though 'experience is the most significant determinant for clinical judgment and response' (Read 1983).

A reflective approach would be for practitioners to 'tailor make' their own standards to reflect their vision and practice. This approach would enable practitioners to take responsibility for their own practice and quality.

Standards of care offer a reflective approach to managing quality by focusing on discrete aspects of practice. Although standards of care can be imported from a validated external body, I am interested in developing standards of care constructed by practitioners themselves. This approach generally follows the development of standards of care at Burford Community Hospital between 1989 and 1991, an approach based on the Royal College of Nursing Standards of Care project (Kitson 1989).

A standard of care reflects a local practice situation that is professionally agreed, and both desirable and achievable. A *local practice situation* is a statement of practice applied to the particular practice unit. For example, in relation to the standard 'Patients are cared for in a safe and therapeutic environment', a midwifery unit may interpret this in a very different way to a surgical unit yet both will pay attention to research and policy that determine what is therapeutic and what is safe.

Professionally agreed means all people involved in meeting the standard of care: nurses, doctors, paramedical staff, cleaners, cooks, pharmacists, etc. The idea of 'professionally agreed' goes against the grain of setting patient-centred standards of care – can professionals and ancillary staff adequately set standards for patients and families? Do patients or patient representative groups need to be involved? At Burford, we invited Age Concern to 'vet' our standards as most of our patients were elderly. At the hospice where I work, we involve volunteers who have experience of caring for dying relatives as part of the shadow clinical governance committee that oversees the quality initiative.

There is a natural tension between what is *desirable* and what is *achievable* that captures the essence of quality. Quality is what is real, what is in front of you. I can feel the fabric of my shirt and sense its quality. However, quality is also something relative or comparable to other shirts, i.e. quality has a desirable element to it. Clearly, standards of care have to be achievable otherwise they would never be met and the hospice would fail its annual review and be closed down. Yet standards also need to reflect desirability, as something to move towards.

A standard of care reduces the practice situation to structure, process and outcome criteria designed to be monitored.

Criteria

- Structure is the resources that need to exist to enable the standard to be met.
- Process is the actions practitioners need to take to meet the standard.
- Outcomes are the relevant indicators that confirm that the standard has been met.

Strucural criteria are very diverse – staffing levels, attitudes and skills of staff, e.g. the complementary therapist ensures 12 hours of professional development yearly, number of syringe drivers, colours of walls, number of single rooms, maintenance contracts and so on. Practitioners often get confused between structure and process criteria and to some extent they do overlap. For example, a policy is an example of structure, as is an organisation's mission statement.

In contrast, a formulary or protocol is an example of process – actions that practitioners must take usually in a specified order of action, for example mouthcare. So a process criterion might read: 'The practitioner assesses and responds to each patient's mouth as per mouthcare formulary'. The formulary would be appended to the standard. One might argue that the existence of the formulary is a structural issue but it is really just a summary of various structure and process criteria. Structural things would include toothbrushes and various mouthwashes stored appropriately.

Nutrition

One of the standards of care we wrote at Burford Hospital concerned nutrition. It is a significant standard to consider in light of criticism that patients do not receive adequate nutrition in hospitals.

The standard statement – 'Patients can enjoy a nutritious meal' – recognises two elements of eating: nutrition and enjoyment. For many patients at Burford and indeed, for people everywhere, meals structure the day. They are social events. For people who are ill, nutrition is an important ingredient in getting well. Yet often when people are ill, their appetites are diminished – hence the significance of nutrition although the quality of hospital food and service has often been criticised. I am sure most readers have first-hand experience of hospital food, as a patient, friend or care worker.

So, what might be relevant indicators to inform practitioners that the standard statement 'Patients can enjoy a nutritious meal' has been met? The hospital standards group met for 2 hours every 4 weeks to review existing standards and develop new ones. The group is open to all multidisciplinary staff and is chaired by the standards of care facilitator. In the spirit of the learning organisation, all nursing staff are expected to manage at least one standard of care around a topic of interest, to be the 'standard-keeper'.

This person becomes the hospice resource person for that aspect of clinical practice, setting up and maintaining a resource file containing relevant information and research. The resource person is also responsible for ensuring the standard is monitored as designed and reports to the clinical governance group.

Clearly any member of staff whose actions contributed to outcomes must be involved in the writing of the standard. So for nutrition we needed to include domestic staff and cook.

I had identified the issue of nutrition as a standard topic by observing the size of portions served to patients and what food was left on the plate (in the days before we had plated meals). Did staff consider the patient's needs enough? I concluded that some patients when faced with too much food simply pushed the plate away and said they could not eat all that. Some patients ate everything, as if they had always been socialised to 'clean their plate', and some patients ate just what they wanted and left the rest. I put it to the staff that we should serve the amount they needed. Common sense really and yet the pressure to serve meals often meant we were careless at times. The group brainstormed ideas about nutrition and easily agreed the standard statement.

Different members of the group reflected on other situations where nutrition seemed to be a problem in some way. As the dialogue progressed we brainstormed issues onto the flipchart and then made connections between structural, process and outcome criteria. We designed a scan sheet that set out these criteria to monitor meal times (Box 14.1). We decided to ask student nurses on placement to monitor these criteria weekly and feed back the results to the standard-keeper. We felt this was a good way to teach students to

Box 14.1   'Patients enjoy a nutritious meal' scan sheet

	The patient receives a meal:	3 – yes, 2 – so-so, 1 – no score + comment
1	That they have chosen within limits	
2	In an amount they can enjoy	
3	That suits their dietary requirements	
4	At the correct temperature	
5	In an environment conducive to eating	
6	On a clean table	
7	With a drink within reach	
8	That they are not rushed to complete	
9	With assistance as required	
10	Where they are not interrupted	
11	They were prepared for	
12	Where any underlying symptom that might impair enjoyment has been adequately responded to: constipation, diarrhoea, nausea, fatigue, pain, etc.	
13	Other factors – please state	

pay attention to detail around nutrition and other standards and, more generally, quality of care as something that mattered.

In constructing and monitoring standards of care, the relevant indicators are internalised by the practitioner as a reflective framework and so, at meal times, the practitioner is more likely to spot situations where the standard is not being met. Such observations can be recorded in the standard file. Scanning and spotting are observational techniques that are predominantly used simply because they are part of everyday practice. In other words, quality is being lived.

Structural criteria included reviewing meal times, menus, introducing flexible breakfasts, involving the dietician more formally in patient nutrition and looking at more natural ways to ensure fibre in the diet. Process criteria emphasised better appreciation of patients' eating patterns and being more proactive in helping patients to learn better eating habits.

Relatives

Consider the standard statement – 'The family are informed, involved and supported within the caring process'. What relevant indicators might inform you that this standard statement has been met?

At Burford, in response to this challenge, we secured a small research grant and surveyed families. We identified a number of process criteria alongside which I suggest a number of questions that might be asked to get feedback that the process criteria have been met. I like to think that these questions are caring cues that can be unobtrusively slipped into dialogue between the practitioner and family member rather than as a formal questionnaire that demands the family's judgement (Box 14.2).

The logic of monitoring process criteria is simply that if the process is right then the outcomes will be right. Of course, nothing is predictable and the vagaries of the human condition suggest that some family members will never be involved, informed or supported enough.

Box 14.2   Relatives standard process scan sheet

The caring team inform the family who they are and how they can be contacted
Q – Do you know the caring team and how to contact them at any time?

The nurse on duty initiates a 'concerned interaction' with the family each time they visit
Q – Do the nurses approach you when you visit and ask how things are or do you have to approach them?

The nurse responds positively to the family's request for information and informs the relative where she/he,
for whatever reason, is unable to disclose information
Q – Are you adequately informed about the patient's condition and progress?

The nurse is aware of how the family is thinking and feeling about the patient's care
Q – Do you feel the nurses knew how you thought and felt about [the patient's] care?
Q – To what extent were you consulted and listened to in making decisions?

The nurse has explored with the family their desired involvement with the patient's physical care and setting
the limits of care giving
Q – To what extent did you feel welcomed and involved in caring for [the patient]?

The nurse identifies and responds to the relatives' (holistic) support needs
*Q – Looking back, could the care staff have supported you more in any way (physically, emotionally, psycho-
logically, spiritually, culturally, socially)?*

Ask yourself, would the nutrition and relatives scan sheet give you valuable quality information if you were to use them within your own clinical practice? Why not try them out?

The value of standards of care

Standards of care are a true quality assurance tool because they do not just monitor quality but seek to develop quality. In summary, standards of care offer practitioners/the organisation:

- a framework for developing specific aspects of clinical practice
- a change management model
- a way of connecting values with practice
- a process for group reflection and team learning
- a resource management model – the focus on structure creates the opportunity to reflect on resources available and the way resources are utilised
- a means for practitioners to demonstrate professional accountability
- a quality assurance tool
- a means to respond to quality agendas
- a way to integrate quality as part of everyday practice.

A means for practitioners to demonstrate professional accountability

To reiterate, quality needs to be lived as part of everyday practice whereby practitioners take responsibility for ensuring their own performance. The responsibility of organisations is to create the conditions in which practitioners can realise their responsibility – the essential role of clinical governance. Perhaps healthcare practitioners have been passive about quality, seeing it as someone else's business. As a result, quality measures have been top down and imposed on practitioners rather than engaging practitioners in responding to the quality agenda.

The effective (reflective) practitioner takes responsibility for ensuring her own effectiveness and working collaboratively with others to ensure best practice. This is the bottom line. There can be no compromise with this expectation. Indeed, practitioners should welcome and embrace this challenge as the hallmark of professional practice.

A way to integrate quality as part of everyday practice

Again to reiterate, quality is something lived. It should not be viewed as something outside everyday clinical practice but as something integral to everyday practice. In other words, quality is something that practitioners need to be mindful of within practice. As such, it is important that monitoring tools are designed to be integral with caring, as part of everyday practice. Of course, whether the tools are perceived as caring is a reflection of the person who uses them. As I shall illustrate in the examples of standards of care below, monitoring tools are observational or asking the patient or family specific questions. Observation tools include scanning and spotting. Scanning is a planned monitor of the standard of care using a designed scan sheet, usually a set of criteria that can be observed. Spotting is simply opportunistic observation of criteria during the course of the day, for example noticing that an immobile patient does not have a drink within easy reach at meal time.

Setting a monitoring schedule is always tentative, especially in the first instance. Perhaps weekly or monthly depending on the particular standard and the extent to which it is 'spotted' as failing its criteria.

Who should monitor? As I suggested with the relatives standard, monitoring techniques that involve asking patients or their families are best slipped into normal conversation as part of caring. For example:

- 'Did you sleep OK last night?' (sleep standard)
- 'You seemed restless in your sleep last night?' (sleep standard)
- 'How was the meal today?' (nutrition standard)
- 'What is this drug for?' (self-medication standard)
- (to a relative) 'How do you find Bill today?' (relatives standard)

Obviously questions that suggest judgement on care processes require sensitivity. Visitors may be especially reluctant to give negative feedback when still visiting (Nehring and Geach 1973). As such, questions are better designed as open rather than closed questions.

In Box 14.3, I set out a checklist for writing a standard of care. The last point is rather hopeful because although practitioners are positive about quality as an ideal, in practice they struggle to accommodate this approach with issues of owning quality, time and technique. It sounds easy but in practice standards are a difficult concept to embrace, difficult to write and even more difficult to monitor because of time. Hence, the organisation must invest in a standards of care facilitator and create the space for this work to be accomplished. It is vital work.

In summary, standards of care are a reflective and versatile approach to managing quality that contribute to developing the learning organisation by creating an opportunity

Box 14.3   Checklist for writing standards

- Reflects agreement by all practitioners/workers involved in meeting the standard statement
- Reflects consumer rights and needs
- Reflects optimum quality, i.e. the tension between what is desirable and what is achievable (within resources) (but always has a creative edge)
- Reflects organisational outcomes
- Reflects professional values and ethics
- Reflects relevant theory and research (evidence-based practice – ensure an index of literature explored)
- Resource file established
- Monitoring strategy designed and review date set (agenda for standards group)
- Avoidance of ambiguous statements or unnecessary jargon
- Has identified pragmatic monitoring tools (usually observation or questions to ask) and set monitoring schedule and review dates (this will be tentative in the first instance)
- Subsumes relevant policies
- Has converted process criteria into protocols or care pathways for 'best practice'
- Has been fun!

Box 14.4   Key points in developing a standard of care

1   Identify an appropriate topic for writing a standard of care; for example, 'patients are comfortable with their pain'; this topic may be a reflection of a current issue or part of a comprehensive list of standards that need to be developed (for example, to respond to the National Care Standards Commission's core and specialist standards of care)
2   Write the topic in the centre of a flipchart
3   Engage the group to brainstorm ideas that relate to this aspect of practice and cluster on the flipchart
4   Accept all contributions non-judgementally
5   After approximately 10 minutes discuss each brainstormed idea led by initiator
6   Reflect on the experiences of patients around the brainstormed ideas – grounding the activity in actual practice rather than as an abstract idea
7   Consider all relevant sources of knowledge that might inform the standard (theory, research, policy, etc.); this will almost certainly require a literature search and review at a later date
8   Draw relationships between the brainstormed ideas
9   Reformulate ideas as structure/process and outcome criteria
10 Write the definitive standard statement
11 Check list for writing standards

for focused multiprofessional group reflection around specific aspects of clinical practice with the intention of understanding and realising best practice. Key points in writing a standard of care are set out in Box 14.4.

Conclusion

Ensuring quality is the professional responsibility of every practitioner. As such, the reflective practitioner lives quality as part of their everyday practice. Reflective practice can be structured through clinical audit and standards of care that enable a focus on discrete aspects of clinical practice.

Lazell's reflection illuminates how quality issues can be determined at a strategic level that bypasses the practitioner. Lazell recoils from this imposition and seeks to exercise her responsibility to be involved in such decisions where they fundamentally alter the nature of her therapeutic relationship with women. So whilst on one hand practitioners need to take responsibility for ensuring quality, on the other hand, organisations must create the opportunity for practitioners to engage in such activity in meaningful ways.

In Chapter 15 I pursue this agenda through clinical leadership.

Read through Lazell's reflection again. Ask yourself:

- What makes this such effective reflective writing?
- Is it reflexive?
- Is she transformed through the experience?
- How is this transformation made explicit?

Chapter 15
Transformational leadership

Chapter 14 shared Lazell's reflection on ensuring quality as part of her journey to become a transformational leader. The plot of her narrative was more concerned with her realising leadership than ensuring quality *per se*. Reflection by its very nature is transforming, and so to be a transformational leader is to be a reflective practitioner. Transformational leadership is moral leadership that facilitates dialogue towards creating better worlds for patients and for staff. It does this by cascading leadership through the organisation, so each person becomes a leader of self and others, taking responsibility for working collaboratively towards realising shared vision as a lived reality. Transformational leadership is investing in collaborative relationships with people, investing in people, acknowledging people, persevering with people. It is being authentic, vulnerable, present, humble and available to others. It is being 'of service' to others – the lubricating oil that makes things work for people. Yet it is also being tough, focused and challenging.

Transforming leadership was developed by Burns (1978), whereby 'one or more persons engage with others in such a way that leaders and followers raise one another to higher levels of motivation and morality' (p19). Burns viewed leadership as a mutually empowering type of relationship that is moral. Yet, if organisations are primarily concerned with meeting strategic objectives, the moral landscape can quickly become obscured, the human factor lost in the machine. Building on the foundational work of Burns, Bass (1985) developed transformational leadership that was related more to organisational leadership than Burns' wider social agenda. Bass identified four inter-related essential aspects of transformational leadership.

- Idealised influence – is leadership based on genuine trust built on a moral foundation?
- Inspirational motivation – does leadership provide meaning and challenge for engaging others in working collaboratively towards shared goals and success?
- Intellectual stimulation – does leadership liberate the creative and responsive spirit in followers to fulfil their individual and collective aspirations towards overcoming problems in realising a shared vision?
- Individual consideration – does leadership invest in each person towards enabling the person to fulfil their potential and needs, leading to higher achievement and growth?

These aspects offer a broad reflective framework for leaders to view and reflect on their transformational leadership. What follows are two examples that illuminate the way reflective leadership has been developed through guided reflection. These have been edited from assignments that Sally and Susan undertook whilst on the Masters in Leadership programme.[1] They offer the reader the opportunity to critique Masters level reflective writing. Sally and Susan are both deputy ward managers working within NHS hospitals. Sally's reflection is on managing conflict from a transformational leadership approach, whilst Susan's reflection is concerned with establishing a learning organisation through implementing clinical supervision.

As you read these two narratives, reflect on the way the writers frame their emerging transformational leadership. Are the aspects suggested by Bass visible?

Sally writes: a little voice in a big arena

It is an ever-demanding society. The National Health Service (NHS) endeavours to provide modernisation and change to meet the needs of society. Policies and protocols are multiplying, targets and deadlines are everyday phenomena and 'budgets' have become the new buzzword. Front-line staff struggle to maintain the focus of a patient-centred service where, every day, there is the constant battle with the system to provide holistic care.

I work as a deputy ward manager within an elective orthopaedic unit in an acute hospital trust. This reflection exposes issues of conflict that arise within my role and how I am learning to respond in ways congruent with my values as an emerging clinical leader.

As a deputy ward manager my role can be one of confusion and difficulty. I am viewed as a leader but not completely let off my reins to explore. When those reins are sometimes dropped I find I'm pulled back with the understanding I wasn't ready to go it alone! My role is ward based, which enables me to maintain patient-centred contact whilst experiencing management and leadership within the NHS. I work along side my ward manager and aim to maintain high standards of care in a professional and organised environment.

Within my role I come up against daily issues of conflict. The pressures placed on the NHS today are filtering down to ward level where the cracks are beginning to show and leadership within this environment is becoming an uphill struggle. As Cope (2001) notes:

> Within organisations we see managers struggling to come to terms with new demands on their managerial and leadership style. We have shifted from a position where control is managed by virtue of a formal badge of office (manager, patient, director, etc.) to one where we have to lead people through the use of more intangible and flexible forms of leadership. (p1)

Following on from Cope's view, I feel leaders of today find they have to focus not only on themselves and the workforce but the surrounding issues, where difference and non-conformity are beginning to become valued, where expression can be an open forum and vision is developing into a natural phenomenon. The NHS is experiencing a change in leadership styles and moving forward from the transactional forms of leadership, which

---

[1]See Chapter 17

Schuster (1994) discussed as being hierarchically driven using status and influence to abuse power.

As I work towards creating the learning organisation (Senge 1990) within my own practice I find myself developing new strings to my bow. I am becoming a designer, a steward and a teacher. I feel my commitment and responsibility to enable people to expand their skills and clarify their vision. Burns (1978) expresses transforming leadership as 'being committed, having vision of what could be accomplished and empowering others with this vision so that all would accomplish more with less. The leader meshes with followers on deeply held values' (p28).

Such words are brain food, feeding my own vision, but it is only brain food. I must live such words.

As a deputy ward manager I am a puppet with many strings providing quality to my work, as a teacher, adviser, supervisor and expert. I work alongside my colleagues supporting, focusing and respecting them and the organisation as a whole. We acknowledge protocols and policies in our everyday work and strive to create and maintain a vision for our future.

With new government initiatives being continually developed there are ever more pressures placed on the organisation to meet targets and deadlines and deliver cost-effective healthcare, contributing to a rapidly changing environment. Leaders have to balance the reality of maintaining quality of care on a reduced budget with reduced resources. Klakovich (1994) shares this view: 'For some time, staff nurses have been pressured to *do more with less*, that is, to maintain high productivity without sacrificing quality' (p42, my italics).

Do more with less – the klaxon call at the factory gate. Because of the pressures being placed on the health service and each department managing their own resources, issues of conflict inevitably arise. Barriers are erected, protocols and policies are barraged around and common courtesy becomes a thing of the past.

Taylor and Singer (1983) suggest that, through tension, companies' capacity could grow as long as the people involved can survive the stress. They discuss that without a certain amount of tension within the working environment, barriers for change would not be broken down. However, tension can cause upset and barriers to be extended, not broken down; then staff can become demotivated, demoralised and unsatisfied. I feel this is reflected within the work of Benner (1984), who discussed that pressures placed on nursing teams can cause the nurses to originally cope with the challenge but in reality they are providing 'too little too late'. My reflective intention is to hold the tension creatively.

Through one such lived experience I became entangled in a conflict situation involving the placement of a patient arising from pressure within the organisation. Since the government introduced the traffic light system for bed management, 'red alert' has become an everyday event in my hospital. Working within an elective ward environment, we have a rapid turn-around of patients and on some occasions are left with an empty bed. We often assist the organisation by accepting non-orthopaedic elective admissions and minor trauma admissions to assist with the tight bed management of the hospital. We have strict guidelines on what we accept due to our rapid pace of work, the experience of our team and the infection risk to our elective patients.

On the occasion in question, the bed manager approached me regarding a gentleman who had been admitted to the accident and emergency department with severe head injuries. He had been brutally assaulted and the police were treating it as attempted murder. His condition was unstable and he required a nurse to special him. As the assailant had not been being caught, he was deemed at risk and would also have a police guard.

I was surprised at the bed manager's request to place this gentleman (whom I shall call George) within our ward environment. I felt the environment to be inappropriate, the staffing was already tight and there was no room for movement to create a nurse special. The ward was busy and there were several acute postoperative patients being monitored and there was also the very real issue, due to the open ward environment, of risk to the patients and staff. I expressed my concerns and stated my case in a 'professional manner' to the bed manager, who accepted the situation and the admission was refused.

Even as I use the words 'professional manner', I realise I am uncertain what I mean … it feels like defensive learnt behaviour I retreat behind. Enough to just note it now.

Two hours later I receive another phone call from the bed manager. This time, in a uptight and forthright manner, he states, 'There is nowhere to place George and pressure is now being placed on me to have George moved from accident and emergency. It has been discussed with the hospital manager and hospital administrator and George will be admitted to your ward!'.

The wind is taken from my sails, I take a deep breath and restate my case, detailing the ward policy and stating the ward would be unsafe in the event of George's admission. My outrage ripples through me … outrage that discussions have been held without my input and decisions made without one of the managers entering the ward to see the environment, the workload and the staffing levels. No respect for myself and my staff, no reasoning or compromise, just a very dictatorial attitude.

An assembly of senior management appears on the ward – the bed manager, the hospital manager and the hospital administrator. They approach me and tell me that George will be brought to the ward shortly and they are providing a nurse from another area to special George for the shift. I feel in awe and overpowered by the situation. I manage to question why the sitaution has been handled in this way and why there has been no discussion with myself and my team over the appropriateness of this patient's placement. My questions are not directly answered; the hospital administrator states the ward staffing has not been affected as they are providing cover for the next 12 hours and the situation will be reviewed in the morning. Although I can see that to resist further will be to no avail, I express my unhappiness with the situation, the lack of communication involved. The managers leave the ward and George arrives with his nurse and police guard. My shoulders feel heavy.

An hour later, now late evening, the chief executive of the hospital appears on the ward. She approaches me and acknowledges the situation that has occurred with George's admission. She explains the difficulty in finding an appropriate placement for George and acknowledges the issues I have raised. She thanks me for the co-operation of my staff and myself and asks to be made aware of any problems.

I was left feeling bruised by the situation but the chief executive had eased the swelling. Because she had gone out of her way visit to the ward and acknowledge a difficult situation, I did not feel so alone. It may have just been clever and kind words but it gave me an inner strength to review the situation.

Conflict situations surrounding bed management and appropriate placement of patients continue. The situation I experienced touches on issues of conflict manipulation, 'focusing on getting away from what we don't want rather than creating what we do want' (Senge 1990: 157). The hospital managers saw that George's admission to the accident and emergency department had caused disruption and once George's condition had been

Patient's perspective Unknown – probably immaterial	How was decision made? Power/utility won the day	Doctor's perspective – unknown – probably immaterial
Conflict Tension between the organisation's demand (reduced the situation to objects) and my demand to be heard (utility versus autonomy)	Could I have put up more resistance to George coming onto the unit?	Ethical principles: The ward was probably not the best care option for patient but short-term probably didn't make much difference. My autonomy – right to be involved Utilitarian demand to use the bed
My perspective My right to be involved in the decision: Ward staffing stretched Wrong environment for patient Advocate for staff who are resisting	The outcome was not wrong but the process of realising it was – distrust/outrage/demoralisation	Organisation's perspective – need the bed – no other options (expedient short-term option)

Figure 15.1 Ethical mapping grid.

stabilised, their priority was to move him to a more isolated environment. George was a problem which needed to be fixed!

I perceived the need to provide George with a more secure environment but had real concerns that the area of elective orthopaedics was inappropriate and that little would be gained from this transfer. Cavanagh (1991) discussed that a competitive style of conflict management usually occurs when a person follows their own gain to the detriment of others. This can lead to frustration, anger and arguments, creating damage to relationships and not viewing the situation as a whole but with tunnel vision.

I turn to ethical mapping to guide me. Ethical mapping (Fig. 15.1) enables me to view this situation from the different perspectives of those involved and ethical principles. As Johns (1999:289) notes, 'The map helps the practitioner see different and often contradictory perspectives of any situation and to examine the factors that determine which perspectives prevails'. It quickly became apparent to me that the only gain of George being admitted to the ward was that the organisation managed to place their problem patient. I feel that George would have received better short-term gain from being placed within a more secure environment. The high-dependency nursing environment that was required for George was unacceptable and inappropriate within a busy ward.

Abiding by the Nursing and Midwifery Council Scope of Professional Practice, as a nurse I need to have competence and confidence in the care I provide to my patient. 'Acknowledge any limitations in your knowledge and competence and decline any duties or responsibilities unless able to perform them in a safe and skilled manner.' Perhaps this is my 'professional manner'?

As the deputy manager, I feel I failed *in my duty* to act as an advocate for the nursing team; to express our limitations and knowledge to care for such a highly dependent patient. I feel overpowered by the organisation, having been told what I was to do like a naughty school girl rebelling against her teacher.

This transactional form of leadership has left me feeling angry and frustrated. I feel the managers involved were working from a negative short-term vision and not considering all the components involved within their decision. Cope (2001) discussed this as map conflict – conflict occurring when two people view the same situation from different perspectives. Map conflict can lead to tense situations and lines of communication can break down, leading to little or no resolution.

Theorists in the past have believed that conflict situations have a positive effect on ourselves and the organisation, Deutsch (1971), cited by Cavanagh (1991), discussed how conflict could be 'highly enjoyable' as you gain experience of your own capabilities. I feel we have to be aware that a conflict situation does not turn into a game for one or both parties' enjoyment and self-development and we keep the problem in the forefront of our minds otherwise it could develop out of control. Cope (2001) discussed the 'fantasy ladder' where a factual problem becomes modified and distorted, turning into fantasy, which then has a potential for conflict. Both parties can end up being on the fantasy rung of their ladder, causing a gap to develop between them (fantasy canyon). 'The fantasy is built on both sides, the conflict is no longer about anything substantial – it is simply about ego, beliefs, political position and power' (Cope 2001: 116). Conflict then becomes a battle of wills and casualties develop. The opportunity to solve the problem becomes reduced and only concludes because one party intimidates or shouts the loudest.

In guided reflection Chris challenged me – was I always fighting a losing battle that left me demoralised? Maybe seeing the bigger picture, I might have seen that and yielded. But I wanted to make the point. I didn't want to yield! I wanted to resist the autocracy that managers can always do what they want to do, to run rough-shod over everyone. I wanted my voice heard, even if it was a rebellious angry childish voice! But I see Chris's point.

Chris asks – how would a transformational leader respond? I say with integrity, assertively, seeking collaboration, treading the fine line between pushing the point and yielding. The theory spins from me (Johns 2004a). The difference was staying in adult mode rather than reacting and slipping into child mode. But yes, I was right to resist, simply on the basis that I had not been involved in the decision.

My demand to be heard and involved was transformational. It will change the organisation. See if I get my promotion or whether I am now tarred. Using Transactional Analysis (TA) (Stewart and Joines 1987) to position myself in relationship with the managers, I quickly became the child within the situation with the parent telling me what I was going to do.

TA is a way to view communication patterns from the different ego states of parent/ adult/child.

The ideal pattern is adult–adult based on rationality and responsibility. However, when someone becomes anxious they tend to flip into part or child mode as a way of managing their anxiety, leading to crossed lines of communication and communication breakdown unless the other person adjusts to accommodate. As Johns' (2004a) analysis of transactional systems illuminates, managers tend to be anxious and parental, and staff passive and compliant like children.

Although parent–child situations can at times be comforting, this situation became one of a critical response to a rebellious non-conforming child. Taylor and Singer (1983: 71) touched on this view when they discussed a bureaucratic organisation; they stated that a feature of such an organisation 'is that people should obey rules and should know their place'. However, they went on to say, 'contacts with staff in other departments are limited and these people are often seen as competitors for resources or even enemies who do not understand the difficulties and needs'.

Although I do not feel staff are always viewed as competitors and I do not believe this was the case in this situation, I *do* feel I was viewed as not understanding the organisation's needs as a whole, which went on to incite the parent-like attitude of the hospital administrator. If I had been approached in a collaborative way, then I feel certain a compromise would have been reached. I was trying to maintain a 'professional' or adult approach but the response was parental. My 'outrage' reflects my shift into a rebellious child digging in her heels against an overbearing parental attitude. When the pattern of communication is not reciprocated then lines literally become crossed and communication breaks down.

Once George had been placed on the ward my focus was on the staff as I felt I had let them down and allowed the ward to be placed in an unacceptable position. I saw myself as the parent, comforting and nurturing the staff around me, ensuring the staff remained focused on George and his needs and not the negative energy felt towards the situation that had occurred.

Dunham and Klafehn (1990) expressed the dilemma leaders can feel trying to show alliance to two separate groups who expect them to take two different forms of action. Although I had a feeling of guilt for not 'fixing' the situation, I feel that the staff around me showed me allegiance; they were disappointed but did not take the view that my action should have been any different. However, my self-esteem had taken a big knock.

I became accountable for the situation that had developed and I refocused on the position, trying to ensure no harm came to George and aiming to provide a good quality of care. I had an inner fear regarding the situation and the way my position had been viewed. I felt anxious and unconfident in my abilities; I had become a shell of the deputy ward manager who had started her shift. I was trying to save face with my staff and function as if the situation had never arisen.

> Anxiety is our biggest enemy; it holds us back, makes us doubt our worth and ability, makes us worry about losing approval. (Dickson 1982: 147)

I found myself within a coat of armour, protecting myself from possible further conflict from the ward staff. I was afraid of criticism from my colleagues for accepting George's admission. Instead of being impulsive and strong, I became concerned that I had placed us in an unacceptable position and the ward was at risk. All healthcare workers live out the daily tension of balancing what is therapeutic against what is safe. Perhaps practitioners err on the side of safety for fear of criticism if the people in their care come to some harm.

Klakovich (1994: 42) emphasised, 'to preserve the caring practice of the nursing profession in today's healthcare environment, a new leadership theory is needed'. Transactional leadership can have a damaging effect on caring values, which was the effect within my situation. Leadership roles should aim to enhance the caring values of the nursing team in order to gain and provide the optimum care available. Burns (1993), cited by Dunham and Klafehn (1990), felt this had been found in transformational leadership. However, following the work of Kerfoot (1996: 433) who talked of connective leaders as 'those who connect instead of conquer, collaborate rather than compete, entrust and empower rather than control, contribute rather than demand', I feel connective leadership could be the next stepping-stone up from transformational leadership.

Transformational leadership and connective leadership have many similar traits. However, connective leadership has its focus more closely on the 'preservation of care' (Klakovich 1994), nurturing and cultivating the caring attitude of the NHS alongside change management. Although transformational leadership acknowledges the importance of maintaining care, Klakovich (1994) believed there was still some emphasis on competition and conflict.

There are few comparisons made between the two leadership styles within the literature I obtained. This may be due to the fact that the styles are so similar that they are viewed as one and the same. So I propose, does the connective leader develop from a transformational leader through experience or possibly due to the human traits they already have? We can only wait and over the next few years this may become evident within the changing world of the NHS.

Reflecting on the conflict surrounding George's admission and the involvement of the chief executive has opened my eyes to the leadership styles involved. The hospital administrator approached the situation with a transactional leadership style, showing a dictorial attitude oozing negative vision. This clashed with the transformational leadership style with which I had approached the situation. I felt I needed to empower my vision on to my colleagues to allow us to approach the situation together and complete the task ahead. By visiting the ward late in the evening and not on an official timetable, the chief executive approached the situation (me?) using a connective leadership style. She expressed her understanding of my concerns and the needs of the organisation. She offered her support and acknowledged my dedication to my role; she expressed thanks to myself and my team for assisting in George's admission. She showed me warmth and empathy throughout our conversation. This created an uplift of my confidence and my self-esteem, maintaining and cultivating my caring attitude. She was bridging the gap between the organisational leaders and myself. When I shared this experience in guided reflection, Chris proposed that her action was like putting a Band-aid over a raw wound. I hadn't seen that perspective because I was in hurt-child mode and needed comforting. Chris's response in guided reflection puts doubt in my mind as to whether the chief executive was responding as a transformational or connective leader. Perhaps she is a clever politician. I must dwell more on that as I learn through reflection on new experiences. Dickson (1982) says:

> As women develop more familiarity with the skills, they learn how to be more reflective in situations instead of reacting only to the other person. Thinking and consequently acting with more clarity improves self-confidence at a deep and fundamental level; instead of muddling along, feeling generally burdened with worries and concerns, they learn to decide on priorities and to sort out who and what really does matter in their lives. (p159)

There I found myself in the big muddy puddle that exists within big organisations created by power plays, different agendas, breakdown in communication and unresolved conflict. The puddle gives off a bad atmosphere and creates a negative working environment.

What insights have I gained? Most significantly, to see the whole picture. As Senge (1990) poignantly states:

> If you can cut a photo in half, each half shows only part of the whole image. But if you divide a hologram, each part, no matter how small, shows the whole image intact. Likewise, when a group of people come to share a vision in an organisation, each person sees an individual picture of the organisation at its best ... the component pieces are not identical. Each represents the whole image from a different view ... When you add up all the pieces of a hologram ... the image becomes more intense. When more people come to share a vision, the vision becomes more real ... people can truly imagine achieving (the vision). (p212)

Only in seeing the whole picture can I see things for what they are. Becoming emotional, I lost sight and became defensive. Then I either fight or flight. To flight is to accommodate the demand. To fight leaves me beaten up, for the managers are more powerful. Neither is a good way. I must hold collaborative intent and hold my ground and then yield if I must because Rome wasn't built in a day. In this way I hold my poise and vision, and my integrity and do not need so many Band-aids! My little voice in a big arena becomes more powerful, yet powerful in a new transformational language. The leader inside me is unleashed.

Transformational tension

Sally reveals the contradiction or creative tension between two different worlds. On one hand, there is the dominant transactional world, characterised by high anxiety transmitted through its bureaucratic hierarchy, resulting in command and control tactics to ensure its targets are met. In such a culture, people are means towards reaching targets. The humanness factor is lost in the machine, reflected in Sally's metaphor of having only a 'little voice'. On the other hand, there is the transformational world that seeks to create the best environment for patients and staff. One is a machine world where people are a means to an end. The other is a world where humanness is valued. It is as stark as that.

Sally's writing is confessional, cathartic, resistant and empowering. Her reflection reveals the way power is exerted – notably the organisational *force* to have its way – dependent on its position on the ladder of command, with the threat of sanction if Sally dares to resist.

French and Raven (1968) offer a useful framework to reflect on the pattern of force/ power within any experience. They identify five sources of leadership power, either authoritative or facilitative (Fig. 15.2).

Perhaps you can sense the authoritative sources bearing down on Sally and feel the threat of sanction in the air if she resists. She didn't give way, she was simply brushed

Authoritative sources of leadership power Force (emphasised within transactional organisations)		Facilitative sources of leadership power Power (emphasised in transformational organisations)	
Positional (legitimate)	Based on the subordinate's perception that the leader has a right and authority to exercise influence because of the leader's role and position in the organisation	Relational (referent)	Based on the subordinate's identification with the leader. The leader exercises influence because of perceived attractiveness, personal characteristics, reputation or what is called 'charisma'
Coercive (sanction)	Based on fear and the subordinate's perception that the leader has the ability to punish or bring about undesirable outcomes	Expert	Based on the subordinate's perception of the leader as someone who has special knowledge in a given area
Reward	Based on the subordinate's perception that the leader has the ability and resources to obtain external rewards for those who comply with directives	Based on intrinsic rewards that ensue from shared success in realising one's vision of practice as a lived reality	

Figure 15.2 Leadership and sources of power (French and Raven 1968).

aside, leaving her bruised and hurt. But her integrity was intact, She held to her guns and her 'voice' was heard along distant corridors, prompting the chief executive's Band-aid response.

Sally's situation is not unusual. Indeed, it is a scenario played out daily across the healthcare arena, leaving nurse managers like Sally bruised and battered. The metaphor of a Band-aid is very apposite. The chief executive was like the nurturing parent coming to heal her child's wounds. When Sally was acknowledged and valued, it was immensely surprising and healing. Perhaps it should not be surprising. That only reflects the way Sally was perceived as a spanner in the works disrupting the system. At the moment she needed to be supported, she was made to feel more stressed.

It is significant to distinguish between force and power – force being used against someone to ensure control and power being used to create something, as with facilitative sources of leadership power. Sally found herself more powerful as a leader when she invested in collaborative relationships with her staff.

Susan writes: liberating to care

The 1990 NHS and Community Care Act placed on organisations the statutory duty to provide effective quality care. In response, NHS organisations have in recent years implemented a programme of clinical governance as a framework to fulfil this duty (Halligan and Donaldson 2001). Individual practitioners are expected and required by their employers to play an active part in such local clinical governance arrangements (Donaldson 2001). Nurses are particularly aware of their required commitment to the concept of lifelong learning and the statutory duty to maintain professional knowledge and competence (Department of Health 1999, Nursing and Midwifery Council 2002).

Garside (1999) notes a natural tension between the necessary regulatory and professional surveillance culture in the NHS and the equally necessary developmental elements of learning where innovation and risk are welcomed. Garside admits that this tension between regulation/surveillance and learning/development is unlikely to disappear, but she does suggest that they can co-exist.

My vision, as a transformational leader, is to create the learning organisation (Senge 1990) and synthesise the five technologies that constitute it: personal mastery, mental models, shared vision, team learning and systems thinking, as an integrated ensemble (see Box 2.2, p39). Senge describes the learning organisation as:

> One where people continually expand their capacities to create the results they truly desire, where new and expansive patterns of thinking are nurtured, where collective aspiration is set free, and where people are continually learning how to learn together. (p3)

Senge (1990) writes that the state of being a learning organisation never actually exists, since the more that is learnt, the more acutely aware we become of ignorance. Organisations are continually journeying and practising the disciplines of learning with varying degrees of success.

Whilst the desirability of the learning organisation appears incontrovertible, operationalising the concept is problematic. Statutory and regulatory documents seem to assume an innate desire in individuals to learn and indeed, Senge (1990) writes that not only is it our nature to learn but we love to learn. Such assumptions in the current conditions in the NHS may be difficult to support. The reality of today's NHS is that nurse shortages are reportedly reaching crisis point, establishment shortfall is nationally 20%, one-third of all nurses are allocated no study time, and bed occupancy is running at 98% (Hall 2003). In such an environment, Wall *et al* (1997) note that NHS staff suffer considerably more stress than any other workforce, with 28% recording levels above the symptom threshold. Further, few healthcare institutions can be described as learning organisations since, in a system largely dominated by highly structured, hierarchical and historically determined professional demarcations, it is an infrequent occurrence that norms or assumptions are challenged or that the required unlearning or relearning takes place (Garside 1999). The task of managing these tensions and inspiring and motivating people to learn and contribute to the learning organisation in such a difficult, highly pressurised arena is one that I, as a transformational leader, recognise as a considerable challenge.

Senge (1990) writes that organisations learn only through individuals who learn. Individual learning alone does not guarantee organisational learning but without it, no organisational learning occurs. Truly excellent organisations are those that know how to tap people's commitment and capacity to learn at *all* levels of the organisation and therefore a crucial element of the learning organisation is that it pays attention to the role and development of every individual within it. This clearly suggests that the effective transformational leader should display a natural tendency to develop others and facilitate learning wherever staff members sit in the hierarchy of the NHS organisation. Good leadership can influence an organisation to act as an effective learning organisation, one that is responsive and adaptive to changes both from within and without to build an environment for better, safer healthcare (Moss 2001).

Malby (1996) suggests that reflection can lead to new mental models about how to do things differently, and development of the skill of reflective practice has certainly enabled me to know myself more effectively, to frame and contextualise my own mental models and be more available to myself and others to realise desirable practice (Johns 2002). In the context of leading, supporting and developing the learning organisation, I would argue that unless I am truly available and knowing to self, transference of such availability would be problematic. My developed ability to clarify my own personal perspectives on values and ethics through reflective practice, combined with my understanding of the art and practice of the learning organisation, thus has implications for my transformational leadership capabilities within the context of organisational life and learning (Rippon 2001).

An organisation's capacity to learn can thus be no greater than that of its members, and my role as clinical supervisor should enable me to facilitate such individual learning that contributes to the cultural transformation of the organisation into one that embraces learning as praxis (Senge 1990). As Johns (2004a) identifies, clinical supervision explicitly intends to enable practitioners to realise, in collaboration with colleagues, each of the technologies that contribute to the learning organisation.

- To develop personal mastery
- To clarify and deepen our personal and collective visions of practice
- To scrutinise one's mental models and shift these towards realising effective practice
- To review and revise systems towards creating the optimum conditions for effective practice
- To develop dialogue expertise within supervision and practice situations to ensure effective practice
- To generate and sustain creative tension

Utilising the disciplines of the learning organisation as the aims of supervision offers a more coherent purpose for clinical supervision, in that it explicitly aims to establish a reflective culture.

The role of clinical supervision in the promotion of individual learning and the development of the learning organisation seems unquestionable, but many authors have written that its implementation may be fraught with difficulties. Cottrell (1999) notes that nurses' existing views of clinical supervision are all too often of a hostile, pseudo-analytic process of belittlement, criticism, shaming and the attribution of blame. The tensions between emancipatory and technical interests, particularly within bureaucratic cultures, have also been suggested (Johns 2001a). Johns (2001a) opines that the emancipatory, developmental and sustaining roles of clinical supervision will be diminished in any interpretation of clinical supervision as a technical consumer protection methodology. A mandatory clinical supervision agenda within an organisation may suggest surveillance and lead to fear of retaliatory action from managers, and evidence suggests that some nurses covertly seek supervision outside the mandatory provision in these circumstances (Scanlon and Weir 1997).

It seems, then, that though widely espoused by governmental and professional bodies and achieving a form of hegemony among some managers of the nursing profession, clinical practitioners have not embraced the concept with a similar enthusiasm (Bond and Holland 1998, Gilbert 2001). Further, while some research evidence indicating its effectiveness exists, it seems that empirical validation is fraught with epistemological and conceptual problems (Burrows 1995, Lyle 1998, Goorapah 1997).

My role as clinical supervisor within this apparently confused, indeterminate and possibly hostile arena appears loaded with complication. It is here that my skills of transformational leadership need to be clearly demonstrated if the clinical supervision agenda is to contribute to the development of the learning organisation through therapeutic interaction with another. Johns (2001a) notes how the intention and emphasis of the supervisor can determine the nature of the supervisory experience (see also p247).

Working within a transformational paradigm, I am acutely aware that I need to take shared ownership of the clinical supervision sessions that I facilitate (alongside the supervisee) with the consequence that I (we) are in control of clinical supervision rather than being controlled by it. Without such customisation and ownership, there is always the danger that clinical supervision and the intended learning may succumb to the transactional, manipulative, managerial and oppressive agenda that arguably constitutes the reality of the NHS today (Ghaye 2000a). Johns (2001a) poses a challenge when he asks whether clinical supervision can be accommodated to fit the existing culture or whether the existing culture can be shifted to the ideals of emancipatory supervision. For the transformational leader, a quite significant shift in the existing culture appears to be necessary. My desire is to promote and liberate learning from experience within the clinical supervision relationship (the emancipatory element) rather than the production of a worker who can be monitored against specific criteria of what constitutes effectiveness (the technical element). This will hopefully contribute to the development of the learning organisation: one that is holistic, flexible, responsible, proactive and caring and in which contradictions between values and practices are identified and resolved (Johns 2003b, Senge 1990).

I have acted as clinical supervisor for almost 2 years within an advisory clinical supervision system in my current workplace. The organisation provides no formal training or support for clinical supervisors, which suggests that while it embraces the concept of clinical governance publicly, it may be covertly resisting the idea of clinical supervision as an emancipatory learning process for the organisation, since it may perceive it as a threat to established patterns of relating (Johns 2003b). There seems no reciprocal agreement between the individual willing to learn through such supervision and the current organisational culture. While commitment is currently lacking and interpretation and introduction of clinical supervision in my own organisation are minimal, future policy directives may mean that clinical supervision will become a 'must do' in the future (Bond and Holland 1998). My role as a transformational leader will be of critical importance once clinical supervision becomes mandatory within my organisation and I am hoping to influence the clinical supervision agenda, at least in my own work area, toward the emancipatory rather than the technical ideal.

I have been Sarah's clinical supervisor for 6 months. Sarah is a junior staff nurse on another ward and therefore outside the scope of my managerial authority. Our supervisor/supervisee relationship is mutually agreed and voluntary. Many authors write that reflective practice for both the supervisor and supervisee is intimately bound up with the process of clinical supervision (Ghaye 2000b, Heath and Freshwater 2000, Power 1999). Johns (2003a) describes guided reflection as a way of structuring the clinical supervision space and such reflective practice can aid the development of the learning organisation with great potential to leverage quality and effective practice (Garside 1999).

The following discussion and illumination of recent clinical supervision sessions will explore my role in Sarah's learning and demonstrates my commitment to contribute to the emergence of the spirit of the learning organisation (Senge 1990). I had tacitly (and possibly naively) assumed that Sarah did not feel that I was monitoring her clinical performance since we do not work together but reflected recently that Sarah and I have never discussed or clarified this aspect of our relationship. Perhaps this demonstrates my lack of knowledge at the time when we commenced the clinical relationship since I now recognise clearly the need to develop formal contracts with supervisees to clarify roles and meaning in the relationship if learning is to occur (Bond and Holland 1998). I remained undecided about the accuracy of my assumption regarding Sarah's perception (although I had intended to discuss it with her) until the following incident occurred.

It was the end of a clinical supervision session in which a completely unrelated issue concerning drug administration was discussed. As Sarah got up to leave the room, she made some comments which, at the time, appeared almost inconsequential to her but which caused me deep reflection.

Sarah: 'Well, I'd better get back to the ward now. It's not that I don't want to or that I don't care but I just find it so difficult to look after people like Mary with her dementia. She can't do anything for herself – she just lies there all day without doing anything or saying anything to anyone, not even her husband or family. I never feed her – I can't bear it. I always get the healthcare assistants to do it. I can't help feeling that I don't like that sort of nursing – it's so unrewarding but I'd never tell anyone else that, it doesn't seem right, does it?'

Sarah and I parted company without further comment being made. I was immediately concerned that, in 6 months of supervising Sarah, I had not encountered such a forthright expression of attitude from her that I instantly felt so uncomfortable with. I was, however, aware that the prevalence of negative attitudes toward the care of older people among the nursing profession is widely reported (Courtney *et al* 2000, Wade 1999). It seemed that although Sarah sensed a real tension between her professional role requirement and her personal feelings, she felt comfortable enough to express them to me. This signified that she did not see me in a surveillance role but my instant reaction was to feel transactional, with the desire to confront Sarah about her poor performance and attitude, as

I perceived it. However, I recognised that such a stance may change the nature of our supervisory relationship and prove a stumbling block to learning in an unthreatening environment in the future. A further concern of mine was that Sarah's honest expression perhaps signified that she felt I would have no concerns about her statement and possibly shared her opinions, which I did not. I considered previous clinical supervision sessions. Had Sarah and I suffered a learning bind where we had previously missed each other's meaning in the interpretation of our practice and values? Schön (1987) suggests that the ability to escape from such a learning bind depends on the supervisor's ability to reflect on the supervisor– supervisee dialogue and this I did extensively prior to the next session.

When Sarah arrived for her next supervision session I asked her if she would like to talk about Mary, since she seemed to find caring for her difficult. Sarah's immediate agreement signified that this was indeed something that she wished to share. I was acutely aware of the need to suspend my own values and assumptions in order to avoid a trans-actional, technical interest intention in the supervision sessions. I consciously worked hard to manage the creative tensions that existed for me between my own vision of what nursing should be and where I currently saw Sarah's practice and attitudes (Senge 1990). If we assume that the effective practitioner takes responsibility to ensure and monitor their own effectiveness then the role of the supervisor is not to sit in judgement but to enable the practitioner to make such judgements for herself (Johns 2001a). However, within clinical supervision there needs to be an element of challenge but this needs to be managed carefully to avoid a spiral of increasing challenge from the supervisor and resultant increasing resistance from the supervisee (Heath and Freshwater 2000, Smith 2000). I introduced Sarah to the Model of Structured Reflection (MSR) (see p51) as a way of focusing self challenge and to structure her deconstruction of her experiences in order to lead to new insights that could be applied to her practice.

Sarah and I discussed the issues at length and some of her comments were very illuminating.

Sarah: 'Lots of old people get dementia, don't they? I wonder what causes it and if it runs in families? My Grandma had it when I was little. She used to scare me and she didn't even seem to know who I was. I remember her wetting my Mum's settee one Christmas and my Dad got really cross and shouted at her. She ended up in a home and I don't remember seeing her after that. It's frightening to think anyone could end up like that.'

Guided by the MSR, Sarah and I discussed the origin and influence of her mental models at length and explored how they influenced her practice (Senge 1990). Sarah felt she knew nothing about dementia but thought perhaps that she should. She asked if I could recommend anything for her to read. While mindful of the need to avoid the perception that I had greater skills or knowledge than Sarah (often detrimental in the clinical supervision relationship since it may suggest supervisor authority), I provided her with some relevant references without offering any opinion on their value (Power 1999). Sarah left the session professing a determination to think about our discussion and visit the library for more information.

When Sarah attended her next supervision it quickly became obvious that she had reflected quite deeply on our session, undertaken some personal learning and reading and had applied this to her practice. She related her recent experience to me.

Sarah: 'I've got to know Mary and Bill and they seem a really nice couple. Do you know Bill was telling me that during the war he didn't see Mary at all for 3 years. All that time she was looking after their little girl and working in a factory making aircraft parts and at night she did fire watching. That must have been so hard for her. Bill said

Mary loved dancing and really missed it when the arthritis got so bad. I've seen photos of them in dance competitions and she looks lovely with her hair and make-up all done.'

Sarah continued with Mary and Bill's life story which signified that she now recognised and valued their personhood. I asked Sarah if she felt more able to nurse Mary now and Sarah confirmed that she was happily taking a more active role in caring for Mary on a daily basis.

Sarah: 'I think I was scared before because I didn't understand what was happening to Mary but I knew that I didn't feel right about the way I acted. Reading those articles you gave me and talking to my Mum about my own Grandma when she was young made me think that perhaps I'd missed something. It was only when I started to talk to Bill that I realised I'd been avoiding him and Mary. She had been a patient with us for 2 weeks and I knew nothing about her! I've noticed other people acting the same as I did and perhaps I can do something about that. I feel like a better nurse now and I've joined the Care of the Older Person Link Group. I might even go and do a course or something.'

To me, Sarah's most significant statement came at the end of our session – again just as she was leaving the room.

Sarah: 'Thanks a lot – I feel better about it all now and I've learnt a lot but I need to think about things a bit more, don't I? I'm using that *(reflective)* model you gave me now and writing things down. See you next time!'

Through the learning process, Sarah had achieved some control of the creative tension that existed, where the current reality of her practice did not match the vision of her nursing care that she professed to hold. In this way, she had enhanced her own sense of personal mastery and now felt a 'better nurse' (Senge 1990). She had re-examined her vision for nursing and now felt she shared and lived the vision of nursing as a profession. She had surfaced and challenged the mental models that influenced her understanding of the issues through an engagement of self with self-awareness and had accepted an internal locus of self-control and responsibility for her own actions – the heart of professional practice (Heath and Freshwater 2000). Sarah's personal learning had highlighted other learning needs within her team and she had resolved to join a group dedicated to learning about the care of older people and to share this with others. Senge (1990) describes such team learning as vital since teams, not individuals, are the fundamental learning unit in modern organisations.

A transformational approach means that I had avoided the transactional, technical interest intention of clinical supervision where monitoring, surveillance and a focus on role performance are evident. Rather, the transformational skills of effective communication, honesty and empathy, development of others and risk taking, experimentation and learning were all utilised to ensure that Sarah was guided on her own emancipatory learning journey of self-awareness and discovery (Schuster 1994). Sarah is clearly only one person in a very large organisation – one who is not currently particularly in tune with the concept of the learning organisation, and her learning may appear insignificant to some in the larger picture. Yet, organisations learn only through individuals who learn – people like Sarah, a junior staff nurse (Senge 1990).

The NHS has a long history of firmly established traditions and authoritarian practices. A cultural transformation will arguably be necessary if organisational learning which embraces new and expansive patterns of thinking, leading to real service-wide quality improvements, is to be developed (Senge 1990). It would seem that contributing to the emergence of a learning organisation from the current cultural stance poses a considerable challenge and requires real determination from the transformational healthcare practitioner/leader of today. For the transformational leader, the spirit of learning and enquiry is ever-present and my contribution and commitment to the learning of both myself and others are a key aspect of my role, since the active force of any learning organisation must be the people who work there.

Finally, my own sense of personal mastery has developed through this work, since I am aware that both Sarah and I have contributed to the learning organisation. We have created a more effective practice environment by working through an experience, identifying areas for growth, and generating the learning needed to achieve positive results.

Reflection

Susan's narrative reflects the way she and Sarah were transformed through guided reflection or clinical supervision. She sets out the markers of the learning organisation to gauge her own transformation through the technology of clinical supervision. Whilst Sarah set the agenda, Susan's own values are clearly evident, reflecting the way practitioners are unwittingly shaped by the supervisor's horizons. This is not problematic when transparent. These ideas are picked up in the next chapter.

Using the dialogue Susan recorded following each clinical supervision session, she draws the reader into the text. Dialogue gives the narrative immediacy, authenticity and vibrancy. This is in contrast with Sally's narrative that lacks dialogue. Although Sally's narrative is compelling, using dialogue may have helped heighten the tension within it. I must admit that in my editing, I introduced some present tense into Sally's narrative, mixing the tenses to create a greater sense of drama unfolding. The use of tenses gives the narrative an interplay between reflecting back and reflecting within – techniques to draw the reader into the text.

Susan described herself as a rational person. I feel this is reflected in the text with its singular lack of reference to her feelings that gives the text a certain coldness and detachment. In contrast, Sally's text is centred in her outrage – exemplifying how feelings create conflict and drama.

Both narratives lack metaphor and images that might be useful to extenuate and hold meaning, creating a more *visual* text. Lack of metaphor and images reflects a lack of writer's imagination and makes for a less engaging text. Perhaps they did not dwell long enough in the text or felt restrained writing for an academic assignment, having previously learnt that rationality earns more credit than imagination.

In my experience, the more visual the text, the more readers seem to be present within the situation. Sally uses the metaphor of 'Band-aid' – a word I had used with her in guided reflection. Her self-description as a 'naughty school girl' helps to create an image that captures the reader's attention and imagination.

Conclusion

I have used two narratives written by Sally and Susan as examples of developing clinical leadership. A reflective leadership would seem vital for creating reflective environments, within clinical practice, the boardroom or the educational curriculum.

These narratives, like Lazell's (Chapter 14), were written at Masters level. Do you perceive a difference in the scope of reflective writing compared with the undergraduate efforts of Jill, Simon, Jim and Clare through Chapters 9–12? I sense a less descriptive and greater critical depth in the Masters work grounded in insights gained from the reflective process.

Of course, making comparison begs the question – how should reflective writing be judged academically? I have previously set out some criteria for judging the coherence of narrative (Chapter 5) and explore this further in Chapters 18 and 19. In Chapter 16 I pursue the ideas of the learning organisation and clinical supervision.

Chapter 16

Clinical supervision and nurturing the learning organisation

Bumping heads

I am always reminded of the story in Winnie-the-Pooh (Milne 1926: 1) when Edward bear, being pulled along by Christopher Robin, bumps his head all the way down the stairs. Milne suggests that this is the only way Edward bear knows to come downstairs but if he could only stop bumping to consider it, he might just find a better way. In this story (or honey pot) we find the essence of reflective practice – creating space to pause and think about what is happening, why it is happening and ways it might change for the better, yet realising that both creating space and affecting change may be difficult because we are locked into patterns of behaviour and relationships. But then we might not find a better way, recognising that things are not so easily changed. Perhaps it is easier to conform and take painkillers for the sore head!

Clinical supervision offers a legitimate space within clinical practice to stop bumping and consider other, more effective and desirable ways to practise, including our relationships with the Christopher Robins of this world; that is, unless Christopher Robin decides to supervise us – then we have some difficulty.

Revealing woozles

A different, altogether more positive image of Christopher Robin is found later in the book when Pooh and Piglet go hunting and nearly catch a woozle. Piglet joins Pooh as he is walking and round the tree 'thinking of something else'. As they do, they become aware of their own tracks but misinterpret the tracks, thinking that it might be woozles. Round and round the tree they go, becoming increasingly anxious until Christopher Robin, who is sitting up the tree observing, points out to Pooh what he is doing. Pooh realises what has been happening and exclaims that he has been foolish and deluded.

In this story, Christopher Robin might be a guide helping Pooh to see things as they really are and to reassure Pooh. He doesn't tell Pooh what to think or do but points out

Pooh's flawed thinking. Often we get so caught up in things 'on the ground' that we miss the bigger picture, and lose track and panic. We feel stupid, get fearful and beat ourselves up. We all get things wrong from time to time. A guide can help the practitioner put things into perspective and after all, there are more important things … like luncheon!

What might woozles represent?

Clinical supervision

In the previous chapter, Susan reflected on developing her transformational leadership through clinical supervision. In the *Vision for the future* document, the NHSME (1993) sets out 10 key objectives for nursing into the 21st century. One objective was developing clinical leadership. Another was developing clinical supervision, defined as:

> a formal process of professional support and learning which enables individual practitioners to develop knowledge and competence, assume responsibility for their own practice and enhance consumer protection and safety of care in complex situations. It is central to the process of learning and to the expansion of the scope of practice and should be seen as a means of encouraging self-assessment and analytical and reflective skills. (p3)

The NHSME's clinical supervision agenda was a reaction for greater professional accountability or put more sinisterly, surveillance to give the public confidence that nurses' and health visitors' practice was being monitored. Midwives already have a form of mandatory supervision although the clinical supervision agenda created by the Department of Health indicates a more robust approach.

The NHSME's design for clinical supervision was strongly influenced by a psychotherapy and counselling model of supervision reflecting the backgrounds of the authors of a government-commissioned paper (Faugier and Butterworth, undated).

The definition of clinical supervision suggests five key aims:

- to develop practitioner competence
- to sustain practitioner competence
- to safeguard standards of care
- to promote practitioner responsibility (for ensuring effective performance)
- to promote self-assessment (judgement of own performance).

On the surface these aims may seem contradictory. On one hand, the intention of clinical supervision is to open a learning space for practitioners to develop and sustain competence. On the other hand, clinical supervision also suggests a surveillance system to safeguard the public against standards of care. What are these standards? If they exist, then whose standards are they? Who will making the judgement? To view clinical supervision as a learning opportunity, I would need to feel safe to reveal any aspect of my practice. If I considered that my clinical supervisor's agenda was to judge my performance then I might be cautious about revealing my experiences, especially those that exposed my practice as problematic.

The contradiction is mediated, at least in my view, with the intention of clinical supervision to enable practitioners to develop responsibility to reflect on and monitor their own performance within a performance model of professional development.

The learning organisation

In her reflection, Susan implemented clinical supervision as a technology towards realising the learning organisation. To recap, Senge (1990: 3) describes the learning organisation as:

> One where people continually expand their capacities to create the results they truly desire, where new and expansive patterns of thinking are nurtured, where collective aspiration is set free, and where people are continually learning how to learn together.

Inspiring words that also reflect transformational values, reflected in the way Susan translated the aims of clinical supervision into the language of the learning organisation:

- to develop personal mastery
- to clarify and deepen our personal and collective visions of practice
- to scrutinise one's mental models and shift these towards realising effective practice
- to review and revise systems towards creating the optimum conditions for effective practice
- to develop dialogue expertise within supervision and practice situations to ensure effective practice.

Perhaps the most significant of these aims is developing personal mastery – the art of holding and working towards resolving creative tension between a vision of desirable practice and an understanding of current reality. Or in other words, reflective practice. The other aims flow from personal mastery.

A quiet eddy

Imagine clinical practice as a fast-moving river. In the 'busyness' of the day, many practitioners feel they are being swept along in the current, reacting to events as they unfold about them. Clinical supervision is like an eddy within the fast-flowing water that enables the practitioner to pause and observe what goes on in the river. In this way, the practitioner may prepare herself to practise more effectively when she re-enters the current and not be so swept along. The eddy is still part of the dynamic harmony of events, it is not time out from the river itself. Yet the current is strong and the ability to find the eddy requires vision, effort and resolve. The eddy must be seen as a desirable place because the current will not let you go too easily.

Contracting

Clinical supervision needs to be contracted as a formal relationship. Proctor (1988) cited by Hawkins and Shohet (1989: 29), notes that:

> If supervision is to become and remain a co-operative experience which allows for real rather than token accountability, a clear, even tough, working agreement needs to be negotiated. The agreement needs to provide sufficient safety and clarity for the student/worker to know where

she stands; and it needs sufficient teeth for the supervisor to feel free and responsible for making the challenges.

In establishing a clinical supervision relationship, the supervisor and practitioner must always agree on their positive intention to work together within a set of mutual expectations, responsibilities and boundaries. Such issues include differentiating supervision from therapy work, maintaining confidentiality (especially in relation to reporting of unsafe practice), writing and storing notes, termination, pattern of meetings and preparing for each session, which should all be discussed and agreed; for example, the expectation that the practitioner brings at last one experience to share that she has reflected on.

Distinction needs to be made between clinical supervision work and what might be construed as therapy. To some extent, the two issues will overlap. For example, in exploring her feelings about the death of a patient, a practitioner also explores her feelings about her own mother's death. Perhaps, in responding to her anger towards her manager, the practitioner notes that 'he acts like my father'. The astute supervisor will point out the association and transference, but should keep the dialogue focused on the practice event. Clearly, a lot more can be said about dynamics, such as transference and counter-transference, that are beyond the scope of this text. Whilst in principle the agenda should always be set by the practitioner, the supervisor has an agenda to ensure that supervision is developmental.

Four variables of clinical supervision

- Voluntary or mandatory
- Group versus individual supervision
- Single or multiprofessional
- Line managed or non-line managed

Voluntary or mandatory

Should supervision be mandatory or voluntary? What is your gut reaction? Why is that?

My view leans towards a voluntary arrangement because practitioners, who have generally been socialised into subordinate work roles, are likely to view supervision as a form of social control and surveillance (Gilbert 2001) and not as a developmental opportunity, especially if the supervisor is the line manager.

Given that practitioners need to be able to grow and take responsibility for their own performance, then mandatory supervision might create these conditions with non-line management supervisors, as illuminated by Susan in her reflection.

Supervision is promoted as a professional activity rather than a managerial activity and yet clinical supervision is always (in my experience) a top-down organisational approach with very little resource attached to it. How is time created within practice to accommodate supervision when nurses are already stretched? What is intended to ease stress may well contribute to it. Nurses seem reluctant to use their 'own time', as if work is confined to shifts, reflecting a lack of responsibility to ensure their own effective performance. This itself reflects a lack of value in nursing – that it isn't worth investing in.

I wonder why nurses are unable to arrange their own supervision within practice as a professional activity to help them stay 'fit for practice'. Supervision notes are an excellent way to demonstrate professional development. Consider you own attitude to clinical supervision – would this benefit you?

Mark on the line below how positive or negative you feel about supervision.

Positive _____ Negative

What factors influence your mark?

Group versus individual supervision

There are advantages for both individual and group supervision. In groups, although practitioners have less 'air' time, they can relate to the experiences shared by other members of the group. This may benefit less vocal or reticent practitioners who feel threatened by individual supervision. Many practitioners say they learn more by listening and relating to others' experiences than they do by sharing their own. In groups there are more diverse views and more support for practitioners, especially if others do relate to their experiences. However, people can feel more vulnerable sharing their experiences in groups. As such, groups may take longer to gel and create a safe environment, moving through forming norms. Groups should be limited to no more than six people. Groups are also prone to irregular attendance which makes group norming more difficult. Groups that are based on practitioners who work together may feel very vulnerable about sharing experiences that criticise other group members – constructing social norms within the group to ensure maximum comfort. The group guide will need to be experienced with group dynamics to counter game playing. Perhaps under these conditions, groups need a more concrete focus, for example clinical audit.

Both individual and group supervision have considerable advantages and perhaps a mixture of both might be ideal. Despite the forming difficulties of work-based group supervision, I do think that they foster collaborative teamwork, shared vision, team learning, mutual support, role responsibility and quality – all advantages over individual supervision.

Single or multiprofessional

Is single profession (e.g. nursing) better than multiprofessional supervision? In groups I have facilitated, I have observed how normal power structures, for example between nurses and doctors, get played out within supervision, thus reinforcing professional norms that subordinate nurses. Given training in supervision skills, I think peer-led small group supervision is a good model.

To be line managed or non-line managed

My own career as a clinical supervisor commenced in 1989 at Burford Hospital, although at the time I termed it *guided reflection* and subsequently *professional supervision* (Johns 1993). I viewed supervision as an ideal model for clinical leadership. With hindsight, I recognised that practitioners never discussed experiences concerning myself, illuminating that even with collaborative intent and collaborative role modelling, the practitioner still

Table 16.1 Potential advantages of non-line management supervision (incorporating potential advantages and disadvantages of line management supervision)

Potential advantages	Potential disadvantages
When supervisor is chosen by practitioner, it gives a greater sense of control/reduces fear of anxiety about judgement	Many issues the practitioner shares may involve the manager (and hence might have been dealt with at the time). However, these may not have been shared with the manager!
Supervisor likely to be more objective, see things more broadly when outside the situation (less likely to have a practice agenda)	The supervisor does not know the practitioner's practice or have expert knowledge (however, knowledge is not necessarily a good thing because it may lead to partial views, especially if the manager is transactional/overly concerned with the practitioner's performance ('fix it' and 'hurt child' syndromes)
More professional role in line with the ethos of professional responsibility and clearly differentiated from management – therefore less outcome focused or remedial with less risk of manager/supervisor imposing an agenda	Unable to link with practice role as clinical leader and using supervisory relationship to develop collaborative ways of relating in everyday practice rather than be confined within the supervision bubble
The supervisor is more likely to have an emancipatory rather than a technological orientation	Availability and cost of appropriate external supervisors

viewed me with caution. This insight was a revelation, illuminating the way practitioners are socialised into subordinate and oppressive transactional type relationships that are not easily overthrown. Such ways of being have become deeply embodied.

Would practitioners have benefitted more from non-line supervision? A vexing conundrum.

Analysis of supervision dialogue (Johns 1998a, Johns & McCormack 1998) revealed a number of advantages and disadvantages with both line and non-line management supervision. I have summarised these in Table 16.1. Similar advantages and disadvantages may apply to all authoritative supervision relationship such as teacher-student relationships.

Emancipatory or technical supervision

There is a tension between an *emancipatory* and a *technical* approach to guided reflection depending on the intent and emphasis of the guide or supervisor (Johns 2001a). The technical and emancipatory are two of the knowledge-constituted interests as conceived by Jurgen Habermas (1984). The emancipatory is knowing that seeks to liberate people to fulfil their desires. The technical is knowing that seeks to shape people towards performing specific activities competently. Of course, both types of knowledge interests are significant. Ideally guidance relationships are negotiated in which both the guide and learner surface their agendas and agree a mutual path that serves both interests. This is Habermas's *communicative* knowledge interest, a mediating type of knowing.

The 'technical' supervisor sets and manipulates the agenda to produce their view of an effective practitioner. The 'emancipatory' supervisor helps the practitioner set and

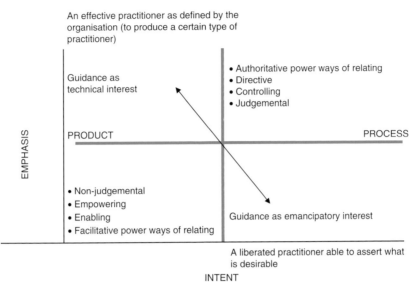

INTENT

An effective practitioner as defined by the
organisation (to produce a certain type of
practitioner)

- Authoritative power ways of relating
- Directive
- Controlling
- Judgemental

Guidance as
technical interest

EMPHASIS

PRODUCT   PROCESS

- Non-judgemental
- Empowering
- Enabling
- Facilitative power ways of relating

Guidance as emancipatory interest

A liberated practitioner able to assert what
is desirable

INTENT

Figure 16.1 The intent–emphasis scale (Johns 2001a).

fulfil her own agenda. It is controversial whether 'technical' supervision can be described as supervision because it is manipulative and yet it fits within the transactional culture that characterises NHS organisations. In other words, because this approach is normal, it is not recognised as manipulative.

This tension can be plotted along an emancipatory–technical axis (Fig. 16.1). Susan claimed an emancipatory stance, viewing supervision as a process to enable Sarah to set the pattern of experience and development. Her agenda was grounded in Sarah's best interests. Significantly she was not in an organisational management relationship with Sarah. The emancipatory approach is easier when not in a line-management relationship simply because the manager tends to be less anxious about the supervisee's performance.

Reflection always intends to be emancipatory, enabling the person to become who they desire to be. That is the primary agenda. Otherwise it becomes a manipulative or perverse form of reflection, where the focus of reflection is set by the guide. Then it cannot be called reflection; it is something else.

So, depending on their emphasis within the guidance relationship, the technical and emancipatory approaches can lead to very different outcomes. An emancipatory stance would intend to liberate the practitioner to pursue her best interests, whilst a technical stance would intend to shape the practitioner to conform to some ideal as imagined by the guide or supervisor. One is essentially liberating, whilst the other is essentially oppressive. However, as I revealed, people who might claim an emancipatory intent often responded from a technical perspective because of embodied ways of being. In other words, they lived a contradiction that was very obvious in their performance as guides. This was particularly evident when the guide had strong values and a vested interest in the other's performance, for example as a teacher or manager.

It is perhaps obvious that guides who lean towards the technical are more outcome focused and tend to use more authoritative patterns of communication whereas guides who lean towards the emancipatory are more process focused and tend to use more facilitative patterns of communication.

Supervisors will never perform effectively if they are anxious about the practitioner's performance, a characteristic of transactional organisations. Anxious people need to control their environments in order to manage their anxiety. Anxiety about outcomes and quality tends to be transmitted down through the system level by level, infecting the workforce. Unit leaders know that they are held to account for what takes place on their units rather than individual practitioners. In the attempt to control this anxiety, unit leaders try to control their environments by responding in parental patterns. The effect is to impose conformity and stifle responsibility. This would be ironic as supervision has the specific aim of nurturing responsibility. The risk is that supervision is viewed in the old sense of the word as ensuring a competent yet docile workforce (Foucault 1979).

There is a real tension between supervision being promoted as a professional activity to benefit individual practitioners yet being implemented as an organisational quality tool – a tension played out along the continuum drawn in the intent–emphasis grid. If you are a supervisee, where do you place your supervisor? If you are a supervisor, where do you place yourself?

Clinical supervision must always be emancipatory, yet how realistic or ethical is it to promote emancipatory action within systems that clearly resist practitioner autonomy to act on new insights to create the conditions where desirable practice can be realised? Is supervision at the level of emancipatory action no more than a furtive subculture of idealism? Do we end up playing in the safe shallow end, afraid of drowning if we step out of our depth where the obstacles of authority, tradition and embodiment wait to snare us (Fay 1987)? Yet even in the shallow end, practitioners do become empowered to act on insights and shift practice for the better.

Despite my emancipatory intent, the fact that practitioners at Burford Hospital did not reveal experiences that involved me was startling. Did the power of bureaucratic socialisation mean that they feared raising issues of potential conflict? I became aware of this dynamic when I commenced guiding people outside my own practice when issues of conflict with management were frequently reflected on.

I suspect that if the practitioner senses any threat she will only reveal 'safe' experiences. If so, both the spirit and intent of supervision will be lost. It will be a sham, a game being played out that consumes time and fosters suspicion. It is the worse image of the 'confessional' (Gilbert 2001) – that the practitioner is expected to confess her 'sins' and will receive guidance and absolution. Under conditions of trust, the confession is an opportunity to reveal and learn through difficult experiences toward realising desirable practice.

With trust, a real advantage of authoritative guidance is the guide and practitioner working together to resolve situations whereas as an external guide, I find myself saying to the practitioner 'You need to explore this with your manager or teacher'.

Peer-led supervision

Considering the previous exploration of who the supervisor should be, my preferred model for clinical supervision is peer group supervision where each person in the group becomes a skilled guide. This approach is desirable because it facilitates a collaborative approach to practice, where practitioners work together towards realising a shared vision, and where each practitioner accepts responsibility for both her own performance and for the group as a whole. As such, it is the most professional model, although as with all 'ideal models', it is subject to domination and abuse.

Laura, a speech and language therapist, shares her experience of an integrated service meeting around a client's experience. Other therapists in the group give her feedback about what they consider as significant. Laura processes and synthesises this information with her own identified significances. With each MSR reflective cue (see Chapter 3) this synthesis continues. Eventually the group considers how Laura might respond more significantly given the situation again. Laura again processes this information against her own views, exploring with the group these alternatives and factors that might prevent her responding in new, potentially more effective ways in tune with the group's vision of practice. Throughout this process the other therapists relate to Laura's experience in terms of their own experiences. It is a rich collaborative learning experience that contributes to developing a learning organisation.

Qualities of the ideal supervisor

What are the qualities of the ideal supervisor? In Box 16.1 I set out some qualities identified with supervisors at UCLH in September 2001. These may help the would-be supervisee to choose a supervisor.

Despite many apparent advantages to line management supervision, I would generally advocate non-line management supervision, although my preference is a peer-led approach. However, the bottom line is the supervisee's preference, acknowledging that clinical supervision is relational. However, I know organisations that impose patterns of supervision which deny the practitioner the option of choosing whether to enter supervision, who might be their supervisor and the mode of supervision (i.e. group or individual) and insist on auditing the outcomes by requiring notes to be made of each supervision session – all, in my view, against the ethos of supervision being a professional model of development.

In principle, practitioners have the right to choose their own supervisor, although this is often logistically difficult. Who are these supervisors? Are they adequately prepared for such roles? Choice may be limited for multiple organisational issues and a compromise may have to be negotiated, yet always within the spirit of supervision.

Box 16.1   Qualities of a clinical supervisor. Who would you want as your supervisor?

Strong sense of vision and purpose about supervision	Authentic/honest	Shares my clinical background
Listener	Open/transparent	Someone who doesn't know me
Challenger	Committed to the supervision relationship	Someone who I feel comfortable with
Non-judgemental	Concerned	Someone who I'm attracted to
I can trust	Compassionate	Someone who I'm not dependent on
Mutual respect	Experienced at reflection and supervision	Someone who I'm not accountable to
Older and wiser	Dynamic and powerful (not over me)	Empathic

Heron's six-category intervention analysis

In the intent–emphasis scale I noted that supervisors with emancipatory intent use more facilitative responses whereas supervisors with technical intent use more authoritative responses. This stems from six-category intervention analysis (Heron 1975) which proposes six basic therapeutic interventions used therapeutically in response to the client or supervisee.

The emphasis is on therapeutic intent and response. Heron contrasts therapeutic with manipulative and perverse type interventions where the practitioner abuses the responses to meet their own agendas. Of course, this would also apply within clinical supervision. The skilled practitioner chooses the most appropriate response to suit the situation, moving easily between each response as appropriate.

In using these interventions, within both clinical practice and clinical supervision, I follow a therapeutic pattern.

When an underlying emotion is sensed, use a *cathartic* response: 'Mavis, you seem angry at Joy'. Or 'Are you happy sharing a room with a male patient?'. The intention is to release and surface the emotion so it can be dealt with. At this level practitioners may fear releasing the emotion because they do not know how to respond to it.

Then, use a *catalytic* response to help the person talk through the issues with the intention of helping them find meaning in their feelings, and by talking through them, to understand deeper underlying reasons for their feelings. In this way the practitioner is helped to release negative energy and begin to convert it to positive energy for taking action.

Confrontation can then be used to challenge, yet always within a supportive framework.

Information can be given but I am always wary of giving advice because it is taking responsibility for the other person. Much better to say 'What options do you have?' rather than 'I would do this', even for novice practitioners who seek direction. When I do think it is appropriate to give advice, I say 'I am going to give you advice' and imagine I have a neon sign over my head that says 'Giving advice' to remind me that this is a power intervention and to remind the supervisee to take it with caution.

Confrontation is always easier when a trusting relationship has been developed because the patient knows you care for them. Evidence exists suggesting that nurses avoided using

Table 16.2 Six-category intervention analysis

Authoritative type responses	Facilitative type responses
Giving information Enabling the other to make a rational decision	*Being cathartic* Enabling the other to express some emotion
Giving advice Helping another see other, better ways of understanding and doing things	*Being catalytic* Enabling the other to talk through an issue
Confrontation Challenging the other's restrictive attitudes, beliefs or behaviour	*Being supportive* Communicating a sense of 'being there' for the other

confrontational, cathartic and catalytic responses, prefering to use giving information, giving advice and being supportive (Burnard and Morrison 1991). These researchers noted that using confrontational, cathartic and catalytic responses involved 'an investment of self which may be emotionally draining for the practitioner'. Nurses are generally not prepared for this type of emotional labour (James 1989). James concluded that this type of work was not valued and therefore not taught, being seen as a natural extension of women's work. Without doubt, working with patients and families is emotional work and, as James (1989) revealed, it is highly skilled. To be an effective practitioner requires the ability and confidence to engage in emotional work, even if it is personally threatening.

Sloan and Watson (2001) distinguish between process and outcome models of supervision. They argue for a process approach based on the work of Heron (1975) and cite my own work as an example of such an approach. Whilst I do emphasise a process approach, I am also mindful that supervision is purposeful towards realising specific outcomes.

Modes of supervision

Another significant process is the balance of high challenge with high support. This leads to growth (Fig. 16.2).

High challenge/low support can create considerable anxiety for the supervisee and ultimately leads to burnout. People do not learn well under situations of high anxiety. High support/low challenge leads to comfort work. This learning milieu may be appropriate for a short time when supervisees disclose experiences of stress but even then challenge is appropriate if thick trust (i.e. trust that is well developed and secure, in contrast to 'thin trust' which is fragile and easily broken (Cope 2001)) has been established. Under conditions of trust, the supervisee knows that even when highly challenged the supervisor remains supportive.

Low support/low challenge leads to apathy. This is probably the predominant mode of development within transactional organisations, reflecting a focus on outcomes and not investment in process.

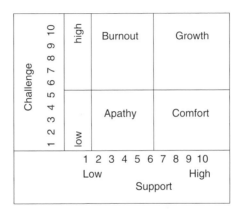

Figure 16.2 Challenge–support axis.

Score yourself and ask your supervisees to score you. Do you get into the high challenge/high support quadrant? Use the grid reflexively as a developmental marker until you consistently hit 9/10 for both challenge and support.

The nine step model

In my efforts to understand the supervision process I developed a linear model of clinical supervision moving through nine steps (Box 16.2). Each of the nine steps is essential to achieve effective supervision.

The first step is 'preparation'. For the supervisee this means having an experience to share in the session. I always contract that the supervisee has 'prepared' the experience by writing a reflection. If not, then I tend to ask the MSR cues, which the supervisee could have done for herself. Clinical supervision is the supervisee's space and she must learn to use it most effectively.

For the supervisor, preparation is ensuring a safe, undisturbed venue, keeping time, ensuring confidentiality, being available, being informed around the issues emerging from the supervisee's reflections.

The second step is 'pick up' – picking up issues from the previous session. This is helped if notes from the previous session clearly identify what action the supervisee should take before the next session (towards realising desirable practice). This step enables continuity through sessions. If I haven't met the supervisee for 4 weeks or more, it might be difficult to remember the issues so the notes are helpful reminders. Writing notes helps the supervisee to reflect deeper on issues explored and reminds her of significant issues that have emerged from the sessions and what actions she has chosen to take. If the supervisee chooses not to act, that's not judgement day, that's simply as it is. Supervision should never be outcome focused. If the supervisee has not taken action as anticipated then that itself becomes a focus for the next session, at least in an emancipatory approach.

The supervision record has four sections.

- Pick up from last session
- What has been discussed in this session
- What has emerged as significant
- What actions do I need to take as a consequence?

Box 16.2   Supervision process – the nine step model

Preparation	Creating the best possible environment for successful supervision.
Pick up	Ensuring continuity of supervision from session to session.
Listening	Listening with intent to draw out significance from the supervisee's story.
Clarifying	Ensuring you have heard correctly from the supervisee's perspective, guiding the supervisee to draw out significant issues, and picking up and feeding back cues.
Understanding	Enabling the supervisee to gain insights into why she feels, thinks and responds as she does within situations.
Options	Enabling the supervisee to see and explore other, perhaps more appropriate ways to respond in future situations and their consequences.
Taking action	Guiding the supervisee to draw conclusions as to how she might like to respond in a future, similar situation.
Empowering	Infusing/empowering the supervisee with courage to act on her insights.
Wrap up	Ensuring the supervisee has summarised the session and feels OK (complete notes).

Notes provide the data for the practitioner to look back and review her reflexive development through the series of unfolding sessions. The practitioner can evaluate the supervision process for its efficacy in facilitating practitioner development using the Supervision Evaluation Questionnaire (SEQ) (see Appendix). The effectiveness of the supervision process should never be taken for granted and must be constantly scrutinised. Evaluation is itself a significant developmental exercise for the practitioner to analyse the supervision process and to give critical feedback.

The third step is 'listening' – I mean really listening to what the supervisee is saying. The art of dialogue, setting aside one's assumptions and judgements to be open to what the supervisee is really saying. Empathic inquiry is the bridge to connect with the other's world. This is the same with patients.

The fourth step is 'clarifying', entering into dialogue, picking up cues and reflecting them back to the supervisee, informing the supervisee that I have heard correctly and am checking out my interpretations.

The fifth step is 'understanding', working towards shared insights.

Steps 6–8 are the same as the looking forward cues within the MSR, enabling the supervisee to anticipate and explore how she might respond in similar future experiences, opening awareness, planting seeds.

The ninth step is 'wrap up' – ensuring the session is summarised and that the supervisee is OK, not an emotional heap in the corner, that emotional issues have been adequately worked through, linking with the MSR cue 'How are you now feeling?'. Perhaps the supervisee can spend the last 5 minutes writing the notes.

Developing professional expertise

Mott (2000) identified three approaches to the development of professional expertise:

- The Update model – what must the professional know to be an expert?
- The Competence model – what must the professional be able to do expertly?
- The Performance model – what is the professional all about? Put another way, this is an approach to developing expertise that looks at the whole performance in context and the person performing it rather than simply knowledge and competence. This approach accommodates the knowledge- and competence-based approaches.

Clinical supervision or guided reflection (these terms are not quite interchangeable because of the specific organisational agenda of clinical supervision) is an example of a performance model of professional development. In other words, it looks at the whole performance, although aspects can be highlighted but always against a background of the whole, enabling an increasingly deeper exploration and impact of systems on performance (see Chapter 1).

The performance model integrates and develops both the update and competence approaches, thus offering a more holistic and adequate model for professional development.

Trudy's story

Trudy is a district nurse. She shared her experience of working with Catherine and Gary in clinical supervision with me over six consecutive sessions. Catherine has terminal cancer and Gary is her husband. This example gives the reader a good impression of the reflexive nature of guided reflection – the way each session picks up and develops the issues from the previous session.

Position my supervision of Trudy along the intent–emphasis scale; what factors support your judgement?

Session 1

Trudy reads from her reflective diary

> Catherine is a 47-year-old woman with cancer in her bowel and peritoneal secondaries. She has a colostomy. Her husband called the clinic at 17.45 requesting me to visit. The message was 'wife unwell/colostomy blocked?' It was taken by another nurse. My dilemma was – do I visit now or do I refer to the evening nurse? I left it to the evening nurse. I rationalised this by thinking that it would be good for her to make Catherine's acquaintance. On my way home I pass nearby this family's house. I was feeling guilty that I had not responded personally, so I popped in. The curtains were drawn upstairs. Catherine was blind, confused, she had 'gone off her legs'. She was lying in the bathroom. I helped to move her onto the bed and she then commenced fitting. Her two sons who were present could not cope with this. They fled. Her husband was shocked. She was fitting for about 15–20 minutes. I called the general practitioner (GP), who suggested I made a 999 emergency call. I resisted this; I was asking myself – 'Do I want her to go to hospital?'. I didn't know the preference of the family about managing Catherine's deterioration and eventual death. This had not become a topic of conversation. The GP arrived and gave Catherine some IV valium which worked although she continued to fit intermittently. Her husband decided on private hospital admission – we had to wait 2 hours for an ambulance to arrive. I stayed with her during this time. Catherine fitted again on the stretcher going into the ambulance. I felt bad because I hadn't spoken to the boys – was my decision to refer to the night nurse the best decision? I felt I didn't have the full facts of the situation and didn't know the situation well enough to make a good judgement.

I ask, 'Could you have rung the husband back to explore what was meant by "unwell"?'
'Yes, I should have done that as Catherine usually managed her colostomy well.'
I pick up on Trudy's comment about eventual death and ask her about her relationship with the family and talking about Catherine's impending death.
Trudy says, 'I have known Catherine for 7 months, she knows her condition is terminal.'
'Are you avoiding talking about this situation with the family?'
'That may be partly true … I need to manage hope and doubt whether I should confront Gary's denial at this time. He is uncomfortable talking about these issues and for these reasons I haven't pushed it. I'm sensitive about a right time to discuss Catherine's death and that right time hasn't presented itself yet … however, I do feel this event marks a crisis within Catherine's illness trajectory … I will explore the meaning of this with Gary and discuss the different options for managing the situation when I visit him on Friday.'
Gently I probe: 'Trudy, do you avoid discussion with Gary and Catherine because it makes you feel uncomfortable?'. Trudy squirms slightly. 'My relationship is largely with Catherine. Gary has always seemed in the margins, seemingly uncomfortable with the emotional issues and focusing more on managing the physical. As a result I don't know him very well … I blame myself for referring to the evening nurse when I know I should have made the decision to visit myself.'

'Maybe with hindsight … we punish ourselves yet maybe at the time that was a reasonable decision. You couldn't have envisaged the way the situation unfolded.'

Trudy challenges herself: 'Yes but did I want her at home for my own needs because I would prefer that?'.

'If that was true, what would it say?

Trudy is silent.

'I sense that Gary and Catherine had different and potentially conflicting needs.'

Trudy asserted: 'Catherine needs good symptomatic control right now but in a private hospital? I'm left with a sense that Gary just wanted her out of the way.'

Taking Gary's perspective: 'Perhaps he can't cope with what's happening with Catherine right now.'

'Yes that's likely. …'

As it is nearing the end of our session I ask Trudy: 'What has been significant about sharing this experience?'.

'Recognising that my guilt is a reflection of the caring trap … thinking I should be there for my patients at all times. I seem to get entangled in these types of relationships. And secondly, my sense of unease with Gary that's against my belief of responding to the whole family.'

Commentary

This was our first clinical supervision session. I held a mirror for Trudy to look at herself. It was a time of connection between us, as I tuned into and surfed her wavelength. I helped Trudy put her feelings of guilt, distress and anger into the dialogic clearing where we could see them for what they were. Why does Trudy feel like this? It was both emotional and intimate, illustrating how powerful supervision can be.

I had given Trudy Ann Dickson's book *A woman in your own right*. In the book Dickson (1982) describes the compassion trap as when the practitioner gets trapped by her caring ethic. Trudy has taken responsibility for Catherine's suffering, indeed she absorbs Catherine's suffering as her own. As a result, she responds on an emotional rather than a rational level to her dilemma – should she visit or ask the evening nurse? The trap awaits the practitioner who lacks the ability to know and manage herself well enough in relationship with the patient or family member. Explanations like the 'caring trap' helped Trudy to see herself – she could see herself within the trap and she could see herself resisting Gary. Such visualisation helps her to understand and shift the negative energy into positive energy for acting on her insights for the journey ahead with this family. Trudy felt the conflict of contradiction within her approach to Gary. She knows she is not available to him, that she resisted him as a threat to her relationship with Catherine. He makes her feel angry and defensive. Yet she knows within the scope of holistic practice that she should be available to him, to feel compassionate toward him.

Throughout the session I was mindful of not absorbing Trudy's suffering as my own, modelling how she might, in turn, respond to Catherine's, Gary's and the boys' emotions in the future.

Session 2

Twenty days later Trudy and I met again. She shares her experience of visiting Gary.

'He said Catherine couldn't possibly come home as she had a catheter, a syringe driver … a stream of problems. I struggled to respond positively to him. I needed to assess Catherine for myself so I phoned the hospital. They were reluctant to give me any information but they said it was OK to visit. Catherine looked really well. If she had been at a NHS hospital they would have discharged her days ago. She had no memory of fitting. She was no longer fitting but had massive oedema of her abdomen and legs. I was questioning her treatment with the staff. She was not on any steroids. I thought the staff had a very limited understanding of Catherine's drugs; for example, they thought nozinam in the syringe driver was for the epilepsy (in fact, it is a broad spectrum antiemetic). It was making Catherine sleepy. Catherine said she wanted to go home. She said this in front of Gary when he arrived. I sensed the conflict between them.

'Could you have responded in other ways?'

'I'm unsure … perhaps ask the GP to speak with the hospital doctors?'

'I sense your anxiety that Catherine's desire to come home should be respected. Look at Gary's perspective and ask yourself whose needs are we responding to? Do you understand and respond to Gary on his emotional level or your own? Can he cope with Catherine's illness? Perhaps his difficulty with coping and emotional distress explains why arranging a support package to support Catherine at home was not enough to persuade him to have her home.'

Trudy is uncomfortable; I feel the balance of my challenge and support as a thin line.

'I feel the hospital is colluding with Gary in terms of his own needs rather than Catherine's – as if Catherine had become some object to talk about and do things with.'

We explore Trudy's options and potential consequences. One option was to involve Clare, the Macmillan nurse, more actively in Catherine's care. It felt like bringing in reinforcements to battle Gary.

I ask, 'Do you want Clare to confront Gary?'

'Clare doesn't know the family well whereas I do. I don't know how Catherine would feel if Clare came in.'

'What you're really saying is that you don't know how you will feel if Clare comes in – will you feel pushed out? Is that your fear? Is it time to confront Gary with the conflict of needs on an emotional level? Could you do that if you felt it appropriate?'

'Say more.'

'For example, "I can see this is tough for you, Gary". He might be feeling guilty about not having his wife at home, so such a response might help him face his guilt. It is not merely a stark choice of either hospital or home to die but to take each day as it comes, to leave the doors open. The cathartic response would make it easier to confront Gary – "What does Catherine want? Should you respect her wishes?"'

'If she came home she could always go back into hospital or the hospice if things deteriorate badly. I haven't really talked with him. I feel concerned that I should be manipulating him toward my views. I accept my sympathies and interests have lain primarily with Catherine.'

'I sense a major issue for Catherine is being in control of her own dying, ensuring that those she leaves behind can cope without her. Issues about her two sons and why she needs to be at home.'

At the end of the session, Trudy says, 'The session has helped me to see things differently, most notably paying attention to Gary's needs and how this is central to getting Catherine home … it has influenced my future actions and helped me anticipate what Gary may be thinking. I will arrange to meet him again! Thank you.'

Commentary

Trudy continues to resist Gary yet struggles with this contradiction of her holistic beliefs. Holism is not a rational technique to be applied but an intuitive way of being. By empathising with Gary, I challenged Trudy to develop her own empathic understanding with Gary's perspective, to tune into his wavelength and understand his own suffering. This was vital if she was going to shift her perspective of Gary as adversary and become available to him. How do we sense what the other is feeling and thinking at such moments? Only when Trudy can work through her resistance to Gary can she truly empathise with him. Trudy's emotional entanglement with Catherine is revealed in her anxiety about Clare's involvement. It illustrates how judgement is blurred by her own concerns.

Trudy moves on in her journey with this family. We have revisited issues surfaced in the first session and yet, just because we can see things differently does not mean we can easily shift our emotional responses or change our embodied responses. Learning through reflection is a holistic process of knowing and transforming self. Yet, we cannot simply shrug off who we are.

Session 3

Forty one days later, Trudy picked up the threads of her unfolding experience with Catherine and Gary.

'I did visit and confront him with the prospect of Catherine coming home. He was uptight. He said "I know I am being selfish but I've got a life to lead, and the boys as well. If Catherine is coming home then someone has to be here all the time". He was adamant and said that he had to return imminently to work in Indonesia. I didn't pursue it because I could see it was making him more uptight. I contacted the hospital. They said Catherine could be kept on insurance funding because she had a syringe driver which counted as treatment. I offered to look after her if she came home. But after that I didn't hear from them or Gary. I became despondent about it. Then, this week, she was sent home for the day. Gary informed me and I went to visit her. She was downstairs sitting at the kitchen table. She looked well. No syringe driver, no catheter. She was eating and drinking. Walking up and down stairs. Her legs were less swollen although her ascites remained and made her look 9 months pregnant. She said "I feel really well". Gary interjected, "You're not well, are you?". He was challenging what she could do, getting up and down stairs. I asked her when she was coming home. She said she was working on it, pulling a face at Gary. He said that she was not ready to come home. I asked her what I could do to help you when you do come home?

And today?! I heard she is coming home on Thursday ... a phone message from Gary. The insurance funding has dried up. He has got to come to terms with it now she's returning home. I have arranged a package of care for her. She's really determined. She said that she had forced herself to eat to make herself better. There was no explanation for the epilepsy. They didn't do a brain scan and she isn't on any epileptic drugs. Perhaps it was a reaction from the nozinam? She was on dexamethasone but now there is friction between them about coming home.'

'Trudy, how do you feel about your involvement with Catherine?'

Trudy looks me in the eye: 'I know it's going to be tough when Catherine eventually dies. Gary's comments are off-putting for Catherine. I know I need to be supportive toward

Gary rather than confronting him with his persistent negative attitude because he may be feeling guilty about not wanting her home. I do feel more in tune with Gary … sense how he's feeling more easily, and hence more available to him. After I last saw him, I let it go. I feel guilty about that. I saw him in the shops and I went off the other way rather than face him. I began to feel awkward pushing it for her. Often at home I would think how she was. I couldn't understand why they had kept the syringe driver going. Her body is covered with abscess sites from the driver – they had to change the site every day. She's on MST now … I can see how I have been drawn into an emotional web, entangled and pulled between them. Talking it through with you I am less entangled … I feel it differently now.'

'That's a good image – visualise yourself in this web and pull yourself out. Here, let me help you…'

I pull on an imaginary rope, pulling her free. Trudy laughs. I help her frame her involvement with Catherine and Gary using the nurse–patient involvement theory of Morse (1991) and Ramos (1992). Trudy identified with the Morse 'type' of 'over-involvement' – 'yes, I've been there!'.

'We all need to experience emotional entanglement, because only then can we recognise the place. Perhaps entanglement is an inevitable consequence of holistic relationship because it's so hard to resist the suffering of the other. It is like a tidal wave that we must learn to surf and control yet without relinquishing its exquisite intimacy and beauty. It's OK to be vulnerable but like the expert surfer we can learn to ride it. Maybe we do get swept away sometimes but that's just another experience to learn from. That's where reflection can help us.'

Session 4

Thirty days later. Trudy is late. 'Sorry … I've been to a funeral and then an urgent visit.'

'Not Catherine's funeral?'

Trudy exclaims, 'No! She's up and well. I'm seeing her twice a week. She's been having some difficulty with her son. He has problems with drugs and also a recent court appearance because of stealing.'

Picking up the cue, I inquire, 'Have you helped the sons talk about what's happening to their mother?'

'No. Gary has not returned to Indonesia yet. He's saying he has got to go next month but he's also said that someone needs to be with Catherine the whole time.'

'Is this necessary?'

'I don't think so, at least not 24 hours a day because if someone has 24-hour care she can't live a normal life, can she?'

'If you're waiting to die, can you live a "normal life"?'

'Well, she struggles to do the housework but she can wash and dress herself, etc.'

'You're responding to her in terms of things she can physically do; what about her responses on an emotional level? Is she coping on this level?'

'She doesn't seem to want to talk on this level although she does give cues such as "living on borrowed time"… it's difficult to talk to her because her husband and sons are often there and they don't want to talk about it.'

'Maybe they don't know how to talk about it?'

'I have another Catherine, who is also dying yet very open to what was happening to her … she needs to resolve issues such as who was going to look after her 5-year-old son. Of course, how people feel and what they think about their impending death can never be predicted. The wavelength becomes a roller-coaster!'

'Perhaps Catherine is ambivalent? As you said, she is not in denial. She accepts she is going to die but she also needs to cope and protect her boys. Perhaps she is trying to be brave? Imagine yourself in her shoes – what sort of things would you need to be doing?'

'Well, sort out my children, put my house in order.'

'Do you remember the message from *Final gifts* (Callanan and Kelley 1991) – that the primary task for the dying person was to ensure that those they left behind were able to cope?'

'I do, that was very powerful ... the other Catherine is "coming to terms"... even things like changing internal doors in the house, things that she had wanted to do. She is now quite peaceful with everything sorted out.'

Pursuing the point, I suggest, 'Perhaps we can see that Catherine is trying to cope with chaos. Perhaps she does need confronting in order to help her sort things out. Perhaps you are avoiding this for your discomfort and uncertainty about her ambivalence.'

'I accept your point ... I just don't feel with this family that they are ready to talk about it. I don't feel her physical deterioration has become that marked where her dying has really become an issue. They are a "difficult" family; I have a number of people who are dying where talking about death is not a problem.'

I take Trudy back to the beginning of the session: 'All this came out of me asking – was it Catherine's funeral!'

Trudy laughs and then says seriously, 'We have had a lot of people dying – nine recently. It's stressful. It doesn't help having conflict with the doctors ... one particular situation over drug dosage made me fume. The doctor wasn't listening to me ... I didn't back down and asserted my point of view. She was short with me but she didn't bawl me out of the office.'

'The intimidating factor – being short.'

Trudy laughed: 'Some patients have commented on her manner – her new year's resolution is to be less short!'

'It's promising she has insight! Maybe she's changing. It doesn't help when work is tough to have oppressive relationships within the team.'

We pause.

I continue: 'Last session I challenged you to consider the balance of being challenging and being supportive with Gary and Catherine.'

'My stance towards Gary has changed. I now see their relationship differently. I see that maybe he couldn't go to Indonesia because he couldn't leave Catherine at home and that being with her was an emotional rather than a physical thing. Could he focus on work knowing she was as she was?'

Commentary

Trudy contrasts Catherine with other dying patients she visits in her effort to make sense of her struggle with Catherine and Gary whilst trying to position herself within the tension of confronting the family's reluctance to talk about Catherine's imminent death. What would be for the best? To know is to tune into the unfolding patterns of shifting wavelengths. My guidance is to make Trudy more mindful of this tension, indeed pushing the point. Other issues that impinge on Trudy's ability to be available emerge, such as the conflict with doctors.

Session 5

Twenty one days later, Trudy says: 'Gary is letting me in now and I'm responding to my intuition that it's now the right time to talk about dying. Catherine's in the terminal stage of her illness ... I went in following a phone call from Catherine that her colostomy was obstructed. Up to this time I had been going in twice weekly. She had been self-caring so I went in to discuss what had been happening to her. On this visit she was in bed. She said she had great abdominal pain. I sought the GP's advice. The GP had prescribed a suppository but this hadn't worked and had since prescribed normacol. Because of the pain I advised Catherine not to take this. I also referred her to the night nurse so she could get help if she needed it.'

'What treatment do you think might be best?'

After considering palliative approaches to Catherine's bowel obstruction, Trudy says: 'Gary was downstairs during this visit. I had informed him that the colostomy was obstructed and that this was a sign of things worsening and her imminent death. Gary said it wasn't fair to keep her alive. Why were we giving her all these drugs? That we needed to put an end to all this! I asked him if Catherine was talking about dying. He said that he wanted to look after her at home and not to go back into hospital. I thought he might be strapped for cash but he assured me that wasn't the reason. She didn't want to go back in and he had accepted that. The elder son didn't want to stray too far in case anything happened to mum. No talk of the younger son, he was still having his troubles. I'm now visiting every day.'

'Trudy, why are you visiting every day?'

'Because my enrolled nurse is no good at counselling. She "whips in and out". Both Catherine and Gary made this observation. She's a good nurse but prefers going in and doing something physical. I need to monitor the colostomy and to respond to her symptoms on a daily basis and to help the family through the crisis.'

'Being there for them?'

'Yes, that's right. I had two other patients who were similar to Catherine with obstructed colostomies. One lived for 3 months after it had become blocked. She would vomit every day. In the end, faecal matter, not very pleasant. I have told them about such possibility. Catherine is struggling to eat just a little. She has requested some HiCal drinks to keep her strength up ... I can tell by the look she gives me that she knows she has deteriorated, but she doesn't want to talk about that. She feels the lumps in her tummy ... still hoping the tumour will go away.'

'It must be hard for you to see her suffer like that, her grief all bottled up inside ... when you know it would help her to share it with you'

It was a poignant moment to dwell in that truth, in silence for a moment. I broke the spell by challenging Trudy over her team leader responsibilities – 'What do you need to do when you know that members of your team are not responding appropriately?'.

Trudy says, 'I find it hard to tackle such issues because I don't like conflict even when I know it compromises patient care ... I want to talk more about Gary. Gary is out of control, feeling helpless, very anxious and angry. He tested out the night nurse to gauge her response – which was OK! This is going to be tough, especially when she becomes more physically dependent, vomiting, etc. I feel OK, not over-involved. I feel happy because Catherine is quite happy. Things are under control. I enjoy visiting them. Before I wasn't in control.'

Commentary

Trudy felt that the dynamics had changed with Gary because he now accepted that Catherine was going to die at home although he clearly struggles with his feelings. The situation is very tense.

Focusing Trudy's attention on the situation with her enrolled nurse was misplaced in that her mind was wrapped up with Catherine and Gary. Yet her avoidance of the topic reflects her avoidance of the issue in practice.

Session 6

Forty six days later, Trudy noted how busy she was and the pressure she felt under just now. She picked up on Catherine.

'Catherine … her death. She was fighting to the end. She was on a massive dose of diamorphine – 500 mg in her syringe driver. She had another massive fit. I'll read from my diary.

I visited Catherine Monday morning early; the Marie Curie nurse had rung me to say that Catherine had a very restless night and was not responding to oral commands and there was a steady trickle of black fluid running from her mouth. I decided to assess the situation and rang the GP from Catherine's house. As I entered the bedroom I was shocked by what I saw. Catherine was groaning and rolling around the bed. Gary was trying to hold her onto the bed. She rolled from side to side, legs hanging over the edge of the bed, her catheter tube kinked and twisted around her leg, her tubing from the syringe driver had become detached. Clearly Gary was distressed.

Catherine lay across the bed, her huge abdomen hard and contracting, her swollen legs looked heavy and shiny, her face, arms and shoulders so thin that you see her bones protruding. I sat on the bed, reconnecting the syringe driver and checked the light was flashing. Gently I talked to Catherine, holding her hand. She was calm for a minute and then she began to groan again, vomited and started to fit. Gary and I rolled Catherine onto her side in the recovery position. I called the GP to come straight away and rang the clinic, asking the reception staff to bleep my nursing auxiliary and ask her to come to Catherine's house urgently. While we waited Gary and I talked; I admitted to Gary that I had never witnessed anything like this before in all my nursing experience.

Catherine's strength was amazing, on occasions rolling onto her enlarged abdomen. All kinds of emotions were spinning through my head. I felt sad for Gary witnessing this, Catherine's loss of dignity; what an awful death and I was helpless to do anything. I had no valium to stop the fit and no injection available to calm Catherine. I spoke to Gary and said the only good thing about this was that Catherine doesn't know what's going on. The GP arrived – he was visibly shocked and passed me a valium enema which I inserted into Catherine's colostomy. Within a few minutes Catherine was calm. I asked the GP for another in case she fitted again and asked him if he had any midazolam 20 mg that I could use to sedate Catherine as she was very agitated and restless. He wrote the medication and Stuart, Gary's son, went to collect the prescription. Ann, my nursing auxiliary, arrived and we washed Catherine, talking gently to her, comforting her, cleansed her mouth and put a clean nightie on and clean sheets. By this time Stuart had returned and I could give the midazolam intramuscularly

262 Becoming a Reflective Practitioner

into her thigh. Within 10 minutes she was asleep. Gary, Ann and I sat around the bed emotionally drained, just looking at Catherine. I knew I could not leave Gary alone. The situation was frightening for him. Gary thanked us both and felt reassured that he was not going to be left alone. He was happier that she was asleep.

Trudy puts her diary aside and asks herself, 'What was I trying to achieve? My main concern was for Gary who was visibly distressed. Catherine would have been horrified if she could see herself, nightie up around her breasts, legs and bottom exposed, rolling around her bed, groaning, complete loss of dignity. Gary was distraught, unable to restrain her almost falling out of bed. I was frustrated that there were no drugs prescribed that I could have given. When Catherine was asleep and calm, Gary could manage. He rarely touched Catherine – he always stood at the foot of the bed or sat in a chair. I never saw him hold her hand although he always talked fondly of her. I came to the conclusion that he was afraid and it would be less stressful for him if Ann assisted me in all nursing duties. I've learnt so much from this but I never did get to grips with Gary. I said to him "it won't be long" and queried whether he wanted her family present. He said that they can come at any time but he didn't want them staying. He said "I don't think of her death, I think of the future". He never shed a tear. I went to the funeral. Her father was heartbroken as his wife had died of cancer as well.'

I acknowledged Trudy's feeling: 'This must have been very traumatic for you … you moved a long way to accommodate Gary within your sphere of care.'

'That's been my real learning – to see and respond to the whole family. It's true, I do normally identify with the woman in the situation which often leaves me feeling angry at the spouses, as with Gary, because he seemed to interfere with helping me to help Catherine meet her needs.'

Commentary

Trudy had written a truly astonishing description of Catherine. I felt the power of her writing as she unfolded the events. It was a story of becoming, of coming to know self and the impact of self on the way events are grasped and interpreted. The contradiction between her holistic belief and her practice was evident from the beginning. I was touched by the symbolic moment as they sat around the bed – Trudy and Ann by Catherine, and Gary alone, isolated in his suffering at the foot of the bed. It reflects the impression painted by Trudy that Gary was an intruder, even to the end. So I wonder to what extent she was transformed through this experience. It was not a perfect ending but such situations rarely are. Issues such as supporting the boys were left relatively untouched.

Mayeroff (1971) notes that: 'I am in-place because of the way I relate to others. And place must be continually renewed and reaffirmed' (p69).

Trudy seeks to be in-place within her caring relationships: a place where she can dwell with the other secure with her intimacy and vulnerability. Reflection was a mirror held for Trudy to reveal herself to herself in the context of her experience with Catherine and Gary. Her honesty was profound and enabled her to find new meaning in being a holistic practitioner, more aware of self, more mindful of her impact on others and, as a consequence, more able to manage herself within her relationships with patients and families. Perhaps less so with colleagues, hinted at as problematic within the text yet never fully focused on, and yet which seemed significant in her everyday practice. They are dangling threads for us to pick up on as appropriate.

Reflection helps her to work out the discomfort so she can know her dwelling place and dwell there more easily. Blackwolf and Jones (1996) say:

> Perhaps you have begun your path of change and are experiencing the pain of previous pains, as you open the cover to the book of your own life. The cover, which up to now has been carefully sealed up. Like the leaves of a head of lettuce, you are beginning to peel back one blemished leaf at a time, to reveal the you of quiet peace. Hidden beneath your polished presentation to the world, your injuries have been waiting for you to acknowledge their existence. It is time to view your injuries and feel your bruises. Through the experiential (reflective) process, we become real. We really become. (p22)

Trudy did not view herself as injured or bruised because such wounds, as with most of us, are masked by the need to cope. Yet, as the dialogue revealed, Trudy's masks were gently revealed, enabling her wounds to be tended. Perhaps 'wounds' sounds dramatic, yet the metaphor of the wounded healer seems common to most nurses. Trudy not only made connections with her deeper self, she also connected with me, as her guide. I was a clearing where she could unwrap herself and touch her deeper self. It is caring. I must shine a gentle light to help Trudy and others like her, for we are strongly defended. It was her love for Catherine that allowed her to reveal herself. In an outcome-oriented healthcare culture, the temptation may be to shine a bright light that frightens the practitioner caught in the glare.

Conclusion

In this chapter I have explored clinical supervision as an expression of clinical leadership and creating the learning organisation. Clinical supervision is a formal approach to guided reflection promoted by government to reinforce professional accountability. It has been widely implemented within nursing in the UK from an organisational approach and is being adopted by other healthcare professionals.

In Chapter 17 I explore the relationship between reflection and chaos theory within the context of developing leadership.

Chapter 17

Reflection as chaos theory

Lazell writes

This narrative concerns a scenario at work which came to my attention as a supervisor of midwives when a patient who had a risk factor for birth asked to exercise her choice in the way she wanted to deliver her baby. This example is used to highlight the influence of Newtonian body-as-machine thinking in the clinical and organisational culture I work within. In doing so, I explore chaos theory as a way of understanding leadership challenges, and the ways in which chaos might be applied in a meaningful way to be a leader, creating an enriched environment, where excellence and creativity in practice and learning can take place.

Newtonian thinking: the failed machine

Some months ago, I was approached by a supervisory colleague, Sally, to comment and offer further advice as to the best way forward to support Harriet who was 30 weeks pregnant. This young woman wished for a water birth in hospital. She did not want continuous fetal monitoring, because she wanted to avoid restricted mobility in labour, and she felt the water would be relaxing and reduce the need for epidural or opiate analgesic. Harriet was expecting her second child. She was motivated because her first birth had culminated in a caesarean section due to *'failure to progress'*. Her previous caesarean section placed her in a risk (small at 0.5–1%) position of a possible scar dehiscence in a subsequent labour. Some units round the UK offer water birth as an option after a caesarean (Garland 2004) yet in our unit, water birth would not be 'allowed'.

There is little current evidence for or against water birth after a caesarean (Garland 2004, 2006). Under our maternity unit protocol for management of birth after a caesarean section, continuous monitoring is advocated, although NICE (2004) recommends it should be 'offered'.

Harriet's community midwife had directed her to speak to the labour ward manager, also a supervisor of midwives, because her request for her forthcoming labour placed her outside hospital policy for management of birth after caesarean section.

When I see the words 'failure to progress', this language depicts a machine that has failed. The words have little connection to a woman. In these words, she is disconnected from her body, a machine failing to move the baby through. There are numerous clinical examples of how a woman's body 'fails': the use of oxytocin accelerates *dysfunctioning* labour, prostaglandin stimulates the woman's body *failing* to go into labour, epidural *numbs* the sensations of labour. Obstetrics is littered with examples where the body is seen as a machine that is inherently imperfect and untrustworthy, needing to be managed or fixed (Davis-Floyd 2001).

Newtonian knowing: the machine in parts

In my work as a community midwife, pregnancy and birth is now a measurable process of separate parts that would be controlled or made linear by increasingly familiar and routine medical procedures and screenings.

Disconnection of the woman from her body parts begins early in pregnancy. The booking visit identifies many possible risks, in order to process the woman's pregnancy and to exclude or monitor deviances. I find myself apologising for the interview appearing so depressingly focused on what can go wrong with her body and baby rather than sharing with her a celebration of new life. After my visit, the woman is soon aware that both body and baby are capable of going seriously wrong (but my detective work and interventions just might keep it all from falling apart!).

Obstetric language defines the compartmentalised notion of the act of birthing. We speak of stages of birth, first, second, third, parts to be defined and measured by graphs depicting time and progress. Defining stages fragments and disconnects the flow, the continuum, of the way things might naturally need to be in birth. Wheatley (1999: 120) says the process of linearising nature's non-linear character blinds scientists to life's processes.

Women in managed technologised hospital births are *disconnected* from their own intuitive life/birth processes and 'knowing' their body. They are away from their familiar surroundings of home, yet *connected* and *tethered* to technology, the hospital and the obstetrical domain.

I reflect upon a recent experience of a woman transferred into hospital from a home-birth, having pushed hard for 2 hours at home. Totally exhausted, she yielded to augmentation of her labour contractions and a Ventouse extraction of the baby. The doctor's words ring in my ears: 'Now you are here, we will get you some decent contractions and get you pushing properly'. I wonder how much of a failure she felt then.

Davis-Floyd (2001) paints a graphic image of the intravenous line as symbolic of the woman's tethered dependency to the medical institution, like the baby's umbilical dependence on the mother in the uterus. Davis-Floyd describes technocratic societies' metaphorical fusion with technology, with women no longer believing in their own human capability to birth.

I wrote the following words sometime ago, after I was struck by the similarity of how my clients do not believe in their body's capability; the words offer my impression of the effect of technological dependence, in this case women's dependence on ultrasound scanning to 'know' all is well and to 'believe' in themselves.

> What will make it 'feel real', Anita?
> Seeing your baby on a screen,
>   black and white, squirming, throbbing bud?
> Didn't it 'feel real',
>   when that little clump of cells became one with you,

and made you sick, and made you spit?
Couldn't it, didn't it, 'sink in' then?

Could you just for once, imagine, and feel,
that private dark place,
of water and blood sound,
pulsating with life,
where your baby grows and knows
in a safe cocoon
of your body and love?

When did the world
take that sense from you Anita?
with its prying eyes,
needing to know,
and show the world everything,
to fix the bits that didn't work,
and throw the bits it didn't want.

When did we stop 'feeling real?'

Newton's scientific discoveries resulted in a world where explanation, prediction and control were proposed as possible, and his understanding of physical mechanics was the basis for the Industrial Revolution. Davis-Floyd (2001) writes of the idea of body-as-machine as an echo of these industrialising periods of history. Newton explored nature with the abstract tools of mathematics and made possible the triumph of the machine. Whittemore (1999), writing of the historical background to natural science, says of the effect of Newton's discoveries: 'The mechanistic deterministic reductionist spiritually void perspective of the world was born'. In short, Newtonian thinking means that by studying the component parts of things, we can understand, know and control.

Wheatley (1999) writes that viewing the world using the imagery of a machine results in things being fragmented into component parts. In this way, within this domain of obstetrical compartmentalised knowing, Harriet is no longer seen as a whole person; she becomes a malfunctioning uterus. An 'it'. Yet understanding and knowing Harriet as a 'whole' rather than her uterus as a component or 'it', as described, brings to mind Wilber's four quadrants of knowing (Johns 2006:50). Wilber identified sources of knowledge offering only partial views of the truth, of that which is known.

Objective knowledge is one such paradigm of knowledge and has been adopted by medical science as the dominant way of knowing. It is a linear and seemingly measurable way of knowing. For example, objective knowledge measures and 'knows' that a standard cervix will open 1 cm per hour in labour if we measure it every 4 hours: 'it' knowledge. Subjective knowledge would be that which I or 'we' know.

Intuitively and experientially, 'I know' labour, or indeed the person as whole, as essentially complex and chaotic. The way of labour defies explanation at times. Intuitive midwifery knowledge about birth as an unpredictable non-linear process is reflected in Belenky *et al*'s work (1986:63). Of subjectivism, Belenky writes, truth is personal and private and intuited. In my practice, it is often based on 'gut feeling' or gained through experiences of seeing, hearing, touching or encountering something familiar or similar. It often has no basis in books or other received knowledge; sometimes I just do not understand what I feel, yet I know. The throaty noises of a woman approaching the point of birth or the baby that 'just doesn't look right' come to mind.

Torbert (1978) writes:

> For the past several centuries, Western society has been enchanted by its supposed value-free exploration of the power of methodologies in the world of knowledge and technologies in the world of action. Unfettered these powers enhance man's manipulative capacity and diminish moral capacity. The twentieth century illustrates increasingly vividly the ecological political ethical and ontological horrors and dilemmas to which such a narrow preoccupation with efficient impersonal causes and effects leads.

Complexity, learning and knowledge cycles

The birth process is not linear; it is frequently not predictable and often immeasurable. As Harriet's previous birth demonstrated, a cervix does not always dilate at a standardised rate, and neither do contractions always increase or strengthen in a measurable way.

Complexity theory acknowledges the unknowable, the links and webs of connections, impacting and influencing the whole birth process, the woman, as far as we can see 'the whole'. Complexity theory acknowledges midwifery intuition; the knowledge of the effect of co-creation of 'what is', even in minute acts of observation, knowing and presence. Each time we measure/observe something, we interfere. As Wheatley (1999: 67) writes:

> There is no objective reality; the environment we experience does not exist 'out there'. It is co-created through acts of observation, what we choose to notice and worry about … conflicts about what is true and false would disappear in the exploration of multiple perceptions.

Thinking about Harriet's situation, and how empirical knowledge influences much risk management decision making, as a supervisor and community midwife, aiming to lead best practice for mothers and babies, I wonder if it is possible to integrate learning that birth is a complex phenomenon (as a component of the creative learning organisation) with an empirical science demand that Harriet's birth might also be understood and known in some measurable way.

Of complexity and chaos theory in relation to the unpredictability of birth, Downe (2004:15) asserts that labour *can* be 'understood', using multiple paradigms of knowing, integrated into research. By building on the complexity theory of labour as a *connective* phenomenon, Downe (2004:17) asserts that the usefulness to childbirth of understanding this connectivity (and for me as a transformational leader) is knowing that complexity is underpinned by simple rules and cyclical processes working within parameters, i.e. complex feedback mechanisms and bounded instability. This requires a shift in thinking about there being 'one way of knowing' but using empirical evidence as a partial aspect of 'evidence' within a wider complex cyclical system of knowing.

This understanding not only implies the complexity and supersensitivity of the birth process; as a leader it invites me to embed the idea of the small interconnected effects of transformational leadership as a force for change. An awareness of the magnifying butterfly effect of small imperceptible actions and ways of being not only on pregnant and labouring women but the effects and impact of the way I lead on my working environment.

Wheatley (1999:139) writes: 'A system is composed of parts, but we cannot understand a system by looking only at its parts. We need to work with the whole of a system, even as we work with individual parts or isolated problems'.

My supervisory colleague, Sally, the labour ward manager, had met with Harriet and explained the hospital protocol and the small known risk of scar dehiscence. Harriet was informed that her choice would place her care outside usual hospital protocol. The Nursing and Midwifery Council (NMC 2002) states that when a woman rejects the advice that the type of care she requests may cause harm to her or her baby, the Supervisor of Midwives should provide guidance to the midwife caring for the woman, ensure correct documentation has taken place and then the best possible care should continue to be given to the mother. Indeed, a recent government document, *Maternity matters* (DoH 2007), states women *should* be given choices about the place of birth. This document places *choice of place of birth* as a key component of its recommendations for maternity services by 2009.

Choice

As a supervisor I felt Sally had given Harriet adequate information and acted appropriately to give the client the opportunity for informed choice. I felt we should now continue to care for her as best as we could in her wish for normal birth in water.

Along with several of the other supervisors, including myself, Carol, the Head of Midwifery, responded to the circulated email regarding Harriet. She stated that Harriet would *not* be 'allowed' into the pool, as it was outside hospital policy. Midwives would be unable to enforce continuous monitoring but the midwife *must not* turn the taps of the pool on. If she did, she would not be covered by the trust's vicarious liability were there to be an untoward event. The midwife would be seen to be colluding with the mother's outside-of-policy choice. If the woman chose to birth at home, she could birth in water.

More emails circulated. Supervisors and consultants were divided on this point. Some felt Harriet's request placed her in danger; it was an unknown. Some felt her request should be supported. Chaotic indeed!

The following week, I had to attend a standard review meeting with the Community Midwife Manager and the Head of Midwifery. Carol thanked me for my many articulate emails concerning Harriet which she said she had read and considered carefully. I wondered if she considered me mad, bad and dangerous for my views. I suggested that Harriet might unwisely choose a water birth at home if we refused to offer her one in hospital. Did we want to encourage that? I still felt passionately that we must support this woman to birth naturally in hospital. Carol's stance was, 'If we agree to one, the flood gates will be open'. She wanted to give a clear message, it seemed! In here and conform, or out and do what you want!

I remember one of my clients some years previously, so distraught by the prospect of being tied to a bed by monitors, having had a caesarean section with her first child; she remained at home labouring, without planning a homebirth. She delivered, her labour unattended, as the midwife arrived at the house. It was unsafe, although all was well in the end, and I reminded my Head of Midwifery of this incident.

I asked Carol if she might approach the hospital lawyers or the risk management team. Yet again, she 'put her manager's hat on', behaved authoritatively and was not going to budge. She stated she was risk averse and the case would not be defendable if things went wrong. *Still* fighting the cause, I suggested if we gave Harriet no option but to deliver at home to birth in the way she wanted, she might take action against the trust if there was an untoward event at home.

It seemed the trust was saying 'do what you want at home, but in here you *conform*'. The threshold of the hospital doors, where medical knowing and power reign, is where Harriet's choice ended.

Canter (2001), cited in Hewitt-Taylor (2004), states that the dominant paradigm of medicine sets up a situation where the healthcare worker can coerce and control by use of reward and punishment. In this way, Harriet was presented with a stark choice: home and do what you want (punishment, perhaps, as less safe for her after a caesarean?) or hospital and do it our way, equates, arguably, as a reward because it was safer for her.

I yielded. I felt I was banging my head on a hard brick wall. I asked myself, what did patient choice mean? I wondered if patient choice could ever exist as a reality. I didn't feel I could make any difference.

Freire (1972) states that individuals or organisations with significant power do not readily give it up. Hewitt-Taylor (2004) continues to argue that whilst government directives suggest power should shift from healthcare staff to patients, the realities of power equations are complex.

Arguably true patient choice might mean patients asking for treatments or investigations detrimental to health or merely for reassurance or 'soft' qualitative purposes. Here, Harriet was asking for a choice encompassing the quality aspect of her birth, perhaps not a quantifiable or valued aspect of the obstetric domain. Once again, the complex issue of what constitutes *valued knowledge* is apparent. As I have explored earlier, the dominating empirical scientific knowledge of best practice means that the most important outcome seems to be a physical measurable benefit that becomes 'the truth'. A contrasting holistic approach to knowing 'what's best' would, in this case, be Harriet hoping for an outcome that is more emotionally and spiritually beneficial. This is *her* truth rather than a generalised empirical truth. Johns (2006) writes of the tendency to validate 'it' knowledge as 'truer' than 'I/we' knowledge in healthcare settings, which has led to a denigration of subjective knowledge.

Maps, strange attractors and learning through leadership

Advocating patient choice is a highly complex cultural matter. Canter (2001), cited in Hewitt-Taylor (2004), says statements relating to shifting balances of power from healthcare staff to patients are generally made in a manner which that suggests power (in this case power held with those who sanction or decline patient choice) is an object that can easily be shifted. A neat transfer of power is not easily achievable and therefore a culture of honesty about the basis of knowledge reality, limitations, differing views, and acknowledging boundaries of power is the first step in achieving a shift.

As a leader, conflict of values, knowledge base and ideals, all of which might be 'known to be the truth' by each of the individuals involved, presents challenges when the system is faced with complexity of patient choice. In this situation, Harriet, the supervisor, the midwife, the manager, the doctor, the trust and the Nursing and Midwifery Council might all express differing stances on this dilemma. As referred to earlier, complexity suggests that the effect of observation and presence always affects the 'whole'. Wheatley (1999:67) says leadership in organisations is responsive to similar quantum effects.

Data is recognised as a wave, rich in potential interpretations and completely dependent on observers to evoke different meanings. If such data is free to move, it will meet up with many diverse observers. As each observer interacts with the data, he/she develops their own interpretation. We can expect these interpretations to be different, because people are. Instead of losing so many of the potentials contained in the data, multiple observers elicit multiple and varying responses, giving genuine richness to the observations. An organisation rich with many interpretations develops a wider sense of what is going on and what needs to be done.

Being honest about knowledge base, differing views and limitations to shift entrenched power bases might emerge as rich learning (Canter 2001, cited in Hewitt-Taylor 2004). Similarly, Cope (2001:108) describes the potential for creativity within situations when there are differing viewpoints, attitudes and conflict over of what constitutes the best way or 'truth'.

In leading midwifery practice, as Mycek (1999) states, I see 'an edge between two eras', two cultural mindsets, two ways of doing things (I suspect we have more than two). Reflecting Mycek's stance of 'teetering on the edge of chaos' and finding creativity within this space, Cope (2001:104) recommends comparative mapping in understanding differences, through recognising the acceptable and unacceptable, and the driving forces creating the maps. Mapping exercises mirror complexity as a model for working transformationally in relationship with clients and colleagues, creating a learning organisation when faced with multiple ways of 'knowing'. Somewhere between all the diverse and rich map terrains here, mutual values can be revealed. These values might be the 'strange attractors' that bring meaning and order from such diversity. Or 'the rich interpretation and awareness of what needs to happen'(Wheatley 1999).

For Harriet's request, midwives, doctors and supervisors, and the patient did *not* think collectively. Bohm's work cited in Senge (1990:265) is informed by the idea of wholeness of systems, systems thinking and team learning. He writes of 'fragmentation' and 'pollution of thought' yet through dialogue, a group who have shared terrains and access to a pool of common meaning can explore complex issues and reveal incoherence of thought.

In this way, I once again see map-shared meaning and dialogue as the strange attractor of complexity theory, bringing order from the edges of chaos, our values and meanings, forming a cyclical body of meaning, understanding and learning. Envisaging this with a fresh lens, I can see a clearing for transformational leadership to align the often scratchy, professionally divisive edges of the clashes of empirical and subjective birthing knowledge and how to share success with clients.

Bohm (1980) compared dialogue to 'superconductivity'. 'Electrons behave coherently at cooler temperatures rather than as separate parts, flowing round obstacles, creating no resistance and with high energy.' The goal of dialogue is to create high energy and high intelligence. Dialogue lifts assumption, and allows free flow of meaning to occur.

I felt extremely frustrated by Carol's stance. The decision to prevent Harriet getting in the water to birth was not, in my view, a very intelligent one, because it sent out a negative butterfly effect to the ever-present, risk-averse culture and did not enhance organisational learning.

A week later, there was a supervisor meeting. Again Harriet's situation was discussed. I felt Carol heard the views of the few midwives who quietly supported Harriet's wishes, but she had made her mind up. I felt disappointed in the supervisors that risk had became the overwhelming focus.

Carol visited Harriet at home and persuaded her to come into the hospital and give birth on dry land. Harriet went into spontaneous labour some weeks labour and delivered normally without continuous monitoring.

Conclusions: where chaos and leadership fuse

Frustrations as a transformational leader, trying to work with women and lead best, woman-centred practice, have emerged in this work, as I felt I was up against a Head of Midwifery who had a risk-averse stance towards offering women choice in labour.

After meeting Carol, Harriet bowed to the hospital regime of safer hospital birth on dry land. She was 'rewarded' by being allowed to mobilise without continuous monitoring, but was denied her choice of a water birth, despite lack of evidence to suggest a water birth was less safe.

Carol managed autocratically. She controlled and commanded transactionally in this situation. The supervisory group had her ear for the afternoon but she had made her mind up and she took a risk-averse stance towards the issue of patient choice. In wishing to keep Harriet's care controlled within the hospital, Carol demonstrated her fear of midwifery spinning into uncontrollable anarchy were we to send out a message that 'anything goes'. Mycek (1999) speaks of the natural human instinct to retain control in an ever-changing and rapidly changing healthcare system. Yet as an organisation we claim to want to increase normal birth and empower women to make choices about birth.

Again Torbert (1978) adds perspective:

> The organisation requires the vigilance of all its members to determine whether its purposes are hazy and whether its specific structure implementing behaviours and the products of its services are congruent with its purposes. But members' charges of organisational incongruities may well be untrustworthy as long as members are unaccustomed to searching for incongruities among their own presuppositions, strategies, practices, and effects ... charges of incongruity may mask an unwillingness to face personal incongruity.

Carol's thinking was not congruent with what we as midwives, and as a maternity unit, espouse to believe. In keeping with the idea of connectivity and quantum effects, Senge (1990) says once people accept a stereotypical way of thinking, the 'thought' becomes active in shaping the person's interactions with others, and the individual they have the view on.

Could this be a cause of the growing global culture of monitoring and trying to exclude every possible risk in many other society arenas?

A butterfly effect of thinking and acting out of a shadow map or, as Torbert would assert, the 'organisational incongruity', left unchallenged, means clogged learning (Cope 2001) and cultivates fear amongst the group.

Bohm's (1980) words about thought read strikingly true here: 'Thought presents itself and pretends it does not represent. We are like actors who forget they are playing a role'. Bohm continues: 'We become trapped in the theatre of our thoughts (the words "theatre" and "theory" have the same root, *theoria*, to look at). This is when thought starts to become incoherent. Reality may change but the theatre continues'.

The reality is that patients *are* increasingly asking for choice and yet our theatre is the puppets and slaves we have become, controlled and dominated by policy and procedure and risk management.

But, we *did* teeter on the edge of chaos.

> Some people approach the edge, become fearful and retreat to the safety of an old and familiar surface. Other people get reckless and fall off the edge into despair and ruin. A few brave travellers use the edge as a launch platform to leap into new possibilities. (Mycek 1999)

Litigation when things go wrong in maternity care is a costly reality. I understood Carol's map in this way, and yet I sense we might have leapt into new possibilities, rather than 'sticking with the knitting, playing it safe, and staying inside the comfort zone' had we shared our maps, engaged in dialogue and worked as leaders together as a group (Cope 2001).

I am presently taking small steps as a transformational leader to make learning come out of complex situations such as these. I want to lead midwifery practice in a meaningful way in tune with my personal vision. So although I yielded to Carol's command, I still hang onto my vision and values and have a much clearer picture of reality.

Choice is prominent in the new *Maternity matters* document (DoH 2007). My prediction is that we will encounter increasing requests for alternative styles of birth that may sit outside hospital policy. So, it is not acceptable, as an organisation that espouses to offer choice but is actually risk averse, that these women might be coerced by default and use of power into homebirths when this may not be the best place for them to deliver. Nor is it acceptable that we are resistant to the demand for change. This situation demonstrates a need to change a culture of control, command and 'do it our way'. We will see more of the same. It is yet another example of the butterfly effect and, for Carol, the flood gates may eventually open!

Complexity theory offers a clearing on a hazy horizon of uncertain terrains, for me as a transformational leader to work *with* the reality of risk and varying paradigms of knowledge about birth yet still offer patient choice. This challenges all levels of leadership working within maternity services to dialogue about alternative ways of knowing/understanding birth, values, limitations, fears and shared purpose. The idea of mapping, to work *with* complexity, illustrates the need for a shared and fused vision and is a vital component of the learning organisation, bringing direction, purpose and meaningful ways to practise. Senge (1990:234) speaks of harmonised energies when alignment and commonality of direction occur in teams.

I am currently working with other supervisors to bring shared vision to our group. Senge (1990:236) says team learning encourages dialogue and flow of shared meaning. My conversations with Carol and other midwives will have created a small butterfly effect in the system. Even though it feels I make little difference and my voice is lost in the big machine, connection with these events, communications with others, just taking the stance to support Harriet as I did, will have affected what happened in some unknowable way, in the bigger picture that I cannot see.

> Nothing happens in the quantum world without something encountering something else. Nothing exists independent of its relationships. We are constantly creating the world – evoking from it many potentials – as we participate in all its many interactions. This is a world of process, the process of connecting, where 'things' come into temporary existence because of relationship. (Wheatley 1999:69)

As I finish this assignment, as if emerging from sleep, sensations filtering through, I am aware again of the spring and my bursting, untended jungle of a garden outside. I have been shut away writing for so many days! I have resisted the urge to go out there and be in it, amongst it, rather than do what I must for this course.

Throughout this writing, I sense a theme of a need for nurturing relationship and connectivity with clients, colleagues, systems we work in, the world, indeed the cosmos that we do not fully understand. My garden and nature are examples of order emerging from complexity and chaos, the beauty and creativity when working *with* systems in harmony. By appreciating connections and relationships rather than trying to control or upsetting the gentle balance, it flourishes. Often, the less I *try* to do and control in the garden, the lovelier it gets and the fewer problems I have with bugs and weeds. Cyclical patterns of order, emerging from the chaos perhaps.

Reflection

In her narrative, Lazell positions her practice within chaos theory to frame and make sense of her organisation's difficulty with risk taking and in doing so, failing the woman and the idea of woman-centred care. Becoming mindful is to embrace chaos as a creative force patterned around strange attractors, for example caring, rather than view chaos as random and a threat to order. Indeed, practice is self-organising, order constantly unfolding patterned around strange attractors.

She reveals reflection as essentially empowering, that in working through an oppressive issue, she finds meaning and resolve to take action. Her eloquent writing is also a call to other midwives to take action to maintain the integrity of midwifery vision of being with woman.

Lazell is a very talented reflective writer. This reflective account reflects the development of her reflective writing style. She breaks up paragraphs as if they are separate yet connected pieces. She is no longer interested in a conventional academic-style flow ... she seeks to find her own style, bringing in quotes, images, poetry to weave her narrative into a coherent and reflexive whole. Consider this as you read the narrative.

Reflection opens a door into the messy world of everyday practice that apparently seems chaotic. Organisational life is hell-bent on controlling things, imposing order but only creating more chaos, because imposing order doesn't work. Order follows its own patterns around meaningful attractors. Chaos theory teaches us that we can 'let go' and go with the flow and order will emerge as a self-organising force. Chaos theory also informs us that we must always pay attention to the whole to see the pattern of relationships and the way things are shaped through conditions. Reflection is 'messy playfulness' – as Wheatley and Kellner-Rogers (1999:18–39) write: 'All this messy playfulness creates relationships that make available more: more expressions, more variety, more stability, more support ... patterns emerge as we connect to one another'.

Conclusion

Lazell's narrative offers us another example of narrative writing. Note the development of Lazell's narrative form from her previous narrative (Chapter 14) as she seeks to find her own narrative rhythm.

Narrative is a way of finding meaning in chaos, writing attracted by the quest to find meaning.

In Chapter 18 I consider the reflective curriculum, opening learning spaces structured through guided reflection and creating the curriculum conditions to enable reflection to flourish; a similar idea to creating the conditions of clinical practice in which reflective practice can flourish. It might seem obvious that the educational curriculum is always a learning organisation yet teachers, like everyone, are caught up in socialised practices that actually impede learning.

Chapter 18
The reflective curriculum

Running in place

Charlotte Joko Beck (1989:123) writes:

> Suppose we want to know how a marathon runner feels; if we run two blocks, or two miles or five miles, we will know something about running these distances, but we won't yet know anything about running a marathon. We can recite theories about marathons; we can describe tables about the physiology of marathon runners; we can pile up endless information about marathon running; but it doesn't mean we know what it is. We can only know when we are the one doing it. We only know our lives when we experience them directly ... this we can call running in place, being present as we are, right here and now.

We can only know when we are the one doing it. I might add mindfully doing it. Running in place, being where we need to be so as to live our vision. Beck identifies three stages to running in place in our practice. By 'practice', Beck refers to zazen or Zen meditation practice. However, this can be interpreted as mindful practice or being mindful as I go about my daily clinical practice.

The first stage in practice is to recognise that we're not running in place, we're always thinking about how our lives might be (or how they once were). What is there in our life right now that we don't want to run in place with? Whatever is repetitive, dull, painful or miserable: we don't want to run in place with that. No indeed! The first stage in practice is to recognise that we are rarely present: we're not experiencing life, we are thinking about it, conceptualising it, having opinions about it. It is frightening to run in place. A major component of practice is to realise how this fear and unwillingness dominates us.

If we practice with patience and persistence, we [can] enter the second stage. We slowly begin to be conscious of the ego barriers of our life: the thoughts, the emotions, the evasions, the manipulations can now be observed and objectified more easily. This objectification is painful and revealing; but if we continue, the clouds obscuring the scenery become thinner.

And what is the crucial, healing third stage? It is the direct experience of whatever the scenery of our life is at any moment as we run in place. Is it simple? Yes. Is it easy? No. We grow by being where we are and experiencing what our life is right now. We must experience our anger, our sorrow, our failure, our apprehension; they can all be our teachers, when we do not separate ourselves from them. When we escape what is given, we cannot learn, we cannot grow. (Beck 1997:123–4)

The words *If we practice with patience and persistence we can enter the second stage* reflect the effort, commitment and time required to learn to run in place. For the Zen practitioner such learning is lifelong. Such learning is focused on the process – *We grow by being where we are and experiencing what our life is right now* – not the outcome. Such is the nature of mindful practice in three stages.

Simple? Yes. Easy? No. As I advocate strongly, we need our guides to help us journey well.

At the core of a reflective curriculum are the stories shared by students and teachers. Within each story is the essence of practice. Each story is a microcosm of the whole. Different aspects of the story can be pulled out from the story canvass and explored against the story's contextual and wider theoretical and philosophical background. A community of storytellers in dialogue seeking to learn through these stories more about being and becoming an effective practitioner, regardless of the discipline.

May 2008. I am attending the Toronto Reflective Practice conference, 'Refresh, reflect, renew – connecting through reflective practice across disciplines'. To commence my end-note paper, I pose the question: WHAT has been going on here at the conference? I note the prevailing themes of story and narrative, and situating such approaches to learning meaningfully and skilfully within curriculum. To emphasise the significance of this theme I read:

> In cultures throughout the world, the figure of the storyteller, encircled by a crowd eager to know what will happen next, is central and vital. In stories and tales, myths and legends, a culture recognises itself and identifies its needs and its ideals. On an individual level too, through these narratives, we recognise the deep and inchoate stirrings within our own hearts. Our strongest memories of stories may be associated with childhood, but the hold of storytelling in our hearts did not really leave us when we grew up; it took on new guises. In our culture, scientists and the manipulators of the media may appear to be the purveyors of truth, but it is still to stories: films, novels, even computer games, that we turn for a more satisfying version of reality. Stories have the power to cut through our mental chatter and hold us spellbound, strangely attentive to the fate of imaginary or long-dead characters. And when we emerge from the compelling world of the imagination, in some mysterious way we seem able to make more sense of the ordinary world that we experience day to day. (p1)

These words, written by Karen Stout, open the editor's preface to 'Parables, myths, and symbols of the White Lotus Sutra' from a series of lectures by Sangharakshita, collected together in *The drama of cosmic enlightenment* (1993). The Buddha decided to teach through stories because conceptual explanation had failed to convince his audiences.

As if to make the point, I then read the following story.

> A student nurse once wrote in her journal ...

> Bill was sad
> I felt his sadness
> I sat with him
> and then the staff nurse asked me to help
> she pulled me away
> my mouth opened to resist
> but no words came out
> passively I complied
> anger filled me
> Bill's eyes said it all
> He has lung cancer
> Later I confronted her

I asked why?
My anger barely contained
spilling out
'Why?' she asked, rising on her heels, clearly ruffled,
'Because you can't sit around all day as you feel like it.'
But Bill?
'There's time for that stuff later when the work's done!'
I am despondent
I want to quit if it is like this
Is this nursing?
Is this the horizontal violence I read about somewhere?
I mentioned it to Gill
she said something like that happened to her last week
I am not alone
but that is no consolation
The tutor says 'it's tough out there'
Sympathetic gestures as if it is my problem
What sort of response is that?
Whose side is she on?
or does she squirm uneasily on the fence in her ivory tower?
The dog at home is so bruised
What's the point of being awake?
What's the point
What's the point.

The audience nod and feel the story's message touch a deep collective consciousness; this story is known and lived. Its truth is self-evident deep within the shadows of our psyche, a reflection of a seemingly universal truth. Such stories are transgressive. They intend to disturb the smooth surface of things to reveal the inner turbulence, embodied, out of mind. Some may take offence or become defensive. Sometimes we do not want to face our truth. Reflection brings us face to face with our failure to stop such situations happening. We squirm with guilt. I do not intend to accuse or suggest this story is each reader's reality. You will know this for yourself. I simply point my finger to the moon.

The turbulence settles. I move onto the question SO WHAT? I ask my audience to take a blank sheet of paper and to imagine and doodle the shape of a truly reflective curriculum, perhaps using ideas gleaned through the conference. At this point of closure I want to stimulate people so when they move away they are awake, open to possibility, more likely to act. For about 5 minutes they toy with their pencils. I do not ask to see these shapes. I share my own (Fig. 18.1).

I am asked about history – I say it is the contextual moment situated in history – a personal, social, cultural, professional, political, environmental, professional, gendered history. In other words, everything that constitutes this moment in time. It is also recognising our roots, that nursing, or any profession, evolves from its history, its tradition.

Teacher identity

Earlier that morning, I had attended Laura Hegge's[1] concurrent session 'Narrative and imagination in reflective teaching practice: recognizing and rewriting frozen stories

---

[1] lhegge@oise.utoronto.ca

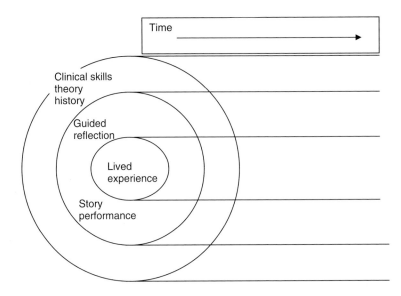

Figure 18.1 My doodle.

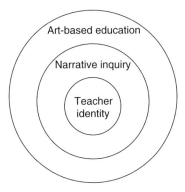

Figure 18.2 Laura Hegge's doodle.

of teaching'. She had drawn a similar shape of a teacher-based narrative curriculum (Fig. 18.2).

I am struck and excited by the resonance with my own doodle. The idea of 'teacher identity' at the core resonates with lived experience, perhaps giving lived experience more focus with its emphasis on outcome. The teacher identity is like a jewel representing one's true self – and the curriculum is designed to enable the teacher or nurse to find her real or true self beneath the layers of assumptions and defences that have built up like silt over time. Only then can she be liberated to realise her therapeutic potential.

Narrative inquiry is reflective practice. Art-based education is intrinsic to narrative inquiry. By stating clinical skills, history and theory, I make the education more explicit. I resist a dichotomy between art based and science based; there is only practice or praxis, suggesting that practice is skilled, informed, purposeful and reflexive.

Tripods

In the concurrent session before Laura, Jasna Schwind and Gail Lindsay, in their session 'From relationships to experience: narrative reflections on nurse-teachers', had shared their idea of a camera tripod. The camera was the nurse's practice. One tripod leg was doing nursing, another leg was knowledge and the third leg was caring. They felt that the knowledge and doing legs were well developed but the caring leg was short and stunted, leaving the nurse unbalanced. The camera is lop-sided, the lens distorted.

The message is obvious: nurses need to be balanced to practise or what Suzuki (1999) terms having the 'right posture' (see Chapter 1). Therefore, the curriculum itself must be balanced to enable this. If the curriculum is unbalanced the nurse will not develop the right posture and cannot nurse effectively.

The image of the tripod resonated with the way I and Alison Leary had imaged the nature of caring within Lydia Hall's theory of therapeutic nursing (see Fig. 18.3). We envisioned a foundational tripod of what it means to be a nurse (the ontological), what it means to do nursing (the epistemological) and the values/purpose of nursing (or any other discipline), for example my clinical vision to ease suffering and enable growth. The fusion of these aspects creates an inner tripod of compassion, craft and wisdom. Wisdom is the dialogue between phronesis or practical wisdom as known through reflection on the particular moment with the wider universal wisdom or philo-sophia. This is the third dialogical movement (see Chapter 4). Craft is the application of wisdom as praxis – it is what nurses do. Compassion is compassion, generally not understood, valued or taught in itself.

The camera lens is 'caring unfolding mindfully' captured through the lens of reflection. This model patterns the curriculum. Of course, it is only a representation and yet it has a compelling attraction.

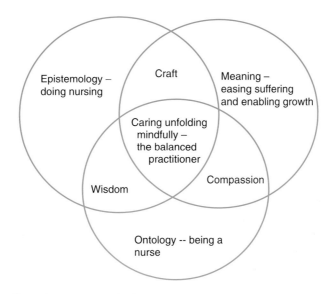

Figure 18.3 Conceptualising the nursing curriculum.

Frozen stories

Laura shared her own story that had become frozen. She hadn't known how to move the story on. And then, with guidance, she found a possible resolution, a fantasy, if faced with a similar situation again. Her imagination was the key to break some of the patterns to move the story on.

Perhaps one value of the archetypal story is that it offers a safe place to imagine solutions to the student nurse's predicament, even though it is not our own story. A kind of simulation in preparation for when the real thing comes along, as it will inevitably do. The story is also a simulation for teacher-guides and mentors. Why did the staff nurse and teacher act as they did? What forces have shaped their responses and how might these forces be shifted? *What is the point!?*

I then pose the third question – NOW WHAT? I challenge the audience – if you truly desire a reflective curriculum, what would constrain you from realising it? What action do you need to take towards realising a truly reflective curriculum?

We do not have time to explore this question. It is left simmering to slowly cook. And yet it is such a vital question because a reflective curriculum requires a sharp turn of the head, moving from the paradigmatic gaze of the traditional curriculum to a reflective one. No easy turn.

Teaching through reflective practice

To reiterate: at the core of the reflective curriculum is a rich vein of guided reflection, a space where students bring experiences from clinical practice to dialogue. It is not enough to tag reflection on to conventional programmes – it needs space to fulfil its learning potential. For example, on a pre-registration diploma or degree programme, I would have reflective practice as the core throughout the programme, at least 4 hours a week, to enable the students to reflect on clinical placements:

- to appreciate and work towards resolving the contradictions and feelings that practice reveals
- as a way of integrating theory and practice
- as a supportive self-development programme
- to become a reflective practitioner.

The idea of integrating the curriculum through a continuous core reflective thread (portfolio) is now incorporated into the pre-registration programme at the University of Bedfordshire. The guide meets with every cohort twice a module (nine modules) for 3 hours. The students must support their learning through the module practice placement with four reflections. Not quite 4 hours per week but a toehold.

Camp-fire teaching

I dialogue with students by sitting with them around the *camp-fire* where we share our stories of practice, seeking to learn through our shared experiences to transcend and expand the horizons of our understanding. My stories trigger others' stories – to capture meaning and evoke the imagination, and to take them deep within themselves. Within any story is the whole curriculum. It is simply a question of drawing out specific aspects from the whole but always against a background of the whole. Holistic teaching to develop holistic practitioners.

Through story we learn about therapeutic relationships, about ourselves, about compassion, about empathy, about ethics; we review our interventions and develop clinical judgement; we learn about quality and relationships with other professionals; we learn how to deal with anxiety and conflict; we learn to hold creative tension and to understand and resolve the tensions of everyday practice; we learn to take responsibility and be assertive; we learn to critique and assimilate theory within our practice; we learn to become mindful and wise; we learn to be available to our patients. To learn to become who we need to be as nurses and other health professionals, we learn our craft. And we learn in imaginative and creative ways.

To succeed, teachers must become reflective practitioners. They need to strengthen their links with clinical practice to construct their own clinical stories and also to become mindful and reflexive on their own teaching craft. Teachers must also move into collaborative dialogical relationships with their students and colleagues, to view themselves as a resource to enable students to succeed. No easy mandate for petrified teachers.

Petrified:
1. make someone so frightened that they are unable to move
2. change organic matter into stone by encrusting or replacing its original substance with a mineral deposit.

The teacher is a guide, leading the students to learn through their experiences, shifting the milieu of the classroom from teacher centred to student centred. The teacher must let go of the life raft of control to flow with what is unfolding. It's OK to be thrown from time to time … becoming a master requires practice, vulnerability, humility and courage. If we who teach ask this of our students then we must ask it of ourselves.

A word on masters:

> The ancient masters
> didn't try to educate people
> but kindly taught them to not-know
> When they think that they know the answers,
> people are difficult to guide.
> When they know they don't know,
> people can find their own way.
> (Lao Tzu 1999:65)

However, sharing stories is not unproblematic, nor should it be if it is to constitute the core of the curriculum. Such activity must be carefully constructed as the first step to creating the conditions for a critical pedagogy within a community of inquiry based on dialogue and 'high challenge, high support'. First and foremost is the construction of trust as *a group responsibility*. Ask yourself – what creates the conditions for thick trust within the classroom?

Trust

Cope (2001:152) identified five attributes of trust that offer a way of reflecting on the factors that contribute to trust (Box 18.1). Each attribute can be given a score of 10. Thick trust would have a total score of 40. Thin trust would be less than 25.

Box 18.1   Five attributes of trust

Truthful	The extent to which integrity, honesty and truthfulness are developed and maintained
Responsive	The openness, mental accessibility or willingness to share ideas and information freely
Uniform	The degree of consistency, reliability and predictability contained within the relationship
Safe	The loyalty, benevolence or willingness to protect, support and encourage each other
Trained	The competence, technical knowledge and capabilities of both parties

Guided reflection groups are contracted in much the same way as clinical supervision, ensuring that every person takes responsibility for self and the group as a whole. Reflective practice and the rules of dialogue are taught.

Teaching reflective practice is straightforward.

- I share my own story; this role models what a story might look like and my risk of sharing it.
- I ask the group what is significant about the story and ask them to relate it to their own experiences.
- I then ask the group to write a description of an experience – just 15 minutes non-stop writing (see p49).
- I then introduce the MSR and systematically move through the cues, using my own story as an example.

This is enough for a first session. I ask the students to develop their own text using the MSR, before we meet again.

- When we meet again I illustrate how the text can be broken down into single lines to open up the spaces between the lines where meaning often lies hidden and other significances are revealed, developing poems and using images and art.
- I then ask them what insights they have gained and how these might be framed using the framing perspectives (see p77).
- When the group next meets we share our insights and how these might relate to another experience that I ask them to bring to the next session.
- I use examples of theory to consider how theory can inform our emerging practice.

And so it continues within the reflexive learning spiral, year in, year out.

The teacher-guide works hard at ensuring a collaborative approach within the rules of dialogue, checking self at every turn so as not to fall back into a 'dominant teacher' mode of being. When hegemony has been the norm, diversity must be actively worked towards. It can never be assumed simply because we might say 'this group is collaborative, based on mutual respect'. Fine words 'out there' but they have to be lived and at first we may not know how to live them. Saying a classroom is safe doesn't make it safe.

The starting point for organizing the programme content of education or political action must be the present, existential, concrete situation, reflecting the aspirations of the people. Utilizing certain basic contradictions, we must pose this existential, concrete, present situation to the people as a problem which challenges them and requires a response – not just at the intellectual level, but at the level of action. We must never merely discourse on the present situation, must never provide the people with programmes which have little or nothing to do with their preoccupations, doubts, hopes and fears – programmes which at times in fact increase the fears of the oppressed consciousness. It is not our role to speak to the people about our own view, not to attempt to impose that view on them, but rather to dialogue with the people about their view and ours. (Freire 1972:24–5)

In sharing of stories it is vital that I problematise myself, critiquing myself in terms of not just what I do but my background behind it. In doing so, I model story sharing and open the space for a critical listening.

Because stories are so personal there is always a risk that people will avoid being critical for at least two reasons. Firstly, they listen more with their hearts than with their heads to identify with the trauma of the story as if *ganging up* against the alleged oppressors. It is difficult to be critical of storytellers when their stories are emotional and oppressive. The natural response of listeners is emotional: to sympathise, rather than be critical.

Secondly, it is a collusive strategy to make the space more safe. In my response as a guide I always seek to hold the space between the head and the heart. I always ask the storyteller to explore the assumptions behind the story, to ask 'What assumptions govern this story?'. Teaching in this way inspires students to write their own stories and in doing so they become more aware of themselves within their practice and pay attention to the subtle nuances of caring that make the difference in effective care.

Sometimes I light a candle, especially if my stories concern someone who has died. Lighting the candle is a way of honouring the person and introducing ritual into the classroom. It is also symbolic of the camp-fire, the fire that draws us together in a sacred space. No need to rush.

> We must slow down or we will miss all that has meaning. Meaning is revealed only when you pause, when you stop, when you pay attention. Learn the lesson of tribal people. Put your busyness on pause, eliminate distractions, and allow the meaning of life and living to return to you. Slow down in order to connect with the meaning of life. (Blackwolf and Jones 1996:90)

Stories can also be performed. Imagine students working together to write and perform a play about caring for a stroke patient or someone who is depressed or giving birth. Performance enables students to embody theory and practice as praxis ... and engage their audiences on a sensual level. Being engaged, people learn. And not just students. Reflective teaching opens the door for the teacher's own learning; by listening to stories, the teacher must also reflect and consider the words in terms of his or her own experiences.

Judging reflective writing

I recently explored with a group of third-year adult branch nursing students their experience with reflection. I had read the group one of my stories. One student exclaimed 'That's just how I see reflection but when I wrote like that I was told it was too descriptive'. They complained that teachers constantly say 'the work is too descriptive'.

They were expected to use a model for reflection (such as the MSR) and yet the depth of the cues had not been explored with them. It is superficial and possibly harmful to expose the students to self-inquiry and then let them swim about in the murky depths of their consciousness, and then to say their effort was inadequate.

Academic reflective writing should focus on one specific criterion: 'What insights/ learning have I gained embedded within a wider philosophical/theoretical and cultural literature (reflexive movement)?'. Academic writing should not be focused on the reflective process, although description of the event and specific reflective cues will naturally be used within an exploration of insights/learning gained. When academic work involves presentation of texts using art and drama then such work always requires a commentary in which insights are clearly set out.

In 1992 I set up the first reflective practice module at the University of Luton (now Bedfordshire). The programme was 60 credits at level 3 (50% of the required modules for an Honours degree). The programme was delivered over 30 weeks (two semesters) meeting for 20×3-hour sessions as a mixture of workshops and guided reflection sessions. It was a truly innovative programme that accepted nurses and midwives across diverse backgrounds. Their shared experiences were relevant to the whole group because they tended not to be about technical or clinical knowledge as evidenced by the students' work.

In this programme students had three assignments.

1. Write up a reflection on a single experience, using the MSR and critically exploring the insights gained.
2. Develop a personal theory of reflection based on theories of reflection and your own experience during this programme.
3. Reflect on the reflexive development of your expertise during the programme, drawing on (at least) three experiences reflected on during the programme.

An analysis of assignment (3) consistently demonstrated the extent of learning achieved through this programme, as evidenced in the narratives written by Clare, Jim and Simon Lee (Chapters 9–12). Other published narratives are Johns and Hardy (2005), Morgan and Johns (2005), and Johns and Joiner (Johns 2002:73–82).

In assignment (2) one typical student wrote:

> Reflection is transforming my practice in so many meaningful and profound ways ... I have never felt so free to care and to be true to what I consider to be ideal practice ... Reflection had enabled me to contextually refocus on the individual. My interactive skills are being sharpened and I am rediscovering the therapeutic value of establishing a close relationship with clients. Until now I have never been able to find an approach to nursing which recognises the true potential of this unique relationship ... My first few reflections were triggered by a feeling that I had failed to achieve my goals in some way ... guided reflection had enabled me to make use of the creative energy of conflict. I have been challenged to stoke up a far more challenging style of practice. I have become empowered to provoke and maintain the contradictions I feel between my goals of desirable practice and actual practice. Just as there are no limits to my expanding consciousness ...

This programme ceased in 2006, to be replaced by a 'developing a clinical effectiveness portfolio' (30 credits at level 3). This programme has 10 sessions spanning 30 weeks. The students' portfolio is designed using the Model for Reflective Inquiry (see Fig. 3.3, p61). The student is required to reflect on eight experiences, applying insights from one reflection to the next in a reflexive spiral of developing effectiveness. The portfolio is a core module within the BSc palliative care programme to create a space for the students

	Semester 1	Semester 2	Semester 3
Year 1	Leadership in organisations Leading change (project)	Managing conflict ———————▶	
	Dissertation – narrative of being and becoming the leader the person desires to be		
Year 2	Alternative perspectives on leadership Ensuring quality (project)	Leading in a chaotic world ———————▶	

Figure 18.4 The Masters in Health Care leadership reflective programme.

to apply learning/knowledge gained from 'taught' modules. Yet even 'taught modules' are taught through story.

Postregistration degree students could choose to use guided reflection as a process of self-inquiry and transformation for their BSc dissertation, some of which have been published – 'Finding a new way in health visiting' (Latchford 2002:144–68), 'Working with deliberate self-harm patients in A&E' (Groom 2002:169–86).

This reflective approach was incorporated into the Masters in Health Care leadership taught modules and dissertation. The student leaders are required to construct a coherent and reflexive narrative of being and becoming the leader they desire to be, commencing from the beginning of the course. The dissertation is the core thread that integrates the programme as a whole (Fig. 18.4). I am currently preparing a new book, *Becoming a transformational leader*, that analyses the first 24 of these narratives and includes seven edited leadership narratives.

In summary, teaching through reflective practice can claim a number of advantages.

- It is grounded in a philosophy of genuine student-led practice, based on the students' own practice – thus ensuring that learning is both practical and meaningful.
- It is holistic through stories where theory and ideas can be seen in context of the particular moment, and the relationship between things can be seen as a whole.
- It is 'whole-brain' teaching, enabling the development of right brain attributes: intuition, perception, imagination and creativity, notably through art.
- It introduces theory in relation to emerging issues – hence the student will find theory more relevant and meaningful and thus assimilate it within personal knowing, what Ausubel (1967) described as 'having a hook to hang your hat on'. This approach to learning deals immediately with any notion of the 'theory–practice gap'.
- It develops learning on an intuitive level and thus may seem more suited to experienced practitioners. However, it also enables the development of intuition.

- It accesses the 'swampy lowlands' where real issues lie rather than focusing on the 'hard high ground' of abstract concepts. Many students may struggle in the real world because of the complexity of practice; reflection gives direct focus to their experience and enables them to make sense of contradictions and develop problem-solving and survival skills. It also acknowledges and accepts their difficulties.
- It values and honours everyday practice as the ground for learning, as befits a practice discipline.
- It is values based, constantly challenging and clarifying vision and purpose, balancing 'being a nurse' with 'doing nursing', addressing such issues as ethics, relationships, compassion and knowing self that are not traditionally taught within a theory-led curriculum.
- It is based in the real world, seeking understanding and meaning of why things are as they are.
- It is problem solving, focusing on areas of contradiction, ethics, politics, tradition, power and change, enabling practitioners to become political, empowered and assertive.
- It makes a difference to practice through its reflexive focus of gaining and applying insights to new experiences. In this way we get 'joined-up learning'.
- It is supportive, dynamic and engaging. And fun!

Disadvantages

- Perhaps some students may feel threatened by the intense gaze, particularly if they lack commitment to practice or study. It is less prescriptive and therefore more 'adult' and requires more responsibility and self-direction.
- It is harder work than conventional learning because it requires the critique and juxtaposition of theory with practice.
- The teacher or guide may not be good enough – stuck in traditional modes of teaching, leading to issues of control or viewing reflection as an educational technology rather than an organic evolving process.

As a result of the Toronto Reflective Practice conference, I have put in motion a new book, *Developing the reflective curriculum*, an organic book growing through initiative developing, emerging, expanding over the next 3 years. The ball is rolling, gathering pace, gathering ideas and examples.

Marcia Ring emails me from the University of Vermont (22 August 2008).

> I can't believe this is the first time I am writing to you since June when you graced us with your presence and wisdom. Some of the MEPN students found your work and conference life altering. I even changed the final assignment for the MEPN students in psych to allow them to do their final Interpersonal Process Recording utilizing your method. Only one took advantage of that but it was truly stunning. If you like, I can find out if I can send it to you. You'd love it. I think she should publish it.

Marcia begins to restructure her Masters in expanded psychiatric nursing to accommodate reflective practice. As she says, the results are stunning. I feel the ripple across the ocean. This student's work, alongside others, and Marcia's own reflections will be published in the new book. Just one example within a new world-wide collaboration to develop a truly reflective curriculum. Opening the doors of perception towards a brave new world.

Conclusion

The reflective curriculum is a vast subject. I have merely outlined one or two ideas. Essentially it turns the relationship between theory and practice on its head following Schön's (1987) reversal of the epistemology of professional practice, using the students' experience as the data for learning and linking theory to that experience in meaningful ways, what Ausubel (1967) termed 'having a hook to hang your hat on'.

In Chapter 19 I explore the performance turn as a natural development from representing lived experience as narrative to presenting experience as performance.

Chapter 19

The performance turn

Introduction

Constructing coherent and reflexive narratives is challenging and stimulating. Two of my recent books reflect 4 years of continuous journalling. *Being mindful, easing suffering* is a narrative of my time as a complementary therapist working in a hospice between September 2000 and 2002. The narrative commences with my experience with meeting Iris and ends shortly after her death.[1] The focus on Iris gives the narrative a sense of continuity interwoven with my experiences of working with other patients within the chronological unfolding of my experience. During this time I was learning both my therapist and narrative craft.

The book *Engaging reflection in practice* presents my narrative from October 2002 to September 2004. The narrative is different from *Being mindful, easing suffering*. Firstly, it has no central figure extending through the text. Secondly, it is written as a series of 'case studies' rather than in strict chronological time. Thirdly, I paid more attention to narrative structure and as such, it is less spontaneous than *Being mindful*. That doesn't necessarily make it a more accomplished narrative. There is a poignancy to the stories in *Being mindful* that is not, at least in my opinion, so obvious in *Engaging reflection*. I sense that a preoccupation with narrative theory or technique can obscure presentation and inhibit expression.

I have come to know what I suspected all the time, that narrative writing is learnt through doing and reflecting on it. The core of narrative is the plot, a reflexive unfolding of my effort to know and ease suffering or, put another way, to be most available to the people I interact with. Reflexivity is evidenced through a series of experiences, usually adopting some framework to measure one's emergence against, such as the being available template. The idea of narrative coherence was discussed in Chapter 5 within my exploration of autoethnography as a significant influence on my approach to narrative design.

The performance turn

I have become involved in exploring what I call the 'performance turn', a shift from representing lived experience as narrative to presenting lived experience as performance.

---

[1] I have since rewritten the Iris part of the narrative, based on my deeper understanding of the nature of narrative writing. I have yet to publish this revision.

My recent conference papers have involved reading or performing narratives that illuminate a particular aspect of my practice as evidenced through the narratives presented in this book. To reiterate, in reading a narrative my primary intent is to focus on some transgressive point about practice. My secondary intent is to open a space for listeners to reflect on their own experiences. My third intent is to illuminate the impact of narrative to support these intents and to develop the craft of narrative and performance research towards enabling people to realise desirable practice.

I first became aware of the difference between someone reading a narrative and listening to the same narrative when I gave a paper at the Institute of Reflective Practice[2] workshop in 2005. Several members of the audience were given the narrative to read prior to the conference. It was clear that listening to a narrative and reading a narrative were different experiences. Reading was, as might be expected, more 'head stuff' and listening more 'heart stuff'. I had experience of this when submitting narratives for publication that had been well received when read. The head begins to censor, to take offence, to demand explanation – 'What is this about?'. In listening, the listener senses what it is about as a heart response if the narrative is engaging enough. Indeed, any writer's explanation of what the narrative might mean would get in the way of experiencing the narrative.

October 2008. I am a visiting scholar at Florida Atlantic University. I perform a narrative entitled Trevor. The reading takes 15 minutes. One doctoral student comments that she had read my stories but listening to them is such a different experience. She felt as if she was there in the situation. It was emotional, deeply moving. She had felt the issues, the drama unfolding, rather than thinking about it.

Other students agree and it is a response I know from past performances, reinforcing the idea that messages heard primarily with the heart leave stronger traces than when heard primarily with the mind.

Just as my approach to narrative has been inspired by autoethnography, so my turn to performance has been inspired by performance ethnography, in particular the demand that performance be a form of social action, revealing and displaying oppression for its impact on constraining the realisation of social good.

Denzin (2003:9–14) notes: 'Performance is an act of intervention, a method of resistance, a form of criticism, a way of revealing agency … Performances make sites of oppression visible'. Denzin's perspective fits within the critical social science remit of critical reflection – that reflection doesn't change just the reflective practitioner but also the reader, listener, audience or co-performers of narrative with the intention to move people to social action and change through participation and dialogue. Dialogue by its very nature seeks to move people towards consensus for creating better worlds. This is the moral root of reflective practice.

Performance is more confrontational than narrative. For example, my autoethnographic narrative of being with my mother the day before she died is a deeply evocative criticism of her residential nursing home. It was entitled 'Reflection on my mother dying: a story of caring shame'.[3] My intent in writing the narrative was to be critical, damning even, to confront uncaring practice and raise social consciousness so other mothers do not suffer such indignity when 92 years old and helpless. Dying should be a state of grace. When I read the narrative to two audiences in New Zealand in September 2008,

---

[2] www.reflectivepractices.co.uk
[3] This narrative is published in *Journal of Holistic Nursing* (in press). At the time of writing it has yet to be performed although it has been read twice.

I was very emotional; feelings of being with my mother rushed back and at times my voice was close to breaking. And yet, it was my emotions that transformed the simple reading into something more, into performance, even though I do not describe it as such. My feeling of contained outrage engaged the audience. Their tears were my own. This is where messages are heard and impact. Caring *is* emotional and heartfelt. I was asked whether I might produce audio-recordings because the listening was so powerful. Perhaps a DVD would be even better.

I prime the audience (as with all my readings) to consider the significance of the narrative in terms of their own experiences. Following the performance, I then invite the audience to dialogue with me (the sixth dialogical movement). I do not say how this narrative is significant for me prior to starting the dialogue.

With performance, the listener is invited to:

- enter into a dialogue with the text
- be open to the possibility of what the text has to say, especially in relation to their own practice/life
- suspend expectations of what the text might say
- be aware of feelings, especially hostile feelings towards the text, and consider why this might be.

As Ben Okri (1997:41) writes:

The writer … does one half of the work, but the reader [or listener] does the other. The reader's/ listener's mind becomes the screen, the place, the era. To a large extent, readers/listeners create the world from words, they invent the reality they read. Reading, therefore, is a co-production between writer and reader.

Performance texts

What follows are two performance texts. The first was written by Ruth Morgan based on her final course assignment whilst studying on the Being and becoming a reflective and effective practitioner course (see Chapter 18). At the time of writing, Ruth led a community nursing team in England. We performed it at the 9th International Reflective Practice conference at Robinson College, Cambridge, in 2003. The performance reflects on the impact of Ruth deciding to sit in a different chair one morning at the daily meeting. She did this as a deliberate response to her frustration with the transactional pattern of relationship that existed within the team in her effort to realise a more transformational type of leadership whereby each person of her team is developed and valued to be responsible for self and the group's collaborative practice grounded in adult–adult patterns of relationship. Ruth felt that transactional organisation reduces people to tasks to be done in ways that reinforce hierarchy and subordination. As such, she feels trapped in a parent–child pattern of relationship, always anxious and critical when things are not done as they should be and guilty when she has been critical.

The performance is structured through 10 acts with minimal adjustment to the original text. Course members performed in the various roles. Names have been anonymised, even Ruth's own name.

Musical chairs

Performers:
Ruth: *Ann*
Janet: *Beth*
Chris N: *Chris, Fiona*
Chris J: *Dorothy, Elaine*

Narrator (Ann): The change seemed simple, the effect was devastating. A few weeks ago, I decided, as team leader of the surgery district nursing team, to alter the seating arrangements in our daily work meeting.
(Team enter and sit in their usual six chairs arranged in a small circle around the desk. This seemingly minor change threw the team into turmoil and even threatened to fragment it. Ann sits in chair 1.)

Act 1

Ann: The team comprises six nurses who, for the sake of clarity, I will give pseudonyms beginning with the letters A, B, C and so on, to indicate order of seniority, although this is the antithesis of how I consider we should regard ourselves.
(Each character announces their name)
The daily morning meetings are held to enable the nurses on duty to discuss their caseloads, liaise with GPs (in the surgery), receive messages (faxes, emails) and incoming calls about patients *(Beth picks up phone, growls down it)* and share out the day's work. The nature of the business means these meetings are frequently subject to unavoidable interruptions, particularly by phone calls, although they are kept brief *(Beth makes abrupt call)* and, if possible, dealt with later.
Despite lively discussions and an atmosphere of friendliness in the team, I had been aware for some time of consistent signals of dissatisfaction from Dorothy, a team member who I sense lacks self-worth and feels undervalued. *(Dorothy hangs head)* I had sought ways of supporting and empowering her but comments about her lowly grade and position had continued. *(Dorothy hangs head lower)*
This troubled me and I mentioned to Beth the possibility of changing our rather hierarchical seating arrangements in the morning as a way of helping Dorothy feel less inferior. *(Beth shakes head)*
Unconsciously, we had adopted a pattern over the years which graded position and authority according to the seat we occupied. My casual comment was not pursued by Beth.
Beth: Can't see the point.
But my thoughts were confirmed one morning by an incidental observation from Elaine.
Elaine: I notice we always sit in the same seats (or words to that effect!).
The comment caused me to reflect on the meetings in more detail and I began to recognise the authoritarian style in which work was discussed and then delegated. I felt this was underlined by our 'graded' seating positions. Chair 1, by the computer and the external telephone, was always occupied by the nurse 'in charge' for that day, chair 2, next to the internal telephone, by the second in command, and so on. As a result, all phone calls and emails were dealt with by the more senior nurses on duty each day. Needless to say, the chair beside the coffee table was reserved for the nursing assistant, student or the otherwise lowliest grade of the shift who then served us all coffee! *(Fiona hands round mugs in hierarchical order!)*
As I say this now, I am astonished that we had unwittingly allowed this hierarchical system to develop and alarmed at the hidden messages being given and received. Pease (1981) researched the implications of non-verbal communication, finding that more human messages

were given by 'gestures, postures, position and distances' than by voice. *(Team leave, stacking chairs 3,4,5)*

Act 2

Ann: The morning I first occupied a 'different' seat was explosive.
(Team enter without Chris, pick up chairs and sit down. Ann leads the way by sitting on chair 3. Others are confused. Beth sits in chair 2, Dorothy and Elaine sit, Fiona sits last in chair 1)
I simply sat down in chair 3 instead of chair 1. This forced the other nurses to take different seats although nothing was said. I noticed that the 'second in seniority' (Beth) automatically retained seat 2 and 'my' usual seat (seat 1) was left to the last one entering the room who happened to be Fiona, the nursing assistant. Chris was not on duty that day. Beth's body language became clearly angry as the inevitable phone calls began *(Beth picks up phone a couple of times, growling down it)*, reaching explosion point when Fiona (sitting by the desk) picked up the receiver beside her to take an incoming call. *(Fiona picks up phone and holds it. Beth slams her diary across the desk)*
Beth *(aggressively)*: Ann, will you please sit back in your seat and take that call?
Ann: Fiona is perfectly able to answer the phone.
Beth *(angrily)*: I say she is not and it is your job to answer the phone.

Act 3 (action frozen)

(Ann stands to narrate)
I was astounded by this reaction. I had not viewed the act of answering the phone as a senior or empowering role and therefore had not foreseen the full implications of my chair move. In reality, my action was exposing the hierarchical attitudes within the team, illustrated by this clear division of labour between senior and junior roles. My attempt to remove status from the team meetings could be seen as a challenge to the authority of the higher graded nurses who sat in the 'power' chairs. Lacking explanation, my action was open to confusing misjudgements. I could be seen as abdicating personal responsibility, as disempowering senior team members or as nonchalantly ridding myself of irksome tasks. Brumpton (1998) anticipates fraught times when a team becomes unsure of individual roles and responsibilities and recommends that all members invest time in reaching agreement over team organisation.
In this context, I now recognise that Beth and I view leadership very differently. I note that Beth frequently asks other team members to do mundane administrative work (photocopying, faxing) for her but generally deals with the more complex and interesting issues herself, including dealing with patients and organisations on the telephone. Leigh and Maynard (1995) describe this as a 'controlling' approach with its emphasis on directing and delegating. My approach was instinctively becoming less authoritarian and more inclined to share both the responsible and the more routine tasks. Done well, this would be viewed by Leigh and Maynard as a 'supportive, inspiring' leadership in which 'success comes through sharing your leadership and power'. However, I did not have a clear vision of the changes I was trying to achieve and, through lack of clarity, the team did not understand my objectives as a context for the changes. Ideally, Squire (2001) recommends a 'stepwise communication strategy' to enable staff to understand and 'own' any changes to be implemented and provide a simple structure of change (RAID model) to facilitate this ownership. My experience demonstrates that successful, sustained change takes time, self-awareness and careful planning, involving all those affected. The crucial step of gaining agreement can be a slow, gradual process of creating awareness, then understanding, leading to support, involvement and commitment.
(Ann sits back in seat 3, unfreezing action)

In the event, I did not respond to Beth's angry command to answer the phone and Elaine leapt to the rescue, changed seats with Fiona, and put the long-suffering caller out of her misery. *(Elaine and Fiona swap seats. Elaine answers caller)*

As the call ended I pre-empted an icy silence.

Ann: How does everyone feel about answering the phone?

Elaine: I don't mind answering the phone.

Beth: I don't agree. It's the job of the G grades to answer the phone.

An uneasy discussion ensued in which group members all expressed, somewhat hesitantly, their willingness to deal with phone calls, and also emails, during our meetings. I pointed out the ranking system in the way we sat and why I felt it needed to change. Beth could not agree.

Beth: The team needs a leader.

perhaps revealing her own need for control and status. I reiterated the importance of a leader but expressed the view that effective leadership was about leading and not about hierarchy. Brumpton (1998) views inspiring leaders as highly skilled in enabling, motivating and co-ordinating team activities but without hierarchical attitudes. The atmosphere prickled with disagreement between Beth and myself with Beth stating resentment at the lack of discussion prior to my change of chair. I had not considered the change significant enough to be worthy of preliminary discussion, beyond our earlier inconclusive conversation, and had completely underestimated the reaction. Mullally (2001) states that the smallest changes often have the greatest impact and McClarey (2001) warns that instigating change without consensus agreement is poor practice since 'most changes affect the whole team'.

Fiona's voice remained quiet during the discussion. I attempted to involve her.

Ann: How do you feel about taking phone calls, Fiona?

Beth *(threateningly)*: Tell the truth.

Fiona *(voice flat)*: I don't mind.

I reflect that, in this incident, Fiona, a relative newcomer to the team, had become a pawn in an unpalatable power struggle between Beth and myself. It was impossible for her to answer the tactless question without 'siding' with one or the other. Such unexpressed inability to express her true self was unhealthy for her, and the team, and was frighteningly far from Druskat's and Wolff's (2001) view of the 'emotionally intelligent' group. They advocate effective teams developing norms that encourage a high level of emotional awareness both within individuals and between group members and also between the group and external organisations. Such an awareness, within my team, would have resulted in Fiona's discomfort being recognised and acknowledged at the time. She could have left the meeting feeling supported and cared for rather than undermined. Druskat and Wolff warn that teams suffer and become dysfunctional because of failure to recognise and respond to individual and group emotion.

The uncomfortable discussion ended with an agreement to discuss the whole issue at the next monthly team meeting, in 4 weeks time, with all present. Meanwhile, we would try sitting in different chairs in the mornings and see how we felt. The issue of competence to answer the phones hung heavy in the air, unresolved.

(Ann stands and moves away from chair to narrate)

I left the room feeling battle-worn and frustrated, drained for the remainder of the day. Covey (1989) observes how much negative energy is expended when people attempt decision making in isolation and with their own independent view of the problem and its solution.

(Team leave room)

Act 4

Over the following fortnight, I persisted in trying to change the hierarchical message of our morning meetings by consistently taking different chairs and thus forcing movement from the rest of the team. I noticed that it took longer to settle in the meetings as members shuffled uneasily, uncertain where to sit.

(Team enter, Ann leading way. Ann sits in chair 4. Others uncertain. End up with Beth in chair 1, Chris in chair 2, others occupy remaining chairs)

Once seated, however, phone calls and messages were taken by those nearest to the desk.

(Team leave and re-enter, again uncertain. Ann to chair 5, Elaine to 3, Ann indicates chair 1 to Dorothy who rejects it and takes chair 6, Fiona to chair 4. Others take remaining seats)

By silent common consent, Fiona never took either of the chairs by the phones and I felt concerned about her. Dorothy, whose dissatisfied signals had unknowingly triggered my action in the first place, refused to sit in seat 1 even when invited by me to do so. She was clearly unhappy at being pushed into what she perceived as the leader's position. On reflection, I can see how this would alarm her. Feeling undermined and undervalued made her want to retreat rather than sit in the most prominent and, perceived, powerful seat. Such poor self-perceptions are both frightening and socially disabling. They built a wall of defence against my message that these were simply chairs and that I remained leader, willing to take responsibility, wherever I sat.

(Team leave room)

Act 5

On one particular morning, through force of circumstances, I sat in my previously assumed position, chair 1.

(Team enter, Ann last. Everyone sits in original chairs, as at beginning of drama. Audible sigh of relief from all)

The relief in the air was so palpable I considered abandoning the changes. Everyone was happier and more comfortable in their previous positions, I had just unsettled the team needlessly. Rashid and Bentley (2001) comment that change can have a negative impact by creating insecurities and tension. I reflected that I myself felt more comfortable sitting in chair 1 and recognised that I preferred the position of authority and the status it appeared to give. This attitude, however, no longer felt comfortable as my view of leadership was changing from one of formal authority, with a tendency to control, to a more sharing and supportive style. My opinion of how to lead was altering intuitively because of my perception of Dorothy's low self-esteem. Leigh and Maynard (1995) recommend a balance between being intuitive and systematic as a leader. They describe intuitive leaders as adaptable, often acting on impulse and as visualising total situations rather than specifics. Systematic leaders depend on information and logic and hate relying on gut reaction. My action demonstrated the strengths and weaknesses of intuitive leadership being flexible in style but lacking clarity and attention to detail. No wonder everyone was confused and I was wavering in my resolve!

(Team leave)

Act 6

(Team re-enter, Chris to chair 2, Beth to chair 1, others take remaining seats)

Perhaps the ones most affected initially were the two colleagues next in line to me (Beth and Chris) who, I noticed with some irritation, simply moved up to chairs 1 and 2 respectively. I decided to speak to them privately and explain my rationale more clearly.

(Team get up to leave)

Ann: Beth and Chris, could I speak to you please?

(Rest of team leave)

Chris: I don't think there are any issues in this team. I don't think it's hierarchical at all. I think all this disturbance is unnecessary. I'd rather leave than carry on like this!

Beth: I agree with Chris that there are no issues in this team but if you think it's important to change chairs I'll go along with it.

(Beth leaves)

Chris was clearly comfortable with her position in the team and had not looked at things from the perspective of the more junior members. Unconsciously, her manner, in fact, often empha-sised the hierarchical structure. Junior team members had complained to me many times of Chris's inflexibility about sharing work and her authoritarian manner on Thursdays when she was usually in charge.

(Chris moves to chair 1, Elaine, Fiona and Dorothy enter and sit in other chairs. Chris barks out orders with back to colleagues)

I reflect that both nurses unconsciously demonstrate a reliance on formal authority and control in their style of leadership which Leigh and Maynard (1995) describe as perpetuating a 'them and us' divide, increasingly inappropriate for today's modern teams. They observe that today's leaders get results by giving up control and sharing their leadership and power. Beth and Chris were probably reacting negatively through a natural desire to cling on to the status of their posi-tion and a perception that it was being undermined.

(Team leave)

Act 7

To my surprise, it was Chris who co-operated first, not Beth. On the day following our conversa-tion, she moved out of her chair and proceeded to sit somewhere different each day. The next Friday, Elaine commented to me, in a surprised voice:

(Elaine enters)

Elaine: The team meeting with Chris yesterday was much better than it has been. I think things are improving.

(Elaine leaves)

I was delighted and amazed that something so positive had emerged out of all the discomfort and ripples of conflict that had been present in the preceding weeks. I continued to role-play the change of chair, by sitting somewhere different each morning. However, Beth appeared to be increasingly entrenched in chair 1. I found her stubbornness annoying but, instead of challenging her, allowed myself to burn with inner resentment and anger, an inevitable product, according to Cavanagh (1991), of avoiding conflict. I perceived Beth to be playing power games and therefore threatening my leadership. Kopp (2000) warns that all interactions in professional relationships contain the seeds of conflict, particularly rivalry and style differences, and that deep divisions can be created because some embrace change and others oppose it.

(Beth enters, sits in chair 1)

Friction between Beth and myself built up, predictably, according to Kopp (2000), because our differences remained unacknowledged and unresolved. Eventually, having prickled our way through a work meeting, Beth waited behind and wisely challenged me about what was wrong.

Beth: What on earth is the matter with you?

We found we had completely misunderstood each other! I thought she was reacting to my divestment of status and power by usurping my position. She, on the other hand, appeared to feel that I so disliked sitting in the 'leader's' chair that she was helping me by occupying it instead. Underpinning these reactions was a hidden desire in both of us to be in control and

I still feel that rivalry was not far from the surface. But, as MacMillan (1996) observes, this can be used to positive effect provided those concerned have respect for each other and the common goal. He likens it to competing like acrobats so that the feats become increasingly spectacular so long as serious injury (and indeed death!) is avoided by the competitors and those who watch.

Act 8

Our confrontation became an emotional battleground of seesawing emotions as we angrily and tearfully expressed our views.

Ann (*accusingly*): You're just playing power games.

Beth (*defensively*): I thought I was helping you. I thought you didn't like sitting in the leader's chair so I was helping you by sitting in it for you.

(*Beth leaves*)

I was too caught up in my own agenda to recognise then how my actions were threatening to Beth's own hierarchical position and how she would have benefited from hearing her role in the team valued and reinforced. It speaks volumes for our relationship, and Beth's loyalty, that we were able to conclude this exhausting session with an agreement from Beth to move around. To my relief, she kept to her word and, from the following day, relinquished her usual chair and began rotating where she sat. I expressed my gratitude to Beth and Chris for their co-operation in a humorous conversation in which we coined the phrase 'musical chairs!'

Act 9

I felt there was an improved atmosphere in our morning meetings from that moment on. The three main occupants of the 'power' chairs no longer occupied them and the impression of status and authority was diminished.

(*Team enter, Elaine sits in chair 1, Fiona in chair 2, others take remaining chairs*)

The impact of this was far greater than I could ever have predicted because it impacted on the pattern of communication within the team.

Mullins (1985) graphically describes different types of communication networks, within teams, as the wheel, circle, all-channel and chains (see illustration on p297). These are shown here in diagrammatic form. As a group, we were operating closest to the chains network in which communication flows along a predetermined channel from one end to the other. This is a centralised form of communication, requiring little interaction between group members along the chains. Similarly, the wheel is a centralised network in which information is passed to and from the central person. With high leadership and low group participation, these networks provide job satisfaction for the leader but group members feel peripheral. The circle is more decentralised but inefficient as members communicate between each other in a disorganised way. It provides greater group participation and satisfaction, however, than the wheel or the chains. The highest level of involvement and fulfilment is achieved by the decentralised all-channel network which allows full participation and interaction between all members and leadership is very low. Under pressure, such a group may revert back to the wheel if there is a perceived need for strong direction. As a result of removing the trappings of power, the nursing team now appear to be developing an all-channel pattern of communication, that should result in a higher level of satisfaction for all members.

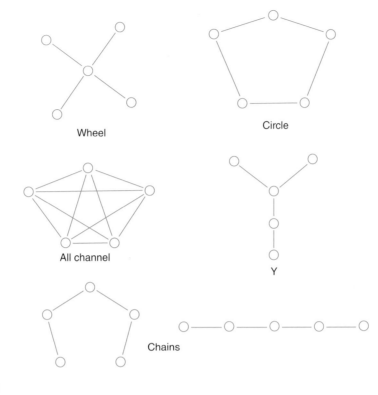

Wheel

Circle

All channel

Y

Chains

(Team leave)

Act 10

Ann: To an extent, the value of this has been recognised by the team. The monthly team meeting at which the seating arrangements were reviewed brought consensus to continue the change. Seven weeks after my first action, the team now moves around more happily and occupies different chairs each day.

(Team enter and take seats. Sit for a few seconds. Rise and reposition in different seats. Sit for a few seconds. Rise and reposition again. On the third time, Dorothy takes chair 1 and Fiona chair 2)

I note that Dorothy took the longest to sit comfortably in chair 1. The fact that she does so now may reflect rising self-esteem. Fiona has proved herself perfectly capable of answering the phone.

(Fiona picks up phone and has longish call!)

I am aware, however, that I only observe the dynamics when I am on duty and wonder how comfortable both nurses are on other days. Next month has been targeted for 'personal appraisals' when I will take the opportunity to gauge individual reactions. The team review, following the appraisals, will provide a forum to gain collective ownership (retrospectively!) for the change.

I have been inspired by the impact of my 'simple' attempt at change. Johns (2004a) suggests 'looking in' and 'looking out' as a means of structured reflection on events. Reversing the order, 'looking out' enables me to understand the lessons to be drawn with greater clarity. The 'significant issues' were the existing team dynamics and my lack of communication in initiating change. I am firmly convinced that the position we started in, with so much power and authority invested in certain chairs, needed changing as soon as possible. I was trying to achieve a harmonious team in which all members felt of equal importance and value. I attempted this by taking action rather than expressing my concerns and allowing areas of conflict to be discussed and change to be agreed. Johns (1992) recognises the pervasive culture, within nursing, of harmonious, rather than therapeutic, teams. He feels that harmonious teams achieve a 'façade of togetherness or teamwork' at the cost of openness and genuine understanding of individual feelings. Johns warns that suppressed feelings within nursing teams discourage openness and authenticity in dealings with patients. My action inadvertently exposed unexpressed emotions and conflicts within the team which now need to be openly discussed and acknowledged in order for us to function therapeutically. I was initially angered and exasperated by some reactions from the group but I realise now I was interpreting their responses wrongly by using my own behaviour as a reference point for understanding. I have discovered the need for agreed aims, objectives and priorities prior to action. The fact that my implementation of change in the end worked successfully was largely due to group members being willing to engage in the communication process part way through! In an article entitled 'Communication is the key', Scott (2001) states that effective working is dependent on active exchange of information and ideas among team members.

'Looking in', I discover my understanding of leadership has broadened and my need for position and authority has waned. My cavalier approach to initially instigating 'the change' perhaps reveals something of my inherent strong desire for leadership and influence. I still 'catch' myself sometimes trying to regain status, especially when working with Beth (the greatest threat to my leadership) but I am challenged by Leigh and Maynard's (1995) timely reminder that the question is not how do I manage to stay in charge? but how can I unlock my team's full potential?

The improved all-channel communication and reduction in formal status has released potential within the team by enabling members to work with greater independence and initiative. Leigh and Maynard welcome this as a sign of success and advise treating the informal power gained by members as an ally rather than a threat to leadership. I have become convinced of the effectiveness of supportive, empowering leadership in preference to controlling and directing. My intention is to increasingly apply those principles to my own position as team leader.

Having worked through this reflection, I now feel equipped to demonstrate to the group the value of what has been achieved in terms of equality and communication within the team.

Chris J reads:

Sometimes when I consider what tremendous consequences come from little things … I am tempted to think … there are no little things. (Bruce Barton, quoted by Covey 1989)

RAW

Performers:
Narrator: *Maria Fordham*
Poet: *Bella Madden*
Therapist's voice: *Chris Johns*
Gill's voice: *Louise Jarrett*

RAW is my first performance text. It is constructed from the narrative of my journey as a complementary therapist working alongside Gill who was having treatment for her breast cancer. The performance captures dramatic moments through the first 2 years of this journey.

RAW was first performed in Aalborg, Denmark, at the 13th International Reflective Practice conference in May 2007 to an audience of approximately 30 people. It was performed again at the University of Bedfordshire in September 2007. The performance is read in four voices against a Power-point background of original images and music.

Session 1: Wednesday 27 November 2002

Chris: A raw early winter's day.
Gill opens the door.
Warmly but nervously she invites me into her space.
She says she has no idea what she's let herself in for.
She might have said 'I have no idea what I've let you in for'.

Her space transforming into our space
space an opening of possibility
no more,
no expectations, or preconceptions,
simply flowing with what is,
no attachments,
no form or permanence,
just unfolding experience
shaped along a healing trajectory
that curves into the mystery.
Gill leans inwards against the kitchen units
and spills her story
her breast cancer diagnosed in September.
An aggressive cancer that required mastectomy
17 lymph nodes removed
Five had been invaded by the cancer.
Breast reconstruction.
chemotherapy – six cycles, one every 3 weeks.
radiotherapy to follow.
The oncologist is happy for her to have complementary therapies …
I whisper under my breath 'and if he wasn't, then what?'.
Listen as the gatekeeper jangles his keys.

Gill: I have cancer … I'm uncertain of the outcome …
She turns her head away and whispers 'Cancer means I will die'. She is depressed, takes an antidepressant, doesn't sleep well. She blames it on the steroids she's taking. The first chemo blast left her blistered.
She feels dreadful. She had no idea what to expect – sickness, mouth ulcers. The flush of chemotherapy drugs swirl in the veins, wreaking their damage like Pac-man, not differentiating between friend and foe. I don't ask the combination of drugs but with hindsight I wish I had.
Gill: I am so tired … I walked up the road the next day and couldn't get back. I had to sit on a wall … I can't do my normal household jobs. I'm anxious about losing my hair. I asked for the cold cap but it went wrong. It started thawing. I was so angry … I have lost some hair … I'm going to the wig shop this afternoon.
Her despair lies thick on the surface, seeping imperturbably into my being.
Her words – *I was so angry* … the careless management of the cold cap adds to her suffering at a time when she suffers so much. She does not mention her breast and I do not inquire.
Her left arm is swollen and aches. Being left handed she has difficulty driving and doing normal household chores. I had noticed the small blue Peugeot in the drive. Normal life patterns thrown into chaos.
She is married to Phil and has two children: Katie is 13 and Chlöe is 19. Chlöe is at university but unsettled because of what's happening. Katie is so difficult. She says 'I hoped she would have been more sensitive to my needs right now. I need her support and understanding. But instead she's angry at me … why? … I've always done everything for her.'

My sympathy ripples. I disclose that my girls are 10 and 13. Charlotte and Aimee …
A point of connection.
Shaping the dimension of space.
I wonder – what does a 13 year old feel under these circumstances? Does she know how best to respond? Perhaps she needs help to understand?
'Maybe Thelma (*breast care clinical specialist*) could help?'
Gill looks down … she doesn't know.
Cancer rips through this family. Tentatively I inquire, 'And your husband? How is he?'
'He's bearing up.'
I wonder about him – his feelings, their intimacy but mindful of not pursuing this issue at this time.
Treading cautiously, careful not to embarrass or threaten her. Careful not to embarrass myself.
Better to swim with the surface waves than tread the deeper currents for the moment. Life too raw to explore its depths.
I venture, 'What if the treatment is not successful?'
Gill turns and looks at me and retorts earnestly, 'Well, I'm not contemplating dying … I can't afford to contemplate that option. I am determined to beat this for my two children … all I want is to see them grow up and be there for them as they do.'
The mother's plaintive cry in the face of losing her children.
I am reminded of Iris who died just a few months ago. Her two children younger than Gill's. I had given Iris reflexology for 2 years at the hospice. I feel the pang of separation and know I must put it aside to see Gill.
I respond, 'That's a good reason to dig in and fight.'
War metaphors of resistance and battle.
'How do you feel about reflexology?'
She says, 'I have no idea'.
I explain: 'Your body is mapped out on your feet. The reflexology is a sophisticated foot massage that triggers reflexes that relate to each part of your body. My aim is to help bring your body into wholeness, balance, energising and relaxing you. Let's try it and see what you think.'
I suggest reflexology rather than massage because of her recent surgery and residual swelling.
Gill laughs nervously: 'OK but I feel strange about feet. I don't like other people's feet touching me'.
I mix essential oils into the reflexology cream. She loves the citrus aroma. She raises her feet onto the footstool. Holding her feet, I encourage her to 'try and relax – your feet are so tense'.
She laughs: 'I wasn't aware I was but I'll try'.
I say 'Let me help you. … close your eyes and become aware of your body, notice any ache or tension in the body, soften around any ache and tension …'
Then, commencing with her scalp I guide her through a body scan, relaxing each part of her body until her whole body is relaxed.
'Now take your attention to your breath, follow your breath in and follow your breath out.'
I whisper, 'Breathing in I calm my body, breathing out I smile. Imagine you are enveloped in a soft healing light. With each in-breath, breathe in this soft healing light until it fills your whole body. Sense the light comforting you, smile at how good that feels. Then, with each out-breath let go of your thoughts and feelings, the worries of the day and your fears … let them drift away on the breath, surrender to this moment and imagine you are a fluffy white cloud in a clear blue sky.'
However, Gill does not relax so easily … and then, her pulse quietens as she quite literally lets go and sinks into the quietened depths as I give the reflexology.
Afterwards Gill says, 'I had these sensations as if some energy was moving upwards through my body. At one point I felt slightly nauseous but that passed off … and it has given me a faint headache.'
She drinks deeply from the offered water.

'Drink plenty of water to help flush the body – the headache is a consequence of easing your stressed body. It's normal but you may feel a bit groggy tomorrow morning but that will pass off … would you like me to visit again?' She does. Stepping out into the warm day, I take a deep breath.

Gill's life is an open wound, raw, still bleeding despite the surgeon's knife being put away. First the physical carnage and now the emotional fallout. She is angry, fearful, sad, agitated to the extent she is labelled depressed.

Depressed – pressed down, hollowed out, as if more than her breast has been scooped from her being. The label singles her out, marginalises her, puts her in a heap, Worse, it becomes self-fulfilling, feeding itself, even a rationalisation for her lowered spirit – 'I'm depressed so it's normal to be like this'. She has not yet begun to find meaning in her experience … our talk reflects the beginning work of making sense and growth even as new trauma unravels – her youngest daughter's response. The young child wants her mother back.

To help is to listen; to listen to her words with empathy, to listen to the silences that ripple between the words, to listen to her body, to feel its ache within, to touch the raw nerve that vibrates angrily.

The reflexology opens a space where she can put down her heavy burden for a moment and be still. A sacred space for healing. A balm for the raw wound. I imagine her response:

Poet:
>   Still?
>   How can I be still?
>   When I feel death taunt me …
>   Haunt me
>   With its whispers …
>
>   Violins scrape across bare metal
>   My teeth grate
>   Nerves on edge
>   The cello's death march
>   All signs spell gloom
>   And yet he led me into a quiet space

Session 2: Monday 9th December 2002 – we meet again

Gill in floods of tears. Gently I ask, 'What is it?'.

Gill: Chlöe has quit university. I know she didn't quit for my sake … she was struggling with her studies and didn't like the university town. Even so I'm angry at her for ditching university. It hurts my pride. She had done so well to get there and now to throw it away like this … she will reapply next year.

Another dent to Gill's self-image even as she seeks to repair the dent, her small fists bleeding against the hard metal. Thelma had informed me that Gill's chemotherapy regimen was aggressive, reflecting the aggressive cancer. Gently I ask, 'How are you?'.

Gill: They've reduced my chemotherapy drugs and stopped the steroids because of the side-effects I was having. I'm better without the steroids, lost that 'spaced out' feeling … I even managed to sleep last night! But I'm anxious that reducing the chemotherapy drugs will make the treatment less effective.

I ask cautiously, 'What did the doctor say?'.

Gill: Maybe I didn't listen carefully enough. I haven't been able to voice my concerns.

Giving people information and advice is one thing. Listening, being sensitive and supportive is another. People are unable to pay attention when distressed. Words flow through them. Her voice silenced in the din. Medical staff are the people of the din.

'Can you contact Thelma or share your concerns when you attend your next chemotherapy appointment?'

Gill simply looks at me.

'Can you?'

I want to inject 'you can' into her numbed mind.

Gill's hair is falling out. She is upset and angry at the hospital for not letting the cold cap thaw before removing it from her scalp … it pulled her hair out when removed. She says, 'Usually I love going out but now I don't want to. I can't bear people to see me like this. Makes me feel like a social leper.'

Her words drift off in despair. 'You were going shopping for a wig?'

Gill cries: 'Yes, I did go to the wig shop and got a wig. I wore it at home but Katie was angry at me … "Don't come near me with that! It looks awful!" I was so hurt by her taunt.' Tearfully she laments, 'I want MY own hair!'.

Tears run in small streams down each side of her face. A proud woman brought to her knees. At every turn something else emerges to taunt her.

'How is Phil coping?'

She says that he is coping fairly well but finds it difficult to talk about what has happened.

Coping fairly well – I have a stereotyped image of a man unable to express his feelings. I want to press her about her husband's feelings when she blurts out, 'I won't have any treatment if this comes back. I want to live for my children. I have doted on them, they are everything to me … but this is too painful. There is no way I can go through this again.'

I ask how she felt about me coming today.

Wiping away her tears, Gill says, 'I wasn't worried either way. My mother has reacted badly to my diagnosis, to the point that I feel I can't handle her just now. I just feel criticised by her … I've been looking after my mother for the past 7 years since father died. That's a picture of him over there.'

We gaze at his picture.

I try and empathise: 'Maybe your mother is struggling with knowing you have cancer and might die. Maybe she's even anxious about losing your support'.

Gill sees that might be true but it hurts to have such conflict just now, on top of everything else.

Through her tears she says, 'I'm sorry …'

Why do people everywhere apologise for the expression of their suffering? I want to hold Gill, comfort her, ease her suffering. The whole family suffers, experiencing their own losses. Gill isolated, alone. Cancer is a family affair. Like a hurricane, it rips a trail of destruction through the family, leaving despair and conflict in its wake. One thing piled up on top of another. Gill in existential crisis. I have stepped into a maelstrom.

Silence between us, as if someone has pressed the pause button.

Poet: John O'Donohue says:[4]

> Sometimes we listen to things but we never hear them. True listening brings us in touch even with that which is unsaid and unsayable. Sometimes the most important thresholds of mystery are places of silence. To be genuinely spiritual is to have great respect for the possibilities and presence of silence.

I move Gill into reflexology mode. Afterwards she says, 'I was intrigued, I could feel areas of my body, especially across the breast scar.'

I remind her that she had a headache after her last treatment

She says it was OK because I had warned her of the possibility of a 'healing crisis'. She had taken some paracetamol and it had gone by the morning. She feels very relaxed, more relaxed than last time although the din Chlöe was making in the kitchen had disturbed her like a white noise

---

[4]O'Donohue, J (1997) *Anam Cara*. Bantam Press, London.

that breaks up the therapeutic rhythm. We choose 10 Bach flower remedies alongside some rescue remedy for when she feels particularly panicky or emotional.

Session 5: Friday 17th January 2003 – a slap in the face

Clear bright frosty morning. Gill's welcoming smile soon dissolves into anguish.

Gill: I saw a new registrar at the hospital … I couldn't communicate with her. She was Indian or something. She said my hair had thinned … *(a knowing look)* … and then she asked if I had thought about a wig! I felt as if I had been slapped in the face. I could have slapped her. I was so angry at her insensitivity. I asked to see the consultant next time.

Gill's outrage overflows. When she needs to be listened to with empathy and compassion, she feels slapped down.

Gill: The chemotherapy unit is always busy and jokey where it's not easy to talk about things. When they ask me how I am, I say 'I'm fine, how are you?'. I've had no contact with Thelma even though she said she would contact me. But then she must be busy. Others must have greater need than me. I'm not used to accepting help. I'm the one who listens … I've taken up so much of your time. I'm sorry …

Chris: That's why I'm here, to help you work through such feelings. It's hard to be alone. Perhaps the chemo suite is not the place for deeper conversations.

But I ask myself – where is Thelma?

Gill says the reflexology gets better each time. She offers me a sandwich. I decline yet I am mindful of her need to give me something back, that caring is reciprocal, especially for someone like her who has always cared for others and struggles to accept being cared for. And yet I sense my emotional distance from Gill, so different from my relationship with Iris. Yet what is different? I cannot put my finger on it. I wonder – do I still grieve for Iris?

Session 6: 12 days later – eyes full of sadness

Gill: I'm so sad, I don't know why. I went to a friend's party. Their daughter had got engaged. I found myself wondering if I would be here for my daughters – this fear is always there. It was also my 48th birthday and I wondered if it would be my last. I'm less optimistic now than I was. Why? I didn't think I bottle up feelings but I guess I do … no-one would tell me about my prognosis and then Dr Cummings, the oncologist, told me I had a 60–70% chance of non-recurrence … I picked up vibes from others that the news was not good.

Gill's face collapses in a torrent of tears. I touch her arm in silent sympathy.

She continues her lament: 'My neighbour came round – she told me that she had lost two friends to breast cancer. Why did she have to tell me that? I only seem to meet people who have had bad outcomes. Not people who have survived. The only glimmer of light was you telling me about your sister-in-law who has survived breast cancer … it's like you live under a cloud.'

Gill had not seen the surgeon. Nor has she spoken recently with Thelma. Thelma knows that Gill struggles, hence her referral to me. Does she assume I pick up the pieces? Even when Gill contacted Thelma once, left a message, Thelma did not respond. What messages does this give Gill? Do they not see her suffering?

Perhaps I should confront Thelma. Yet I know Gill wouldn't want that. I know Thelma is caring but she is also very busy – this makes her reactive rather than proactive to demand. Gill does not demand directly … yet her demand is real if unspoken.

Ironing my frown, I gently inquire, 'Who can you talk to?'.

She says: 'You … I don't talk to anyone else like this.'

I say, 'I *am* here for you … I won't desert you … I will give you reflexology at least until your radiotherapy is finished.' In saying this I commit myself to this woman.

Today is Gill's sixth treatment. I had mentioned six treatments at the beginning and I wonder if she anticipates my withdrawal as loss. I step across an unnamed boundary into a greater intimacy. I feel the shift inside as I move across the distance to hold her.

She remains very tired with the chemotherapy cycles. Fatigue, her constant companion alongside her depressed mood. She was told to put her life on hold whilst going through chemotherapy and radiotherapy. Her life suspended … giving herself time … she does not like being ill, being dependent on people.

Smiling, Gill says, 'On a more positive note, some of my hair is regrowing. I wore the wig out to the party. It was so hot under it but I felt less self-conscious … when I first came home some friends visited but stopped. I've always been a social animal so it's difficult.'

As if having cancer is alienating, irreconcilable with normal life, leaving her estranged, on the outside.

Gill has driven her car a couple of times which caused her left arm to ache and swell. Her small car does not have power steering. Driving the car is a practical issue yet she would be better equipped with a compression support bandage but no lymphoedema referral.

My frustration is barely concealed but who said therapy should be comfortable for either of us!

On a softer note, I say that she needs to be her own judge of what she can or cannot do.

All this emerges out of reviewing agrimony. We review the rest of the Bach flower remedies.

Reviewing cherry plum, Gill laughs and says, 'It does feel like I'm on the edge of a precipice … that's so uncanny to read that – help people cope with panic of being overwhelmed. It feels scary! Better hold your arm in case I fall!'

Instinctively I ask if she has any religion. She says no, she doesn't … and then adds, 'In fact, what faith I might have has evaporated. I'm angry having cancer and the death of my sister from cancer some years ago. It's unfair … what have I done when there are so many evil people in the world?'.

We omit the pine. Gill recoils from an image of self-pity. It implants a negative self-image even though it reflects her reality. We add walnut to help Gill cope with the changes of living with cancer and adapting to a new identity of cancer sufferer. Gill wants to return to normal but she is forever changed. I want to plant the idea of adapting to a new self even though just now the idea of adapting to live with cancer is difficult to contemplate. It is no good glibly saying 'think positively' because she can't.

As Beck (1989) says: 'And that's the problem with positive thinking and affirmations: we can't keep them up forever. Such efforts are never the path to freedom'.

I write Gill a poem:

> Gill, how can I best ease your suffering?
> She replies 'Please journey alongside me,
> touch me to stroke away the stress,
> listen deeply to my cries,
> empathise with my experience
> even as I struggle to voice it,
> name my fears
> so we may face them out,
> sympathise with me
> so I am not alone,
> let me know that you care
> so when I wake in the night
> I can draw on that love
> and not take fright

Session 7: Monday 10th February 2003 – if you're passing and have time

I park the car by the low wall by the side of Gill's front garden. The dustmen have been. Rows of emptied wheely bins stand in random patterns. It's cold. Dark clouds set a gloomy picture, threatening rain.

I remove my shoes at the door, symbolic of entering a sacred space. I kneel at Gill's feet. Her hair has thinned. She flicks off one or two fallen hairs from her shoulders. She confesses she has been so tired.

Gill: Last Friday I just couldn't get out of bed. Eventually I stirred myself to go shopping. Some nausea but that passed off. My left arm aches constantly across the shoulder and across my ribs … I went to the support group. I wish I hadn't. I got stuck listening to a woman who'd been attending for some years talking at me about her problems. I was irritated because I wanted to listen to another woman talking about her radiotherapy treatment. I can't talk about any of my problems at the group. Thelma was there. I invited her to call if she was passing if she had the time but she hasn't … not yet, she must be busy.

I ask if she spoke with other people having chemotherapy.

Gill: I haven't. It's not fair to burden anybody but I did speak to one woman because she had all her hair. I said to her that she hadn't lost her hair. The woman laughed and said that she was wearing a wig! I felt so deflated.

Gill is ambivalent about attending the support group. Part of her seeks support and another part shies away. It has value in terms of appreciating other women's experiences and getting information, for example about her forthcoming radiotherapy. She knows the treatment involves daily journeys to a distant hospital 5 days a week for 5 weeks. She doesn't know anything about the radiotherapy itself or how will it affect her. She knows that travelling each day will be hard and Phil will have to take time off from work. But, at last, she has an appointment to see the lymphoedema therapist in 6 weeks time.

During the reflexology I imagine the Bodhisattva White Tara present as I move my hands about her feet. I imagine that I too am a bodhisattva wrapping Gill in compassion and wisdom, seeking to help ease her suffering so she can emerge as a whole person from this fragmenting trauma.

> We are two deer
> grazing on the high pasture;
> suffering, you turn to
> nuzzle my warm fur
> of life for comfort;
> I pause until you are still
> and can graze more easily.

Session 8: Monday 3rd March 2003 – the problem with honesty

Gill shares how she spoke to a woman today attending for chemotherapy. This woman had a recurrence after $3\frac{1}{2}$ years. Gill had felt shocked: 'The oncologist's words rang through my head about recurrence and here was the proof and only after $3\frac{1}{2}$ years'. What made it worse was that the woman thanked her for being such a good role model because she looked so good when she was feeling such a wreck inside.

She has started tamoxifen.

Gill: I feel bloated as if I've put on weight although I'm not eating well. I still have this metallic taste in my mouth from the chemotherapy that spoils my taste. And I'm not sleeping very well either with all this worry.

Gill was given no information or advice about tamoxifen. Poor communication is becoming a constant theme through this story. Wrapped into their systems, they don't see the suffering woman. As I hold her feet, Gill asks if she has any hard patches. I say she does, around her shoulder area, perhaps indicative of tension. Gill says that she's read on the internet that hard patches on feet are linked with cancer. Intrigued, I inquire what it said. She can't remember the detail.

Afterwards she says, 'I felt as if I had moved into another place where I could see things more clearly … when before I had felt so helpless. It was a place of light and surrender.'

Poet: Touch brings presence home. At the highest moments of human intensity, words become silent. When you are lost in the black valley of pain, words grow frail and numb. Touch offers the deepest clue to the mystery of encounter, awakening and belonging. It is the secret, affective content of every connection and association.

I hold Gill's hand. She folds her other hand over mine and asks me to hug her. I feel her pain tight and hard within her. Holding her helps her to relax, to ease the tight fist of pain.

Later, I reflect on the oncologist's words – 'I am going to be honest with you'. His warning shot of bad news. She had been told that she had a 60–70% chance of 'cure', now she is told she will never be cured. Hope dashed. Gill is trapped in a waiting room, left desolate and fragmented.

> I gather the broken pieces
> holding them together
> yet the cracks give the game away.

Poet:

Audre Lorde writes:[5] I want to write rage but all that comes is sadness … I carry death around in my body like a condemnation. But I do live. The bee flies. There must be some way to integrate death into living, neither ignoring it nor giving in to it.

Session 9: Friday March 14th 2003 – red hair day

I gaze at the clear blue sky. No clouds. My mind equally clear. Gill laughs at my red hair, sprayed for Comic Relief bad hair day. Humour triggers release, lightening the burden if just for the moment.

Gill reveals how she couldn't face attending the breast care support group again.

Gill: All that chatter and I don't like talking about myself. I didn't need it. However, I did speak to my neighbour. It was awkward. She didn't know what to say to me with our reversal of roles. I was always the one to listen to her. She said she had been busy but I know that isn't true.

The tide turns, the shoe on the other foot. Life turned upside down, social roles reversed.

Session 10: Friday 21st March 2003 – the promise of primrose

Gill has read the leaflet I gave her from Cancer Backup on tamoxifen. It was helpful. She has quit smoking. It isn't helping her mood. She's been miserable. She pauses to put on a nicotine patch.

Gill reflects: 'Perhaps it isn't the right time to quit, but at least I'm trying. Taking tamoxifen, I'm waking early, 3 am, sweating. Get up and get a cuppa tea … my head full of thoughts whirring … it's then I crave a cigarette.'

I quip, 'Your usual pattern, a cuppa tea and a fag. Maybe we can create a different ritual? Maybe a warm bath and some oils?'

---

[5] Lorde, A (1980) *The cancer journals.* Aunt Lute Books, San Francisco, p13.

Gill says that Thelma has told her about primrose oil, that using it in the bath can help with the tamoxifen effects. I say, 'I can mix some oils in primrose carrier oil for you to use in your bath'.

Gill: Would you really do that for me? Thank you Chris (she takes my hand and continues) thankfully the metallic taste from the chemotherapy has faded. I can actually taste food again. I'm eating well … on another note Chlöe has been offered places at six universities. I hope she will accept just in case.

Just in case? Just in case of what? Just in case her cancer recurs? Gill desperately wants her daughters to do well just in case she dies. The poignancy of human tragedy. Normal events get blown up. Literally life and death.

Poet:

Audre Lorde writes:[6] Spring comes, and still I feel despair like a pale cloud waiting to consume me … I need to remind myself of the joy, the laughter, the laughter so vital to my living and health. Otherwise the other will always be waiting to eat me up into despair again. And that means destruction. I don't know how, but it does.

Session 13: Friday 25th April 2003 – badly knocked back

Gill greets me with a broad smile.

Gill: I went for my radiotherapy planning on Tuesday. I commence a 5-week course on May 6th. It's going to be a big effort but having survived the chemotherapy I feel I can take this more in my stride. Positive thinking! Must be the patchouli!

But when I suggest that she is more positive, her mask crumbles. Between her tears she blurts: 'I'm so down … I've felt so low since the operation … I try so hard to put a brave face on things but …'

I press her: 'But something's happened. What is it?'.

Gill shrugs her shoulders: 'It's nothing really … OK, I saw the surgeon who operated on me. He was not receptive – he asked me why I had come to see him. I said, because I hadn't seen him since the operation. He was clearly unimpressed with this reply. He asked, what did I want? So I told him I was anxious about the lump below my ribs …'

Gill (touches her ribs and mimicks the surgeon): 'So you do have something to see me about,' he condescendingly retorted. He didn't have a view on the lump. He said, 'I'll be blunt … if the tumour recurs it is likely to be the liver'. He explained that the tumour had been bigger than expected, that it had adhered to some lymph glands and the margin of clear breast tissue was minimal. I was devastated by this news … why do they have to tell you this! It is like a death sentence! I don't mind for myself … dying … but the children … (pause) He then left the room. A nurse offered no support. I saw Thelma … she said she would phone but hasn't … I feel I should be strong.

The wave of irritation ripples through me that Gill should suffer such a careless jibe. It is not easy for me to witness her suffering.

Her flow of tears softens my anger. The surgeon placed Gill firmly in her wounds. He aggravated the raw wound. Gill knows the odds are stacked against her, that the cancer will recur and such thoughts haunt her in the small hours of the morning when she wakes, her head spinning. He snatches hope from Gill's grasp, denting the healing quest. Trust withered on the parched vine. Her suffering piled high. It is perverse she should experience such a lack of care.

I pull the cork, the cathartic pull to release the dam so healing can flow. Gill must express these feelings, this frustration, this anger, this pain so she can move on from it, learn from it, grow from it, converting the painful negative energy that saps her spirit into growth energy. My

---

[6]Lorde, A (1980) Ibid, p12.

impulse is to contact Thelma and express my outrage yet I know Gill would not want me to do that. It is not easy to witness her suffering. After the reflexology Gill looks completely different. She says, 'This stops me from cracking up'.

Later, I write a poem to work out my anger.

> Gill pushed into the waiting room to await the cancer's return
> with its deadly promise of death;
> Hear the unforgiving sneer
> 'minimal margins'
> 'bigger than expected'
> 'likely to be the liver'.
> Life on hold, more in suspense
> frantically pressing the pause button.
> that doesn't work.

Poet:

Audre Lorde writes:[7] I do not forget cancer for very long. I live with the constant fear of recurrence of another cancer. But fear and anxiety are not the same at all. One is an appropriate response to a real situation which I can accept and learn to work through … but the other, anxiety, is an immobilizing yield to things that go bump in the night, a surrender to namelessness, formlessness, voicelessness, and silence.

Session 14: Thursday 8th May 2003 – arms raised

Gill shares her story of commencing radiotherapy

Gill: The first day the treatment took about half an hour. It was uncomfortable with my left arm raised above my shoulder with my head turned towards the right. It felt for ages. My skin feels as if it has been out in the sun for a shade too long. On the second visit, the radiographers were more organised – the treatment only took about 10 minutes. The return journey by car was awful, sitting in traffic. My arm aches a bit more now with the radiotherapy but I was warned that might be so. They told me I'm likely to be tired due to the radiotherapy – don't tell me what fatigue is!! Been there, got the T-shirt! By the way, Thelma phoned me … did you say anything to her?

Chris: No, but I wanted too … I felt so frustrated at your treatment.

Gill is thoughtful: 'I thought you must have said something to her and that's why she phoned. I told her how awful I felt with the surgeon. She was sympathetic, that's all … because my night sweats are such a big problem I asked the oncologist about the other drug … the one that begins with an r?'

Chris: Anastrazole or arimidex?

Gill: Yes, that's it. I feel sure I'm on tamoxifen because of the cost. The oncologist said it was because of the risk of osteoporosis. He said tamoxifen protects the woman, unlike the other drug. I know tamoxifen statistically cuts my chance of reoccurrence by 50% whereas the other drug is 75% – what would I prefer? The greater risk of osteoporosis or increased survival chances? No competition. Plus I wouldn't experience these wretched night sweats.

I glibly say, 'You've been doing your homework. Did he agree?'

She answers no, that he wanted her to stay on the tamoxifen. Adamantly, she retorts, 'I won't accept his decision … HIS decision? Whose life is it?' Her words trail off and then she confesses she is smoking again. She feels guilty about that, angry at herself for being so weak … and now not working, she can't afford to smoke. More worry.

I say, 'Gill, can you accept that's just how it is at the moment? Smoking is how you cope with anxiety but I can see it also creates anxiety with your guilt. A Catch 22 scenario.'

---

[7]Lorde, A (1980) Ibid, p14.

After the reflexology she says she felt something across her liver area and asks if it was a sign. I ask, 'A sign of what?'.

She just looks at me so I fill the silence with words.

'You mean of recurrence? No, I felt nothing.'

The surgeon's words ring in her ears. If I did feel something would I tell her? I give Gill an article taken from the *Sunday Times* about shizandra[8] and its positive impact on cancer. Gill is impressed. She wants to give it a try.

I am uncertain giving Gill this type of information and setting her down a path of pursuing alternative treatments that are costly and largely unproven. I suspect it can become obsessive and counter-productive. John Diamond's snake oil![9] But she can make her own decision, claim her agency to act on such information.

Session 16: Monday 9th June 2003 – bright and breezy

Gill is bright and breezy. Just two more radiotherapy treatments and then it is finished. Her shoulder and arm ache more, which she attributes to the radiotherapy. She does her exercises every day ... it's vital to recover her arm. She's tired but no way as bad as with the chemotherapy.

I ask her whether she is getting enough rest. She looks at me as if I'm from outer space ... a knowing laugh. The daily chore of being a mother ensures no rest. Ironing in particular is difficult but she seeks no help and none is offered. I sense the social patterns of families are not easily shifted. Gill hasn't seen any doctors whilst undergoing the radiotherapy. She's still mad at the surgeon for his attitude.

She's been to the support group again.

Gill: I went out for a meal with them, just four of us. It was pleasant. I tried to get Thelma to get me permission to take shizandra but she hasn't got back to me again! I know she's busy but then she went on holiday! I'm still smoking although I intend to stop. I still need this prop ... I finally quit my old job because of the heavy lifting involved. I fancy a caring role because of my cancer experience ... do something meaningful, give something back ... I did enrol as a cadet nurse but I didn't pursue it but now I would have liked to have been a nurse.

I note that her is hair is thicker. She retorts, 'Yes, but nowhere as thick as it used to be! I've changed a lot over these past months ... my appearance has always important to me *(sighs wistfully)*. My hair is now grey and thin. Not good.'

After the reflexology Gill says how much she had looked forward to the treatment today.

Gill: I've missed you. It's been a while and only then did I realise how important the treatments have been. I'm positive you have stopped me going insane. I believe in all this, you know. I felt my left breast and shoulder more during the treatment. My headache's even gone.

She asks, as she always does, if I would like a sandwich. I say I need to get to the hospice but appreciate her need to give me something in return for my therapy. She seeks to frame our relationship as a social rather than a health relationship, perhaps because she generally has had unsatisfactory experiences with health personnel. Perhaps it is because she needs to be understood as Gill, a person, not a patient.

She has a 'willow tree' angel of learning on her mantelpiece. I have told her I had one given to me by Icelandic nurses in February. She says I am an angel and that receiving mine was no coincidence. I smile and hold her hand yet I feel slightly awkward to receive this gift of words.

---

[8]Shizandra berry helps the body's ability to distribute oxygen. www.sante.uk.com
[9]Snake oil is a metaphor for alleged quack therapies (Diamond 2001).

Why should I feel awkward? Is that some false humility? Do I resist her pull for a more social relationship, anxious that would increase my obligation, pulling me into a compassion trap where I would feel guilty if I withdrew therapy? I need to be more certain of myself.

Narrator: Rachel Remen notes that:

> One of the reasons that many physicians feel drained by their work is that they do not know how to make an opening to receive anything from their patients. The way we were trained, receiving is considered unprofessional. (Remen 1996:254)

Reflections at the kitchen table – Sunday morning, 15th June 2003

I sit at my farmhouse kitchen table reading *Kitchen table wisdom* by Rachel Remen. She reflects on observing Carl Rogers demonstrate unconditional positive regard.

Narrator:

> Rogers conducted it without saying a single word, conveying to his client simply by the quality of his attention a total acceptance of him exactly as he was. The doctor began to talk and the session rapidly became a great deal more than the demonstration of a technique … he began to shed his masks, hesitantly at first and then more easily. As each mask fell, Rogers welcomed the one behind it unconditionally, until finally we glimpsed the beauty of the doctor's naked face. (Remen 1996:219)

I wonder at this art of complete listening and its value to help Gill strip away her masks she clings to. Perhaps in our talk she does begin to reveal her naked face, manifested through her tears.

Narrator: Remen continues by writing:

> Listening is the oldest and perhaps the most powerful tool of healing. It is often through the quality of our listening and not the wisdom of our words that we are able to effect the most profound changes in the people around us. When we listen, we offer with our attention an opportunity for wholeness. Our listening creates sanctuary for the homeless parts within the other person. That which has been denied, unloved, devalued by themselves and others. That which is hidden. (Remen 1996:220)

I resonate with and sense the truth in her words *our listening creates sanctuary* in the way I dwell with Gill. Remen gives form to this sense, helping me become mindful of this quality of being when I am next with Gill. How well do I listen? How well do I communicate unconditional positive regard or compassion?

> I am so engrossed in this idea
> that my scrambled eggs
> and tea have gone cold.

Narrator: Remen continues by sharing her experience of walking in the rain in New York City where she was born. In the vast expanse of concrete it seemed that nothing would respond to the rain and grow. She writes: 'But the important thing is that the rain comes. The possibility of growth is there even in the hardest of times. Listening is like the rain' (p220).

I sense I am the rain that always comes and perhaps, slowly, Gill begins to grow again even in the harsh landscape of her despair. She begins to find patches of green within the grey walls that surround and confine her. Remen guides me to be more mindful of listening; more mindful to listen more intently, with more compassion, more mindful of opening the spaces for Gill to dwell and face her naked self.

Session 18: Monday 21st July 2003 – happy to rest like this

As I arrive the sun is shining yet a few moments earlier I had driven through heavy rain. Gill opens the door. She appears cheerful. She reminds me of the summer weather ... sunny periods interspersed with heavy showers. Vulnerable weather.

She saw the oncologist last Friday. He *is* going to stop the tamoxifen and commence Gill on arimidex after some blood tests to check her bone density. Gill is perplexed at his decision. I ask, 'Did you ask why?'.

Gill: No ... I told him I have severe side effects – hot flushes and now some facial downy hair! *(Suddenly her anger erupts)* Why change now – why not at the beginning? I knew arimidex gives me a better chance of non-recurrence than tamoxifen. I'm confused ... he said something about the menopause ... now that I'm menopausal I didn't need the tamoxifen but the tamoxifen induces menopause?? He said – stop now, but I'm continuing taking them until 3 weeks before my appointment with him in September ... they must be helping although he had said it won't make any difference to my chances of recurrence.

Another storm cloud bursts. Muddled information causes suffering that spills out as anger. Doctors and nurses must realise that women like Gill are informed by the media and the internet and hence they must involve women in a genuine dialogue about treatment options.

Gill's side still hurts and swells where the surgeon pulled the muscle round to form the breast cup for the reconstruction. Relentless ache pulls at her. I wonder if physiotherapy would help but that would require a referral. Gill is adamant she is not seeing the surgeon again for some time because of her previous experience with him. Losing confidence in the layers of the health team is demoralising; do they lose sight of Gill the person, seeing only the cancer body? I struggle to imagine that the care team have this attitude but Gill's experience frustrates and angers her. Gill seems to soak up gloomy news. Perhaps that's why her neck and shoulders are so tight. Underneath it all, like a deep current in the ocean, the fear of recurrence lurks. Such events as the oncologist's decision to change the medication may seem slight, yet small changes in the deep currents create big waves that crash on the rocks of despair.

I realise I am absorbing her frustration. It's not good for me. I sense it but cannot resist it. It floods over me and takes my energy. Holding her feet and using my breath, I regain my poise. After the reflexology Gill is slumped on the sofa as if she has collapsed into herself. She feels 'chilled'.

I step out into the overcast summer's day. The sun is hidden behind dark clouds. Rain threatens. Gill's rollercoaster continues along an unpredictable yet familiar trajectory. Reviews of treatment, more tests, shifts in treatment, unresolved effects of the surgery, all set against the background of an aggressive stage 3 cancer and the fear of recurrence.

Her body has forced itself into her consciousness as something unreliable, something to fear for what might be lurking in its folds. The pattern is set, tilted towards the pessimistic. Gill's life has fundamentally changed even though she looks back to grasp what has been.

Narrator: Young and Cullen (1996:9) noted from their research respondents with advanced cancer that:

> From the time the illness took hold, and increasingly as it bit deeper, their lives were more under the dominion of inescapables, of external forces that were beyond their own control, with death itself looming over all.

I sense how each day is an effort, an accumulative effort that takes Gill's strength and saps her *oak* will.

She tries to turn her head toward a brighter future, yet her body keeps pulling her to glance back, over her shoulder, always wary of 'it' sneaking up and catching her. The appointments, tests, threats of future surgery and treatment to eradicate the oestrogen that feeds the cancer; these external threats dominate her. She cannot relax unless caught off guard. The vigilant sentry at the gate. Alone, high and dry in the valley where demons scream at her. Alone in a cave of imponderable shadows.

Patterns repeating. But the old patterns no longer work. Reflexology holds the space. Holds her as she struggles to weave new patterns. Yet, even as I close the door, I sense the demons move back in. Respite is brief.

Poet: Audre Lorde writes:[10] I must let this pain flow through me and pass on. If I resist or try to stop it, it will detonate inside me, shatter me, splatter my pieces against every wall and person I touch.

Session 19: Friday 1st August 2003 – oak mother

A warm summer's day. I ponder – How will Gill be? What new events have turned her life inside out? Does she feel the sun?

She looks good although she has a cold. Shocked by the TV advert that shows small children breathing out cigarette smoke yet she still smokes. Smoking a release from the stress. As she pulls on the cigarette so the fear eases its pull on her. An ironic lifeline. Yet she is anxious to quit. So she fails and blames herself as weak.

She reveals new trauma.

Gill: I went for a blood test for calcium levels before commencing arimidex. God, it was painful! It was the same girl as before. She's sweet but hopeless. I've been asked to come in again for another test – the first sample wasn't adequate. I'm dreading it will be her again *(laughs nervously)* … I also have a bone scan arranged, then another appointment with the oncologist but thank God no appointment to see the surgeon! The pain in my back is still sore … it doesn't change much. Just aches more through the day. I just have to put up with it … maybe it'll ease with time.

Chris: Perhaps you should complain so other women are not being harmed by this blood-taking nurse.

Gill: Perhaps I should but, no, I couldn't do that … she might get into trouble.

Gill is the protective mother, she would rather suffer the slings and arrows of children than hurt them.

And always the dark cloud of the surgeon lurking. Her new career as a full-time hospital appointee.

I notice the vacuum cleaner standing in the corner. Gill only does a bit here and there. The house no longer spick and span. No help from the family. Phil is a working-class man who has clear ideas about roles. He puts the bread on the table. He is sympathetic but life patterns are engrained. Already he takes time off to take Gill for treatments and appointments. The cancer is also his burden and saps his energy, makes him edgy. How does he feel? What does he think? Is his reaction typical for spouses? Maybe I could help him but he is hidden from me. Gill has no energy or will to prepare for the planned holiday. She feels it will be such an effort. She doesn't want to go. Gill careful not to burden them with her complaints.

The oak mother standing firm even as the roots loosen in the storm. Standing alone. Gill shares her isolation – the neighbour who said 'we don't live in each other's pockets'; her brothers – she has barely seen her nephew who is now nearly a year old. She feels people are uncomfortable with her because of her cancer. Yet it works both ways – she is also uncomfortable with them because of the cancer. It seems the cancer comes between and fragments relationships.

Gill's face crumples, she cries, she apologises for crying. Hastily she tries to rearrange her mask.

She doesn't like to show people her tears. She says, 'I've no-one to share with … You're so calm … that's why I can say these things … what will I do when you don't come anymore?'

I feel the demand. The ethical dilemma of caring – how could I pull the rug away? Perhaps I create the dilemma by dwelling with her. Perhaps I become indispensable. Perhaps if I just came

---

[10]Lorde, A (1980) Ibid, p12.

into the house and did her feet rather than engage on a deeper holistic level, the dilemma would not exist. Perhaps I should have confronted her more with attending the support group and demanding Thelma's support. But Gill does not want to demand. She wants to cope and not be a burden, as she sees it. She does not want to identify with other cancer 'victims'. Like her family, she wants to be normal.

I remind Gill how relaxed she had been after the last two reflexology sessions. Her face brightens, as if remembering the comfort of therapy is itself comforting. She says she didn't realise how stressed she gets until she realised how relaxed she was after a therapy. She felt so good for a while after the last treatment. For a while? She says, 'Several days … and then I forget'.

The benefit of therapy held in the mind as an idea as well as in the body. Memory gradually erased in the immediacy of the day. Yet, perhaps a deeper memory of benefit slowly lightens the landscape so that things are never quite as dark as before.

Gill has been trying to listen to music and relax between sessions, using her breath as I have taught her. But it is not easy, her head full of thoughts.

The irony is that relaxation confronts Gill with her suffering, when her natural inclination is to seek distraction from it. I will bring a relaxation CD to guide her. Perhaps words of guidance will help dispel her crowded mind.

We are interrupted by Phil returning early from work. He puts his head around the door and says he won't disturb us! I meet him before I go. He is reserved and full of cold. My eyes search his, trying to invite him, but they are averted. I sense he suffers and copes silently.

Session 20: Friday 12th September 2003 – that man was not nice!

Gill tells the story of her visit to the surgeon.

Gill: It wasn't good despite Thelma being there. Afterwards he just stood up and walked out. No goodbye. He hadn't listened to my concerns at all. Indeed, he didn't seem to know about the valve he had inserted into me to regulate the saline pouch. Phil said afterwards 'That man was not nice'. Phil has a temper but he contained it. I could see he was getting agitated. I got a letter from him today explaining about the valve … I can't face seeing him again. I told my GP – she's offered to refer me elsewhere … Thelma was supportive … but I could see she was helpless.

Session 21: Thursday 24th September – happy anniversary

Last Tuesday was the first anniversary of Gill's breast lump diagnosis. She exclaims, 'I'm still here!'.

I imagine that making it through the first year is a significant marker. Staring death in the face until death turns away. Gill had previously asked me about becoming a therapist as a career idea where she can help people as I help her.

She recounts her story of enrolling at the local college for the holistic practice programme.

Gill: I ended up joining in a class because the course had already commenced. I was actually given an Indian head massage by a student, which I did not enjoy. All this oil in my hair! No warning. I also felt uncomfortable revealing my body, the scars. I felt I couldn't say no … under pressure from the teachers. Everyone seemed so young. I was sick that evening. It was all too much. Now I don't know what to do!

But Gill had made the effort. She feels liberated being off the tamoxifen. She has more energy and feels more positive, turning her face towards the future even as she stumbles. Yet the pain hasn't eased.

Session 25: Thursday 23rd October 2003 – synchronicity

Gill greets me with her usual warmth but her flatness ripples through me. She is struggling with the side effects of arimidex, especially a sore tip of tongue. Struggling to get some decent sleep. I sit on the floor as we review her Bach flower remedies. When I get to gentian I remind her that gentian is for her vulnerability to getting knocked back. My cue: 'You seem flat today, is something up?'.

As if pressing a trigger, her face crumples. She pours out her anguish. Katie has been playing up. We talk it over, trying to make sense of it all and find a possible way forward.

She looks at me and asks, 'Why do I tell you all of this?'.

'So why do you?'

Gill laughs: 'So why do I?'.

'Because I've been visiting you for nearly a year and you feel comfortable talking to me?'

'I don't talk to anyone else like this … I don't like to share these things.'

Resonance: a sympathetic vibration

Healing is resonance. We are separate but connected. Synchronicity:

- keeping time together
- the bringing together of different parts of the story.

In keeping time together, we journey along our parallel wavelengths tuned by Gill's wavelength and influenced by my presence towards a more healthy trajectory. In bringing together different parts of the story, I guide Gill to find wholeness when she has been so fragmented against the vast, complex and indeterminate canvas of life.

During the reflexology my thoughts drift off. This happens from time to time but today it is constant. I have to keep bringing myself back to pay attention. Technique on auto-pilot. I sense a problem with technique, that technique can easily become mindless, then I am no longer mindful of paying attention to listening and responding intuitively to the person.

This is a significant insight and yet I must also acknowledge a fear of letting go of technique and trusting myself. Pearl (2001:132) notes that *fear is only the absence of love*. Perhaps technique is not conducive to love because the focus is on the technique, not the person. Such insight is profound.

Afterwards Gill says she struggled to relax. Her head full of thoughts about Katie. Resonance of distracted minds.

The flow of Gill's journey has shifted from her illness and treatments to her crisis with Katie. Yet her crisis with Katie saps her energy, lowers her mood, weakens her resistance. Her relationship with Katie in the face of an impending recurrence of cancer and death is vital. Therefore the tension between them becomes more vital. The tension rooted in some part in the cancer. Everything linked together in the web of life, a web that entangles Gill in its complexity. I help to untangle the knots that bind and suffocate so she can breathe more easily.

I write Gill a poem.

Poet:

> Entangled in the web of suffering
> you struggle to break free
> no sooner one leg free
> than the other caught up,
> you cry out with frustration
> at the complexity of the web,
> seemingly no way to escape its grip;

let me gently pull this thread of life hanging loose
and ease you into a space where
the creepers of suffering don't pull so tight.

Session 27: Friday 21st November 2003 – Mr Pipsqueak

Leaves scattered along the lane mark the shifting seasons. Gill's equanimity skittled by the prospect of attending a new appointment with Mr Clint.

Gill exclaims, 'He's so rude … oh, what's the word I want?'.

'Arrogant?'

Gill: Yes, that's it … Phil would have a go at him but he's cautious in case it goes against my treatment … I've thought more about changing consultants but is it really worth it? I have a friend who also sees Mr Clint and has had a similar experience with him. She calls him Mr Pipsqueak! *(laughs)* Yes, that's it, I'm going to sit there and think of him as Mr Pipsqueak!

The tension melts. Turning him into a risible object takes away his power. Yet Mr Clint is buried deep within Gill's wound, making it raw, constraining healing. Despite Gill's suffering I empathise with his predicament. To see and hold a woman's breast is a thing of beauty, of love, of sex, of life. Yet he holds the breast and cuts it off. I imagine him standing in the theatre facing the heap of breasts he has removed. I can see how he must avert his gaze from the woman, to see only the breast, the wound, even as she presses him for recognition – 'see me' – and he must push her away. He has done enough. He is exhausted. Yet he cannot give way for he is also a hero. A god even. He cannot confide or wilt … eventually he cracks open to reveal the void he has become. The crack covered with green wraps.

But Gill does not see his plight. She cannot forget his taunt. Knocked back by the memory.

She fears her first follow-up mammogram. What might it reveal? She looks at me and I sense the dark shadow hover close.

I add gorse to her Bach flower prescription to help her prolonged sense of despair although she has not given up hope. As Bach says (cited in Chancellor 1990:97), 'They [who need gorse] look as if they need sunshine in their lives to drive the clouds away'.

Session 28: Wednesday 17th December 2003 – flabbergasted

Fragments of Gill's talk.

Gill: Mr Clint said, 'How are you? You look well' … I was flabbergasted! It's the first time he's been pleasant. I think Thelma must have had a word with him. I told him about the pain. He said he could take some fluid out of the valve, which he did [inflated with saline solution] … that's helped a bit, less pressure although I can still feel the edge [of the implant] and it constantly hurts. He suggested further surgery may help but I don't know about that. I would rather live with it than do that. I'm seeing him again at the end of January … the mammogram was awful … painful and Phil wasn't allowed to wait with me. He was told brusquely to wait outside. I felt so cross but Phil took it OK. I wanted him next to me to talk to me. I couldn't talk to any of the other women.

Mr Clint shifts his glance and sees Gill, not just a breast he has hacked off. Immediately, a cloud of torment lifts. A world of possibility opens where before was darkness. She feels understood and accepted. She can contemplate a future without trepidation and humiliation.

In contrast, her experience with the mammogram reflects the way staff reduce her and Phil to objects to be processed: being mindless, causing suffering.

Gill: My mouth is so dry … is there nothing that can keep it moist?

Session 30: Friday 9th January 2004 – struggle to be heard

Christmas was OK, yet Gill feels depressed and can't snap out of it, which makes her angry at herself. I tell her that she masks it well for she is always smiling. She recognises herself.

Gill: That's me … that's the way I've always been … people are always telling me. But now I try to smile but inside I'm not smiling … it's partly unresolved anger. I didn't get the breast screen result until Christmas eve, 3 weeks after the screen. I'm angry at Thelma because she promised to give me the results within 7–10 days. She rang the day I got the results by letter. I told her she had promised me. It was clear. I had complained to her about Phil's treatment at the clinic. I asked her if she had done anything about partners attending the breast screen, but she hadn't. I know she's busy but … I'm not angry, just disappointed.

In a few words we have the gist of Gill's story: the struggle to be heard, informed and supported through the nightmare of her cancer journey. At least she is confronting Thelma, spurred by her anger.

Listening to her story, to her unnecessary suffering, I too feel outrage that healthcare fails so abjectly. Gill had been twisted inside with anxiety about this result.

> breathing in, I calm my body
> breathing out, I smile
> breathing in, I lift the weight of despair
> breathing out, I am at peace.

Session 36: four months later, Tuesday 11th May 2004 – comfort the hurt child

Tomorrow is Gill's operation to deal with the persistent worsening pain in her left side. She is positive although she doesn't know what to expect. She assumes she will have a silicone implant to replace the saline pouch and valve.

Gill *(jokily)*: I asked him if I could have the other one done at the same time.

'What did he say?'

'He sort of laughed and didn't say anything … I had some bad news. An old friend recently died of breast cancer – she was diagnosed the same time as me. I know that breast cancer is a very individual disease but her death reminds me that I'm living on a knife edge. It's scary to be reminded like that.

Session 37: Tuesday 15th June 2004 – not so slim

A clear blue sky. A metaphor for life without suffering. Gill is pleased with the surgery. Her arm no longer aches. However, her 'menopausal' symptoms have worsened, more flushes but nothing like with the tamoxifen. She doesn't know how long she'll be on the arimidex and zoladex. I almost say 5 years but hold my tongue. I suggest she seeks this information from her GP when her next zoladex injection is due.

Gill: I am walking each day. It tires me but I've got to get some exercise because I'm getting fat even though I'm not eating very much … I've always proud of my trim figure … I feel angry at the family because they aren't considerate enough. They don't touch me or embrace me any more, I feel contaminated, as if my body repels them. I've always been there for them but am taken for granted all too easily.

Gill's tears are close to breaking. She grieves for her lost figure. Every treatment has a price to pay. No allowances made for her cancer. Perhaps the family do not make allowance as their way of coping so life can seem normal. To lift the lid on normal would be to open a Pandora's box of emotions that slither like vipers.

I wonder about the roots of her sadness. Is it just the threat of recurrence or is deeper than that, in her whole identity as a woman? We have never talked about her relationship with Phil, her husband, in terms of intimacy and sexual relationships. Is she alone at night? Does he give her messages that reinforce her loss of womanhood? Would I intrude into territory that even she avoids? Is it my business? As with Iris, I sense my discomfort with exploring Gill's sexuality. It feels forbidden territory but is that just my projection? Would she lose trust in me if I ventured to explore? Am I being too precious? I have put out feelers before – asking 'How is Phil?'. 'Oh he's OK,' closes the feeler.

Session 40: Thursday 26th August 2004 – facing adversity

We stand in the kitchen talking as Gill prepares Katie's brunch and relates her holiday adventures.

Gill: The holiday in Norfolk was rain, rain and more rain. The rain beating hard on the caravan roof kept me awake at night. The holiday was not as relaxing as I hoped for … I must tell you about when Phil, Katie and me were cycling down a narrow lane in the rain … *(she pauses and laughs)* I tried to cycle around a large puddle but fell off my bike into the pot-hole! I was soaked and covered in mud. Now it's funny. It wasn't so funny yesterday when I fell down the stairs and hurt my side. Now I'm wondering – am I losing my balance?'

She laughs but I sense the threat within her words. She reveals more bleak news of people she knows with cancer. An old school friend has just been diagnosed yet her experience is so different from Gill's. Another school friend now has the cancer in her bones. She goes quiet and says, 'It's 2 years now since I first felt the lump …'. She swallows hard and adds, 'I never thought I would be here today'.

'But you are here today … perhaps you can now turn your head more to the future?'

'It's true. I can't go back to who I was. I am changed, I realise that … that I have to make the best of things. Someone told me I need to stay in the present and not the future …

I respond, 'That might have been me … try waking up in the morning and saying something like "It's a good day to be alive", if that doesn't sound too corny. Gill, what do you want from life?'

Gill goes even quieter and then whispers, 'To see my girls grow up'.

But first Gill must find the secret place inside her, where she can transform her suffering into energy for the way forward; the strength, discipline and self-endurance to sustain her on her journey.

Narrator: Blackwolf and Jones say:[11]

> What sadness still grips at your heart? What anger must you release? What trauma do you have to dance? Honor the trauma of your self. If you have been a victim, please, find someone qualified to hear you, to help you heal and understand your pain. Look to your experience with the soft focus of ain-dah-ing. See the world, honor the questions, and enter into the dark places. Allow the pain of your trauma to help lead you back into the light of peace and balance.

Ain-dah-ing is our home within the heart. It is acceptance and love of self. Can Gill enter the dark places and move through her trauma into the light? She raises again her fear that the girls could inherit the cancer from her. Her fear is natural. I cannot reassure Gill. It is another worm wriggling in her mind.

And so it is. I continue to journey alongside Gill, to flow with her experience, that she may feel understood and cared for. I am balm for her raw wound even as fresh trauma rips it open again and again.

---

[11]Blackwolf and Jones (1996), p100.

Poet: Audre Lorde writes: Maybe this is the chance to live and speak those things I really do believe, that power comes from moving into whatever I fear most that cannot be avoided. But will I ever be strong enough again to open my mouth and not have a cry of raw pain leap out?

Notes

In the second performance we finished the RAW performance silently with a Power point presentation of key insights into the significance of therapy with Gill and other women with breast cancer I have worked with living in the community. This presentation is set against a background of Esmerine's deeply moving grating of cello and violins.[12]

- Having metastatic cancer is highly **stressful** yet largely **invisible**.
- Having metastatic cancer is living under a constant **threat of death**.
- People like Gill are **disenchanted** with health services through **poor** experience.
- People like Gill are **isolated** even within their own families.
- Society **fears** cancer.
- People like Gill experience prolonged existential **crisis**.
- Cancer carries a heavy **financial burden**.
- Children of cancer families can be beyond the **gaze** of health services.
- People like Gill benefit greatly from ongoing, consistent, dedicated social support.
- Yet people like Gill receive **inadequate** support from health services.
- Cancer rips through families.
- Families struggle to face up to the **reality** of cancer.
- Women strive to protect the family from the impact of their cancer at personal cost.
- Reflexology **breaks** the stress cycle.
- **Reflexology** brings immediate tangible comfort and is highly valued.
- Touch is more beneficial than counseling.
- Reflexology needs to be given **at least** monthly.
- The artistry of reflexology is mindfully revealed to me.
- I am therapist, social worker, Macmillan nurse, community nurse, GP, chaplain, psychologist … perhaps even an angel?
- People like Gill **struggle** to maintain relaxational programmes between sessions.
- It costs less than £1000 to support Gill per annum – **what cost is saved**?
- A new **holistic practitioner** is required, skilled in body therapy to **bridge** the gap between health and social care, offered in either a clinic or the person's own home as an ongoing **relationship**.

This roll-call of insights powerfully hammered home the messages that are implicit within the text. In the first performance in Denmark, we left the audience to draw their own insights and dialogue with us. Yet little dialogue evolved because the audience felt too emotional to respond. It is a dilemma whether to spell out the messages or whether to leave it to the audience. What does seem vital is to create a dialogical space, perhaps after a 'cooling down period/refreshment space, to explore audience 'reaction'. I continue to explore this issue.

---

[12] Esmerine – 'Aurora' mada 002-2. www.madronarecords.com

We had invited breast care and cancer charities to attend. They didn't. In fact, they didn't even bother to respond to their invitations. I also invited breast care workers to attend from local hospitals, again with no response. I need to think more about marketing performances. I approached the charity Macmillan to consider funding a project developing holistic practitioners. They declined. Yet my call for social action has not been entirely unheard. The local community NHS trust is considering a project attaching holistic practitioners to its three neighbourhood nursing teams. Watch this space.

RAW has been revised twice on reflection of the performances. Performance is more difficult than imagined. The most problematic aspect was the representation of Gill: how much dialogue to actually say *as Gill*. I wonder if another voice can adequately represent her. Perhaps her voice should be read by me from my journal. As it is, I have reconstructed her words in my journal. I sense a naturalistic dilemma of trying to represent Gill. On stage it just didn't sound right. The intonation was not right. The voice was not Gill.

We had read from scripts – whilst this was fine for me as I was reading my journal, it didn't feel right for Gill's voice. As such, I have now revised the narrative, minimising Gill's voice as read by someone representing Gill. I have left just one or two lines to be read as statements rather than in dialogue with me.

Since RAW I have constructed a second performance, 'Climbing walls', based on my practice with Ann, another woman with breast cancer. I now work with drama and dance teachers[13] to adequately perform (in contrast with reading) the narrative. This second performance was presented as a key-note presentation at the 14th International Reflective Practice conference at Rotorua, New Zealand, 2008. Working with drama and dance teachers shifts the goal posts big-time, demanding attention to performance methodololology.[14]

How might performance be judged as valid? First a warning!

Clough (2000:278) warns that if we set criteria for judging what is good and what is bad experimental writing or performance ethnography, we may only conventionalise the new writing 'and make more apparent the ways in which experimental writing has already become conventional'.

Denzin (2003:123), synthesising the work of Bochner (2000), Ellis (2000), Richardson (2000), Conquergood (1985), Spry (2001), Madison (1999), and Clough (2000), among others, notes that narrative/performance should:

- unsettle, criticize, and challenge taken-for-granted, repressed meanings
- invite moral and ethical dialogue while reflexively clarifying their own moral positions
- engender resistance and offer utopian thoughts about how things could be made different
- demonstrate that they care, that they are kind
- show instead of tell, using the rule that less is more

---

[13] Amanda Price, April Nunes and Antje Diedrich at the University of Bedfordshire – co-supervisors within the School of Guided Reflection and Narrative Inquiry.
[14] This work is explored in depth alongside the work of doctoral students using this methodology in the revised edition of *Guided reflection: advancing practice* (due for publication in 2009).

- exhibit interpretative sufficiency, representational adequacy, and authentic adequacy
- present political, collective and committed viewpoints. (p123–4)

I would add that the sense of the reader being present within the performance and gaining insight are also criteria for coherent performance, emphasising the significance of the sixth dialogical movement. In listing these criteria I reiterate that narrative needs to be well crafted, engaging and transgressive (Okri 1997) (Chapter 5).

Authenticity/speaking your truth

Wilber (1998) notes that the criterion for truth from an individual subjective perspective is authenticity. Put another way, narrative must ring true – the author must 'speak their truth'.

Our speech and thoughts are a reflection of our values, although we might speak untruthfully or with a false tongue. Therefore if I espouse to be caring, compassionate and work in collaborative ways with my colleagues, you might expect my speech not just to reflect those values but in fact be caring, compassionate and collaborative. Anything less would be a contradiction that the mindful practitioner would hopefully acknowledge and work towards resolving. Speaking my truth is being responsible for myself and my actions. Sometimes I may be faced with a moral dilemma as to whether to tell the truth or not, especially if the truth might in my judgement hurt someone. Being truthful involves saying what I *really* think – what is in my heart and mind. Before I can be truthful to others I must be truthful to myself. I have to know myself.

Sangharakshita (1990:68) says:

> If we do not know ourselves, in the depths as well as on the heights, if we cannot penetrate into the depths of our own being and be really transparent to ourselves, if there is not any clarity or illumination within – then we cannot speak the truth.

We may shrink at the prospect of being truthful and if that is so, then we need to face up to the forces that shrink us. If I do not speak my truth or I am careless in my speech then I cannot be fully available to my patients. I may even cause suffering and diminish the growth of the person.

Conclusion

The performance turn takes narrative into another dimension to engage people on a deeper embodied (spiritual, emotional, psychological) level, moving towards using narrative/text as social action to confront unsatisfactory practices. The performance turn extends to the curriculum, a sophisticated form of simulation, where care of patients can be researched and performed by students as learning. I finish the book with a glance at this new horizon I tentatively but enthusiastically move into.

Appendix

Clinical supervision evaluation tool

This tool has been designed to enable you to reflect on the quality of your individual or group supervision. The information will facilitate giving feedback to your supervisor concerning the effectiveness of supervision.

How long have you been in supervision with your current supervisor?	
Is your supervisor (please circle):	Line manager Non-line manager within the organisation Outside the organisation
What is your grade?	
What is the grade/position of your supervisor?	
How frequently did you contract supervision?	Every … days
How frequently (on average) do you actually have supervision?	Every … days

Whilst completing the tool is perhaps time consuming, please complete it carefully and honestly. *In particular please comment on your scores with specific examples.*

Mark along each scale the extent to which you agree with each statement:

5   most strongly agree
1   least agree

1	I felt safe to disclose my experiences	5	4	3	2	1

Comment

2	It was easy to identify experiences to reflect on	5	4	3	2	1

Comment

| 3 | I always came to each session prepared to share an experience | 5 | 4 | 3 | 2 | 1 |

Comment

| 4 | I never cancelled sessions | 5 | 4 | 3 | 2 | 1 |

Comment

| 5 | The balance of challenge and support was excellent (I didn't feel too threatened or comfortable) | 5 | 4 | 3 | 2 | 1 |

Comment

| 6 | Supervision has inspired me | 5 | 4 | 3 | 2 | 1 |

Comment

| 7 | Supervision helped me clarify key issues and gain new insights into my practice | 5 | 4 | 3 | 2 | 1 |

Comment

| 8 | I have become very reflective | 5 | 4 | 3 | 2 | 1 |

Comment

| 9 | I have become more open and curious about my practice | 5 | 4 | 3 | 2 | 1 |

Comment

| 10 | I felt I was being moulded into becoming a 'supervisor' clone | 5 | 4 | 3 | 2 | 1 |

Comment

| 11 | I have become aware of the factors that influence the way I think, feel and respond within situations | 5 | 4 | 3 | 2 | 1 |

Comment

| 12 | I am more aware of/focused on my role responsibility, authority, and autonomy | 5 | 4 | 3 | 2 | 1 |

Comment

| 13 | The input of theory was both relevant and substantial | 5 | 4 | 3 | 2 | 1 |

Comment

| 14 | Work has become more meaningful and interesting | 5 | 4 | 3 | 2 | 1 |

Comment

| 15 | Supervision picked me up when I felt overwhelmed | 5 | 4 | 3 | 2 | 1 |

Comment

| 16 | Reflection has helped me to express my ideas, opinions, and feelings | 5 | 4 | 3 | 2 | 1 |

Comment

| 17 | Supervision enabled me to tackle issues that I might otherwise have avoided | 5 | 4 | 3 | 2 | 1 |

Comment

| 18 | Supervision helped me deal with negative emotions (such as anger, failure, outrage, guilt, distress, resentment) | 5 | 4 | 3 | 2 | 1 |

Comment

| 19 | I am more in control of 'who I am' | 5 | 4 | 3 | 2 | 1 |

Comment

| 20 | My supervisor really listened to me | 5 | 4 | 3 | 2 | 1 |

Comment

| 21 | I was happy with my supervisor | 5 | 4 | 3 | 2 | 1 |

Comment

| 22 | I never felt judged by my supervisor | 5 | 4 | 3 | 2 | 1 |

Comment

| 23 | We constantly reviewed the way supervision has helped me to develop and sustain my practice | 5 | 4 | 3 | 2 | 1 |

Comment

| 24 | We always commenced each session by reviewing the previous session | 5 | 4 | 3 | 2 | 1 |

Comment

| 25 | Supervision sessions were never interrupted | 5 | 4 | 3 | 2 | 1 |

Comment

| 26 | I always knew what I needed to do at the end of each session | 5 | 4 | 3 | 2 | 1 |

Comment

| 27 | My supervisor always wanted 'to fix' the problem for me | 5 | 4 | 3 | 2 | 1 |

Comment

| 28 | My supervisor was overly parental and patronising | 5 | 4 | 3 | 2 | 1 |

Comment

| 29 | The environment for supervision was excellent | 5 | 4 | 3 | 2 | 1 |

Comment

Use this space to make any further comment

Supervision evaluation tool /f – revised March 2002.

References

Alexander, L (1998) Writing in hospices. In: C Kaye and T Blee (eds) The arts in health care: a palette of possibilities. Jessica Kingsley, London.

Alfano, G (1971) Healing or caretaking – which will it be? *Nursing Clinics of North America* **6**(2): 273–80.

Armitage, S (1990) Research utilisation in practice. *Nurse Education Today* **10**: 10–15.

Ashworth, P, Longmate, M and Morrison, P (1992) Patient participation: its meaning and significance in the context of caring. *Journal of Advanced Nursing* **17**: 1430–9.

Atkins, S and Murphy, K (1993) Reflective practice. *Nursing Standard* **9**(45): 31–7.

Atkinson, RL, Atkinson, RC and Smith E (1990) Introduction to psychology. Harcourt Brace, New York.

Ausubel, D (1967) Learning theory and classroom practice. Ontario Institute for Studies in Education, Toronto.

Autton, N (1996) The use of touch in palliative care. *European Journal of Palliative Care* **3**(3): 121–4.

Bailey, J (1995) Reflective practice: implementing theory. *Nursing Standard* **9**(46): 29–31.

Bartlett, H (2000) Quality improvement: will nursing seize the opportunity? *Nursing Times Research* **5**(6): 424–5.

Bass, B (1985) Leadership and performance beyond expectations. Free Press, New York.

Batehup, L and Evans, A (1992) A new strategy. *Nursing Times* **88**(47): 40–1.

Batey, M and Lewis, F (1982) Clarifying autonomy and accountability in nursing service: Part 1. *Journal of Nursing Administration* **12**(9): 13–18.

Beck, CJ (1997) Everyday Zen. Thorsons, London.

Begley, A-M (1996) Literature and poetry: pleasure and practice. *International Journal of Nursing Practice* **2**: 182–8.

Belenky, MF, Clinchy, BM, Goldberger, NR and Tarule, JM (1986) Women's ways of knowing: the development of self, voice, and mind. Basic Books, New York.

Benjamin, M and Curtis, J (1986) Ethics in nursing, 2nd edn. Oxford University Press, New York.

Benner, P (1984) From novice to expert. Addison-Wesley, Menlo Park.

Benner, P (2003) Clinical reasoning: articulating experiential learning in nursing practice. In: L Basford and O Slevin (eds) Theory and practice of nursing: an integrated approach to caring practice. Nelson Thornes, Cheltenham.

Benner, P and Wrubel, J (1989) The primacy of caring. Addison-Wesley, Menlo Park.

Benner, P, Tanner, C and Chesla, C (1996) Expertise in nursing practice: caring, clinical judgement, and ethics. Springer, New York.

Berne, E (1961) Transactional analysis in psychotherapy. The classic guide to its principles. Grove Press, New York.

Betz, M and O'Conell, L (1987) Primary nursing: panacea or problem? *Nursing and Health Care* **8**: 456–60.

Biley, F (1992) Some determinants that affect patient participation in decision-making about nursing care. *Journal of Advanced Nursing* **17**: 414–21.

Biley, F and Wright, S (1997) Towards a defence of nursing routine and ritual. *Journal of Clinical Nursing* **6**(2): 115–19.

Blackford, J (2003) Cultural frameworks of nursing practice: exposing an exclusionary healthcare culture. *Nursing Inquiry* **10**(4): 236–42.

Blackwolf and Jones G (1995) Listen to the drum. Commune-E-Key, Salt Lake City.

Blackwolf and Jones G (1996) Earth dance drum. Commune-E-Key, Salt Lake City.

Bochner, A (2000) Criteria against ourselves. *Qualitative Inquiry* **6**: 266–72.

Bochner, A and Ellis, C (2002) Ethnographically speaking: autoethnography, literature, and aesthetics. AltaMira Press, Walnut Creek.

Bohm, D (1980) Wholeness and the implicate order. Routledge, London.

Bohm, D (ed Nichol L) (1996) On dialogue. Routledge, London.

Bolton, S (2000) Who cares? Offering emotion work as a 'gift' in the nursing labour process. *Journal of Advanced Nursing* **32**: 580–6.

Bond, M and Holland, S (1998) Skills of clinical supervision for nurses. Open University Press, Buckingham.

Borglum, D (1997) The long shadow of good intentions. *Tricycle* **7**(1): 66–69.

Boud, D, Keogh, R and Walker, D (1985) Promoting reflection in learning: a model. In: D Boud, R Keogh and D Walker (eds) Reflection: turning experience into learning. Kogan Page, London.

Boyd, E and Fales, A (1983) Reflective learning: key to learning from experience. *Journal of Humanistic Psychology* **23**(2): 99–117.

Brodersen, L (2001) Creatively capturing care: poetry and knowledge in nursing. *International Journal for Human Caring* **6**(1): 33–41.

Brooks, S (2004) Becoming a transformational leader. Unpublished Masters in Leadership dissertation, University of Bedfordshire.

Brumpton, K (1998) We can work it out. *Nursing Times* **94**(29): 62–3.

Bruner, J (1994) The remembered self. In: U Neisser and R Fivush (eds) The remembering self: construction and accuracy in the self narrative. Cambridge University Press, New York.

Buckenham, J. and McGrath, G (1983) The social reality of nursing. Adis, Sydney.

Bulman, C (2004) An introduction to reflection. In: C Bulman and S Schultz (eds) Reflective practice in nursing, 3rd edn. Blackwell Publishing, Oxford.

Burns, J (1978) Leadership. Harper and Row, New York.

Burkhardt, M and Nagai-Jacobson, M (2002) Spirituality: living our connectedness. Farrar, Straus and Giroux, New York.

Burnard, P (1995) Nurse educators' perceptions of reflection and reflective practice. A report of a descriptive study. *Journal of Advanced Nursing* **21**: 1167–74.

Burnard, P and Morrison, P (1991) Nurses' interpersonal skills: a study of nurses' perceptions. *Nurse Education Today* **11**: 24–9.

Burrows, D (1995) The nurse teacher's role in the promotion of reflective practice. *Nurse Education Today* **15**: 346–50.

Burton, A (2000) Reflection: nursing's practice and education panacea? *Journal of Advanced Nursing* **31**(5): 1009–17.

Bush, T (2003) Communicating with patients who have dementia. *Nursing Times* **99**(48): 42–5.

Butterfield, P (1990) Thinking upstream: nurturing a conceptual understanding of the societal context of health behaviour. *Advances in Nursing Science* **12**(2): 1–8.

Callanan, S and Kelley, P (1991) Final gifts. Bantam Books, New York.

Cameron, D, Phillips, S, Sawh, K and Wadey, P (2008) Expressing voice and developing practical wisdom on social justice through art. In: C Delmar and C Johns (eds) The good, the wise, and the right clinical nursing practice. Aalborg Hospital, Arhus University Hospital, Denmark, pp 59–72.

Campbell, J (1988) The power of myth. Doubleday, New York.

Cara, C (1999) Relational caring inquiry: nurses' perspective on how management can promote a caring practice. *International Journal of Human Caring* **3**(**1**): 22–30.

Carmack, B (1997) Balancing engagement and detachment in care-giving. *Image: Journal of Nursing Scholarship* **29**(**2**): 139–43.

Carper, B (1978) Fundamental patterns of knowing in nursing. *Advances in Nursing Science* **1**(**1**): 13–23.

Carroll, L (1988) Alice's adventures in Wonderland. Random House, London, p26.

Casement, P (1985) On learning from the patient. Routledge, London.

Cattrell, R, Lavender, A, Wallymahmed, A, Kingdon, C and Riley, J (2005) Postnatal care. What matters to women? *British Journal of Midwifery* **13**(**4**): 206–13.

Cavanagh, S (1991) The conflict management style of staff nurses and nurse managers. *Journal of Advanced Nursing* **16**: 1254–60.

Chancellor, P (1990) Illustrated handbook of the Bach flower remedies. CW Daniel, Saffron Walden.

Chang Ok Sung (2001) The conceptual structure of physical touch in caring. *Journal of Advanced Nursing* **33**(**6**): 820–7.

Chapman, G (1983) Ritual and rational action in hospitals. *Journal of Advanced Nursing* **8**: 13–20.

Charmaz, K (1983) Loss of self: a fundamental form of suffering in the chronically ill. *Sociology of Health and Illness* **5**(**2**): 168–95.

Cherniss, G (1980) Professional burn-out in human service organisations. Praeger, New York.

Cioffi, J (1997) Heuristics, servants to intuition, in clinical decision making. *Journal of Advanced Nursing* **26**: 203–8.

Cixous, H (1996) Sorties: out and point: attacks'ways out/forays. In: H Cixous and C Clement (eds) The newly born woman. Tauris, London.

Clough, P (2000) Comments on setting criteria for experimental writing. *Qualitative Inquiry* **6**: 278–91.

Cochran, L and Laub, L (1994) Becoming an agent: patterns and dynamics for shaping your life. State University of New York Press, Albany.

Conquergood, D (1985) Performing as a moral act: ethical dimensions of the ethnography of performance. *Literature in Performance* **5**: 1–13.

Cooper, M (1991) Principle-oriented ethics and the ethic of care: a creative tension. *Advances in Nursing Science* **14**(**2**): 22–31.

Cope, M (2001) Lead yourself. Be where others would follow. Pearson Education, Harlow.

Cotton, A (2001) Private thoughts in public spheres: issues in reflection and reflective practices in nursing. *Journal of Advanced Nursing* **36**(**4**): 512–19.

Cottrell S. (1999) Some current beliefs in the NHS and some consequences for implementing clinical supervision. Excerpt from conference address. http://www.clinical-supervision.com.

Courtney, M, Tong, S and Walsh, A (2000) Acute care nurses' attitudes towards older people: a literature review. *International Journal of Nursing Practice* **6**: 62–9.

Covey, S (1989) The 7 Habits of Highly Effective People. Simon and Schuster, London

Cowling, WR (2000) Healing as appreciating wholeness. *Advances in Nursing Science* **22**(**3**): 16–32.

Cox, H, Hickson, P and Taylor, B (1991) Exploring reflection: knowing and constructing practice. In: G Gray and R Pratt (eds) Towards a discipline of nursing. Churchill Livingstone Melbourne, pp373–90.

Cutliffe, J and McKenna, H (2004) Expert qualitative researchers and the use of audit trails. *Journal of Advanced Nursing* **45**(**2**): 126–35.

Daiski, I (2004) Changing nurses' disempowering relationship patterns. *Journal of Advanced Nursing* **48**(**1**):43–50.

Davidhizar, R and Giger, J (1997) When touch is not the best approach. *Journal of Clinical Nursing* **6**(**3**): 203–6.

Davis, P (1999) Aromatherapy A-Z. CW Daniel, Saffron Walden.

Davis-Floyd, R (2001) The technocratic, humanistic and holistic paradigms of childbirth. *International Journal of Gynaecology and Obstetrics* **75**(**1**): 5–23.

Day, C (1993) Reflection: a necessary but not sufficient condition for professional development. *British Educational Research Journal* **19**(**1**): 83–93.

De Hennezel, M (1996) Intimate death (trans. C Janeway). Warner Books, London.

De La Cuesta, C (1983) The nursing process: from development to implementation. *Journal of Advanced Nursing* **8**: 365–71.

Denzin, N (2003) Performance ethnography. Sage, Thousand Oaks.

Denzin, N and Lincoln, Y (2000) Introduction: the discipline and practice of qualitative research. In: N Denzin and Y Lincoln (eds) The Sage handbook of qualitative research. Sage, Thousand Oaks.

Department of Health and Social Security (1972) Report of the Committee on Nursing *(Chairperson, Professor Asa Briggs)*. HMSO, London.

Department of Health and Social Security (1986) Neighbourhood nursing – a focus for care *(The Cumberlege Report)*. HMSO, London.

Department of Health (1996) Clinical audit in the NHS. HMSO, London.

Department of Health (1998) A first class service. HMSO, London.

Department of Health (1999) Making a difference. HMSO, London.

Department of Health (2004) National service framework for children, young people and maternity services. Department of Health, London.

Department of Health (2007) Maternity matters: choice, access and continuity of care in a safe service. Stationery Office, London.

DeSalvo, L (1999) Writing as a way of healing: how telling our stories transforms our lives. The Women's Press, London.

Dewey, J (1933) How we think. JC Heath, Boston.

Diamond, J (2001) Snake oil. Vintage, London.

Dickson, A (1982) A woman in your own right. Quartet Books, London.

Donaldson, LJ (2001) Safe high quality health care: investing in tomorrow's leaders. *Quality in Health Care* **10**: 8–12.

Downe, S. (2004) Normal childbirth: evidence and debate. Churchill Livingstone, London.

Dreyfus, H and Dreyfus, S (1986) Mind over machine. Free Press, New York.

Driscoll, J (2000) Practising clinical supervision: a reflective approach. Baillière Tindall, London.

Druskat, V and Wolff, S (2001) Building the emotional intelligence of groups. *Harvard Business Review* March: 81–90.

Dunham, J and Klafehn, K (1990) Transformational leadership and the nurse executive. *Journal of Advanced Nursing* **20**(**4**): 28–33.

Dyer, I (1995) Preventing the ITU syndrome or how not to torture an ITU patient (part 2). *Intensive and Critical Care Nursing* **11**(**4**): 223–32.

Edwards, S (1998) An anthropological interpretation of nurses' and patients' perceptions of the use of space and touch. *Journal of Advanced Nursing* **28**: 809–17.

Eifried, S, Riley-Giomariso, O and Voight, G (2000) Learning to care amid suffering: how art and narrative give voice to the student experience. *International Journal for Human Caring* **5**(**2**): 42–51.

Ellis, C (2000) Creating criteria: an ethnographic short story. *Qualitative Inquiry* **6**: 272–7.

Ellis, C (2004) The ethnographic I: a methodological novel about autoethnography. AltaMira Press, Walnut Creek.

Estabrooks, C and Morse, J (1992) Toward a theory of touch: the touching process and acquiring a touching style. *Journal of Advanced Nursing* **17**: 448–56.

Evans, D (2002) The effectiveness of music as an intervention for hospital patients: a systematic review. *Journal of Advanced Nursing* **37**(**1**): 8–18.

Farrar, M (1992) How much do they want to know? *Professional Nurse* **7**(**9**): 606–10.

Faugier, J and Butterworth, T (undated) Clinical supervision: a position paper. School of Nursing Studies, University of Manchester.

Fay, B (1987) Critical social science. Polity Press, Cambridge.

Feil, N (1993) The validation breakthrough: simple techniques for communicating with people with Alzheimer's-type dementia. Health Professions Press, Baltimore.

Ferruci, P (1982) What we may be. St Martin's Press, New York.

Fordham, M (2008) Building bridges in homelessness, mindful of phronesis in nursing practice. In: C Delmar and C Johns (eds) The good, the wise, and the right clinical nursing practice. Aalborg Hospital, Arhus University Hospital, Denmark, pp73–92.

Foucault, M (1979) Discipline and punish: the birth of the prison (trans. A Sheridan). Vintage/Random House, New York.

Frank, A (2002) Relations of caring: demoralization and remoralization in the clinic. *International Journal of Human Caring* **6**(**2**): 13–19.

Fredriksson, L (1999) Modes of relating in a caring conversation: a research synthesis on presence, touch and listening. *Journal of Advanced Nursing* **30**(**5**): 1167–76.

Fremantle, F (2003) Luminous enlightenment. Shambhala, Boston.

Freire, P (1972) Pedagogy of the oppressed. Penguin Books, London.

French, J and Raven, B (1968) The bases of social power. In: D Cartwright and A Zander (eds) Group dynamics. Row Peterson, Evanston, IL, pp150–67.

Friedson, E (1970) Professional dominance. Aldine Atherton, Chicago.

Gadamer, H-G (1975) Truth and method (trans G Barden and J Cumming). Seabury Press, New York.

Gadow, S (1980) Existential advocacy. In: S Spickler and S Gadow (eds) Nursing: image and ideals. Springer, New York, pp79–101.

Garland, D (2004) Is the use of water in labour an option for women following a previous LSCS? *Midwifery Digest* **14**(**1**): 63–7.

Garland, D (2006) Is waterbirth a 'safe and realistic' option for women following a previous caesarean section? *Midwifery Digest* **16** (**2**): 217–20.

Garside, P (1999) The learning organisation: a necessary setting for improving care? *Quality in Health Care* **8**: 211.

Gaydos, H (2008) Collage: an aesthetic process for creating phronesis in nursing. In: C Delmar and C Johns (eds) The good, the wise, and the right clinical nursing practice. Aalborg Hospital, Arhus University Hospital, Denmark, pp163–78.

Ghaye, T (2000a) Colleague centred care: the reframing of clinical supervision. In: T Ghaye and S Lillyman (eds) Effective clinical supervision. Mark Allen Publishers, Dinton.

Ghaye, T (2000b) The role of reflection in nurturing clinical conversations. In: T Ghaye and S Lillyman (eds) Effective clinical supervision. Mark Allen Publishers, Dinton.

Gibbs, G (1988) Learning by doing: a guide to teaching and learning methods. Further Education Unit, Oxford Polytechnic (now Oxford Brookes University).

Gilbert, T (2001) Reflective practice and clinical supervision: meticulous rituals of the confessional. *Journal of Advanced Nursing* **36**(**2**): 199–205.

Gillespie, D (2000) On being silenced. Insights from Foucault and Habermas. In: T Ghaye (ed) Empowerment through reflection: the narrative of healthcare professionals. Mark Allen Publishing, Trowbridge.

Gilligan, C (1982) In a different voice. Harvard University Press, Cambridge, MA.

Goldstein, J (2002) One dharma. Rider, London.

Goorapah, D (1997) Clinical supervision. *Journal of Clinical Nursing* **6**(**3**): 173–8.

Gray, G and Forsstrom, S (1991) Generating theory from practice: the reflective technique. In: G Gray and R Pratt R (eds) Towards a discipline of nursing. Churchill Livingstone, Melbourne, pp355–72.

Green, A (1996) An explorative study of patients' memory of their stay in an acute intensive therapy unit. *Intensive and Critical Care Nursing* **12**(**3**): 131–7.

Greene, M (1988) The dialectic of freedom. Teachers' College Press, Columbia University, New York.

Groom, J (2002) Working with deliberate self-harm patients in A&E. In: C Johns (ed) Guided reflection: advancing practice. Blackwell Publishing, Oxford, pp169–85.

Habermas, J (1984) Theory of communicative action. Vol. **1**: Reason and the rationalisation of society. Beacon Press, Boston, and Basil Blackwell, Oxford, in association with Polity Press, Cambridge.

Hall, C (2003) Nurse shortage in NHS is near to crisis point. Daily Telegraph 29 April.

Hall, L (1964) Nursing – what is it? *Canadian Nurse* **60**(2): 150–4.

Halldórsdóttir, S (1991) Five basic modes of being with another. In: D Gaut and M Leininger (eds) Caring: the compassionate healer. National League for Nursing, New York.

Halligan, A and Donaldson, LJ (2001) Implementing clinical governance: turning vision into reality. *British Medical Journal* **322**(7299): 1413–17.

Hawkins, P and Shohet, R (1989) Supervision for the helping professions. Open University Press, Buckingham.

Heath, H and Freshwater, D (2000) Clinical supervision as an emancipatory process: avoiding inappropriate intent. *Journal of Advanced Nursing* **32**: 1298–306.

Heron, J (1975) Six-category intervention analysis. Human Potential Resource Group, University of Surrey, Guildford.

Hewitt-Taylor, J (2004) Challenging the balance of power: patient empowerment. *Nursing Standard* **18**(22): 33–7.

Heywood, J (2006) 'And those who were dancing were thought to be insane by those who could not hear the music.' Unpublished Masters in Health Care Leadership dissertation, University of Bedfordshire.

Hickman, P and Holmes, C (1994) Nursing the post-modern body: a touching case. *Nursing Inquiry* **1**: 3–14.

Holly, ML (1989) Reflective writing and the spirit of inquiry. *Cambridge Journal of Education* **19**(1): 71–80.

Howse, E and Bailey, J (1992) Resistance to documentation – a nursing research issue. *International Journal of Nursing Studies* **29**(4): 371–80.

Hunt, J (1981) Indicators for nursing practice: the use of research findings. *Journal of Advanced Nursing* **6**: 189–94.

Hunt, S and Symonds, A (1995) The social meaning of midwifery. Macmillan, Basingstoke.

Isaacs, W (1993) Taking flight: dialogue, collective thinking, and organizational learning. Center for Organizational Learning's Dialogue Project, MIT, MA.

James, N (1989) Emotional labour: skill and work in the social regulation of feelings. *Sociological Review* **37**(1): 15–42.

Jarrett, L (2008) From significance to insights. In: C Delmar and C Johns (eds) The good, the wise, and the right clinical nursing practice. Aalborg Hospital, Arhus University Hospital, Denmark, pp 59–72.

Jarrett, L and Johns, C (2005) Constructing the reflexive narrative. In: C Johns and D Freshwater (eds) Transforming nursing through reflective practice, 2nd edn. Blackwell Publishing, Oxford, pp162–79.

Jewell, S (1994) Patient participation: what does it mean? *Journal of Advanced Nursing* **19**: 433–8.

Johns, C (1989) The impact of introducing primary nursing on the culture of a community hospital. Masters of Nursing dissertation, University of Wales College of Medicine, Cardiff.

Johns, C (1992) Ownership and the harmonious team: barriers to developing the therapeutic nursing team in primary nursing. *Journal of Clinical Nursing* **1**: 89–94.

Johns, C (1993) Professional supervision. *Journal of Nursing Management* **1**(1): 9–18

Johns, C (ed) (1994) The Burford NDU model: caring in practice. Blackwell Publishing, Oxford.

Johns, C (1995) Framing learning through reflection within Carper's fundamental ways of knowing. *Journal of Advanced Nursing* **22**: 226–34.

Johns, C (1998a) Becoming a reflective practitioner through guided reflection. PhD thesis, Open University.

Johns, C (1999) Unravelling the dilemmas of everyday nursing practice. *Nursing Ethics* **6**: 287–98.

Johns, C (1998c) Caring through a reflective lens: giving meaning to being a reflective practitioner. *Nursing Inquiry* **5**: 18–24.

Johns, C (2000) Working with Alice: a reflection. *Complementary Therapies in Nursing and Midwifery* **6**: 199–203.

Johns, C (2001a) Depending on the intent and emphasis of the supervisor, clinical supervision can be a different experience. *Journal of Nursing Management* **9**: 139–45.

Johns, C (2001b) The caring dance. *Complementary Therapies in Nursing and Midwifery* **7**(**1**): 8–12.

Johns, C (2002) Guided reflection: advancing practice. Blackwell Publishing, Oxford.

Johns, C (2003a) Clinical supervision as a model for clinical leadership. *Journal of Nursing Management* **11**: 25–34.

Johns, C (2003b) Lecture notes: creating and sustaining an effective practice environment. MA Clinical Leadership 9/04/03.

Johns, C (2004a) Becoming a reflective practitioner, 2nd edn. Blackwell Publishing, Oxford.

Johns, C (2004b) Being mindful, easing suffering: reflections on palliative care. Jessica Kingsley, London.

Johns, C (2005) Balancing the winds. *Reflective Practice* **5**(**3**): 67–84.

Johns, C (2006) Engaging reflection in practice. Blackwell Publishing, Oxford.

Johns, C and Hardy, H (2005) Voice as a metaphor for transformation through reflection. In: C Johns and D Freshwater (eds) Transforming nursing through reflective practice, 2nd edn. Blackwell Publishing, Oxford, pp85–98.

Johns, C and McCormack, B (1998) Unfolding the conditions where the transformative potential of guided reflection (clinical supervision) might flourish or flounder. In: C Johns and D Freshwater (eds) Transforming nursing through reflective practice. Blackwell Publishing, Oxford.

Johnson, D (1974) Development of theory: a requisite for nursing as a primary health profession. *Nursing Research* **23**(**5**): 373–7.

Johnson, M and Webb, C (1995) Rediscovering unpopular patients: the concept of social judgement. *Journal of Advanced Nursing* **21**: 466–75.

Jourard, S (1971) The transparent self. Van Nostrand, New York.

Kelly, MP and May, D (1982) Good and bad patients: a review of the literature and a theoretical critique. *Journal of Advanced Nursing* **7**: 147–56.

Kerfoot, K (1996) World class excellence. *Dermatology Nursing* **8**(**6**): 433–4.

Kermode, F (1966) The sense of an ending. Oxford University Press, New York.

Kieffer, C (1984) Citizen empowerment: a developmental perspective. *Prevention in Human Services* **84**(**3**): 9–36.

Kikuchi, J (1992) Nursing questions that science cannot answer. In: J Kikuchi and H Simmons (eds) Philosophic Inquiry in Nursing. Sage, Newberry Park, CA.

King, L and Appleton, J (1997) Intuition: a critical review of the research and rhetoric. *Journal of Advanced Nursing* **26**: 194–202.

Kitson, A (1989) A framework for quality: a patient-centred approach to quality assurance in health care. Scutari Press, Middlesex.

Klakovich, M (1994) Connective leadership for the 21st century: a historical perspective and future directions. *Advanced Nursing Science* **16**(**4**): 42–54.

Knopf, M (1994) Treatment options for early stage breast cancer. *MEDSURG Nursing* **3**: 249–57.

Kopp, P (2000) Overcoming difficulties in communicating with other professionals. *Nursing Times* **96**(**28**): 47–9.

Kübler-Ross, E (1969) On death and dying. Tavistock, London.

Larson, P (1987) Comparison of cancer patients' and professional nurses' perceptions of important caring behaviours. *Heart and Lung* **16**(**2**): 187–93.

Latchford, Y (2002) Finding a new way in health visiting. In: C Johns (ed) Guided reflection: advancing practice, Blackwell Publishing, Oxford, pp144–66.

Lather, P (1986a) Research as praxis. *Harvard Educational Review* **56**(3): 257–77.

Lather, P (1986b) Issues of validity in open ideological research: between a rock and a hard place. *Interchange* **17**(4): 63–84.

Latimer, J (1995) The nursing process re-examined: enrolment and translation. *Journal of Advanced Nursing* **22**: 213–20.

Lawler, J (1991) Behind the screens: nursing, somology and the problems of the body. Churchill Livingstone, Melbourne.

Lawrence, M (1995) The unconscious experience. *American Journal of Critical Care* **4**(3): 227–32.

Leigh, A and Maynard, M (1995) Leading your team. Werner Soderstrom Osakeyhtio, Finland.

Leigh, K (2001) Communicating with unconscious patients. *Nursing Times* **97**(48): 35–6.

Levine, S (1986) Who dies? An investigation of conscious living and conscious dying. Gateway Books, Bath.

Lieberman, A (1989) Staff development in culture building, curriculum and teaching: the next 50 years. Teachers' College Press, Columbia University, New York.

Liehr, P and Smith, MJ (2008) Story theory. In: MJ Smith and P Liehr (eds) Middle range theory for nursing, 2nd edn. Springer, New York, pp205–21.

Lindberg, I, Christensson, K and Ohrling, K (2005) Midwives' experience of organisational and professional change. *Midwifery* **4**: 355–64.

Lliffe, S and Drennan, V (2001) Primary care and dementia. Jessica Kingsley, London.

Logstrup, KE (1997) The ethical demand. University of Notre Dame Press, Notre Dame, IN.

Lorde, A (1980) The cancer journals. Aunt Lute Books, San Francisco.

Lyle, D (1998) Opinion: is clinical supervision the answer to quality care? *Nursing Management* **5**(6): 3.

Mackintosh, C (1998) Reflection: a flawed strategy for the nursing profession. *Nurse Education Today* **18**: 553–7.

Macleod, M (1994) 'It's the little things that count': the hidden complexity of everyday clinical nursing practice. *Journal of Clinical Nursing* **3**(6): 361–8.

MacMillan, S (1996) Working in a team. *Professional Nurse* **11**(9): 601–5.

Madison, DS (1999) Performance theory/embodied writing. *Text and Performance Quarterly* **19**: 107–24.

Madrid, M (1990) The participating process of human field patterning in an acute care environment. In: E Barrett (ed) Visions of Martha Rogers's science-based nursing. National League for Nursing, New York.

Malby, R (1996) The need for nursing leadership. *British Journal of Healthcare Management* **2**(3): 18–19.

Margolis, H (1993) Paradigm and barriers: how habits of mind govern scientific beliefs. University of Chicago Press, Chicago.

Maslach, C (1976) Burned-out. *Human Behaviour* **5**: 16–22.

Maslow, A (1968) Towards a psychology of being. Van Nostrand, Princeton, NJ.

Mayer, D (1986) Cancer patients' and their families' perceptions of nurse caring behaviours. *Topics in Clinical Nursing* **8**(2): 63–9.

Mayeroff, M (1971) On caring. Harper Perennial, New York.

Mayo, S (1996) Symbol, metaphor and story: the function of group art therapy in palliative care. *Palliative Medicine* **10**: 209–16.

McCaffrey, R (2002) Music listening as a nursing intervention A symphony of practice. *Holistic Nursing Practice* **16**(3): 70–7.

McClarey, M (2001) Implementing NICE guidance. *Professional Nurse* **16**(6): 1145.

McElroy, A, Corben, V and McLeish, K (1995) Developing care plan documentation: an action research project. *Journal of Nursing Management* **3**: 193–9.

McNeely, R (1983) Organizational patterns and work satisfaction in a comprehensive human service agency: an empirical test. *Human Relations* **36**(10): 957–72.

McNiff, S (1992) Art as medicine: creating a therapy of the imagination. Shambhala, Boston.

McSherry, W (1996) Raising the spirit. *Nursing Times* **92**(3): 48–9.

Menzies-Lyth, I (1988) A case study in the functioning of social systems as a defence against anxiety. In: Containing anxiety in institutions: selected essays. Free Association Books, London.

Mezirow, J (1981) A critical theory of adult learning and education. *Adult Education* **32**(1): 3–24.

Miller, L (2002) Effective communication with older people. *Nursing Standard* **17**(9): 45–50, 53, 55.

Milne, AA (1926) Winnie-the-Pooh. Methuen, London.

Moon, J (2002) Reflection in learning and professional development: theory and practice. Routledge, London.

Moore, T (1992) Care of the soul. HarperCollins, New York.

Morgan, R and Johns, C (2005) The beast and the star: resolving contradictions within everyday practice. In: C Johns and D Freshwater (eds) Transforming nursing through reflective practice, 2nd edn. Blackwell Publishing, Oxford, pp114–28.

Morse, J (1991) Negotiating commitment and involvement in the nurse–patient relationship. *Journal of Advanced Nursing* **16**: 552–8.

Morse, J, Bottorff, J, Anderson, G, O'Brien, B and Solberg, S (1992) Beyond empathy: expanding expressions of caring. *Journal of Advanced Nursing* **17**: 809–21.

Morse, J and Dobernect, B (1995) Delineating the concept of hope. *Image* **27**: 277–85.

Moss, F (2001) Leadership and learning: building the environment for better, safer health care. *Quality in Health Care* **10**(suppl 2): 1–2.

Mott, V (2000) The development of professional expertise in the workplace. *New Directions for Adult and Continuing Education* **86**: 23–31.

Mullally, S (2001) The NHS Plan – an action guide for nurses, midwives and health visitors. Department of Health, London.

Mullins, L (1985) Management and organisational behaviour, 2nd edn. Pitman Publishing, London.

Munhall, P (1993) 'Unknowing': towards another pattern of knowing in nursing. *Nursing Outlook* **41**(3): 125–8.

Mycek, S (1999) Teetering on the edge of chaos. Trustee April: 10–13.

National Institute for Health and Clinical Excellence (NICE) (2004) Clinical guidelines. Caesarean section. National Institute for Health and Clinical Excellence, London.

National Institute for Health and Clinical Excellence (NICE) (2006) Routine postnatal care of women and their babies. National Institute for Health and Clinical Excellence, London.

National Health Service Management Executive (NHSME) (1993) A vision for the future. Department of Health, London.

Nehring, V and Geach, B (1973) Why they don't complain: patient's evaluation of their care. *Nursing Outlook* **21**(5): 317–21.

Newman, M (1994) Health as expanded consciousness. National League for Nursing, New York.

Nicklin, P (1987) Violence to the spirit. *Senior Nurse* **6**(5): 10–12.

Novelestsky-Rosenthal, H and Solomon, K (2001) Reflections on the use of Johns' model of structured reflection in nurse-practitioner education. *International Journal for Human Caring* **5**(2): 21–6.

Nursing and Midwifery Council (2002) Midwives rules and standards. Nursing and Midwifery Council, London.

Oakley, A (1984) The importance of being a nurse. *Nursing Times* **83**(50): 24–7.

Ochs, L (2001) This nurse suggests asking before you touch. *RN* **64**(4): 10.

O'Donohue, J (1997) Anam cara: spiritual wisdom from the Celtic world. Bantam Press, London.

Okri, B (1997) A way of being free. Phoenix House, London.

Ottaway, R (1978) A change strategy to implement new norms, new styles and new environment in the work organization. *Personnel Review* **5**(1): 13–18.

Paramananda (2001) A deeper beauty: Buddhist reflections on everyday life. Windhorse, Birmingham.

Parker, M (2002) Aesthetic ways in day-to-day nursing. In: D Freshwater (ed) Therapeutic nursing. Sage, London.

Parker, R (1990) Nurses' stories: the search for a relational ethic of care. *Advances in Nursing Science* **13**(1): 31–40.

Pearl, E (2001) The reconnection. Hay House, Carlsbad, CA.

Pearson, A (1983) The clinical nursing unit. Heinemann Medical Books, London.

Pease, A (1981) Body language. Sheldon Press, London.

Pennebaker, J (1989) Confession, inhibition and disease. *Advances in Experimental Social Psychology* **22**: 211–44.

Pennebaker, J, Colder, M and Sharp, L (1990) Accelerating the coping process. *Journal of Personality and Social Psychology* **58**: 528–37.

Pennebaker, J, Mayne, T and Francis, M (1997) Linguistic predictors of adaptive bereavement. *Journal of Personality and Social Psychology* **72**: 863–71.

Pike, A (1991) Moral outrage and moral discourse in nurse-physician collaboration. *Journal of Professional Nursing* **7**(6): 351–63.

Pinar, WF (1981) 'Whole, bright, deep with understanding': issues in qualitative research and autobiographical method. *Journal of Curriculum Studies* **13**(3): 173–88.

Pink, D (2005) A whole new mind: moving from information age to the conceptual age. Riverhead Books/Penguin, New York.

Pitkin, WB (1932) Life begins at forty. McGraw-Hill, New York.

Plager, K (1994) Hermeneutic phenomenology: a methodology for family health and health promotion study in nursing. In: P Benner P (ed) Interpretive phenomenology. Sage, Thousand Oaks.

Platzer, H, Blake, D and Ashford, D (2000) Barriers to learning from reflection; a study of the use of groupwork with post-registration nurses. *Journal of Advanced Nursing* **31**(5) 1001–8.

Podurgiel, M (1990) The unconscious experience: a pilot study. *Journal of Neuroscience Nursing* **22**(1): 52–3.

Polanyi, M (1958) Personal knowledge: towards a post critical philosophy. Routledge and Kegan Paul, London.

Polkingthorne, D (1996) Transformative narratives: from victimic to agentic life plots. *American Journal of Occupational Therapy* **50**(4): 299–305.

Powell, J (1989) The reflective practitioner in nursing. *Journal of Advanced Nursing* **14**: 824–32.

Power, S (1999) Nursing supervision: a guide for clinical practice.. Sage Publications, London.

Prigogine, L and Stengers, L (1984) Order out of chaos. Bantam, New York.

Puzan, E (2003) The unbearable whiteness of being (in nursing). *Nursing Inquiry* **10**(3): 193–200.

Quinn, J (1992) Holding scared space: the nurse as healing environment. *Holistic Nursing Practice* **6**(4): 26–35.

Quinn, J (1997) Healing: a model for an integrated health care system. *Advanced Practice Nursing Quarterly* **3**(1): 1–7.

Rael, J (1993) Being and vibration. Council Oak Books, Oklahoma.

Ramos, M (1992) The nurse–patient relationship: themes and variations. *Journal of Advanced Nursing* **17**: 496–506.

Rao, MT (1993) Coping with communication challenges in Alzheimer's disease. Singular Publishing, San Diego.

Rashid, C and Bentley, H (2001) Nurse prescribing and professional relationships. *Journal of Community Nursing* **15**(11): 14–20.

Rawnsley, M (1990) Of human bonding: the context of nursing as caring. *Advances in Nursing Science* **13**: 41–8.

Ray, M (1989) The theory of bureaucratic caring for nursing practice in the organizational culture. *Nursing Administrative Quarterly* **13**(2): 31–42.

Read, S (1983) Once is enough: causal reasoning from a single instance. *Journal of Personality and Social Psychology* **45**(2): 323–34.

Reiman, D (1986) Non-caring and caring in the clinical setting: patients' descriptions. *Topics in Clinical Nursing* **8**(2): 30–6.

Remen, R (1996) Kitchen table wisdom. Riverhead Books, New York.

Reissetter, K and Thomas, B (1986) Nursing care of the dying: its relationship to selected nurse characteristics. *International Journal of Nursing Studies* **23**: 39–50.

Reverby, S (1987) A caring dilemma: womanhood and nursing in historical perspective. *Nursing Research* **36**(1): 5–11.

Richardson, L (2000) Evaluating ethnography. *Qualitative Inquiry* **6**: 253–5.

Rinpoche, S (1992) The Tibetan book of living and dying. Rider, London.

Rippon, S (2001) Nurturing nurse leadership: how does your garden grow? *Nursing Management* **8**(7): 11–15.

Roach, S (1992) The human act of caring. Canadian Hospital Association Press, Ottawa.

Roberts, S (1983) Oppressed group behaviour: implications for nursing. *Advances in Nursing Science* **5.4**: 21–30.

Robinson, D and McKenna, H (1998) Loss: an analysis of a concept of particular interest to nursing. *Journal of Advanced Nursing* **27**(4): 779–84.

Rogers, A, Karlsen, S and Addington-Hall, J (2000) 'All the services were excellent. It is when the human element comes in that things go wrong': dissatisfaction with hospital care in the last year of life. *Journal of Advanced Nursing* **31**(40): 768–74.

Rogers, C (1969) Freedom to learn: a view of what education might be. Merrill, Columbus, OH.

Roper, N, Logan, W and Tierney, A (1980) The elements of nursing. Churchill Livingstone, Edinburgh.

Rosenberg, L (1998) Breath by breath. Shambhala, Boston.

Russell, F (1999) An exploratory study of patient perception, memories and experiences of an intensive care unit. *Journal of Advanced Nursing* **29**(4): 783–91.

Sacks, O (1976) Awakenings. Pelican Books, London.

Sangharakshita (1990) Vision and transformation. Windhorse, Birmingham.

Sangharakshita (1993) The drama of cosmic enlightenment. Windhorse, Birmingham.

Sangharakshita (1998) Know your mind. Windhorse, Birmingham

Scanlon, C and Weir, W (1997) Learning from practice? Mental health nurses' perceptions and experiences of clinical supervision. *Journal of Advanced Nursing* **26**: 295–303.

Schön, D (1983) The reflective practitioner. Avebury, Aldershot.

Schön, D (1987) Educating the reflective practitioner. Jossey-Bass, San Francisco.

Scott, C (2001) Communication is the key. *Professional Nurse* **16**(1): 810.

Schuster, J (1994) Transforming your leadership style. *Leadership* 39–43.

Seedhouse, D (1988) Ethics: the heart of health care. Wiley, Chichester.

Senge, P (1990) The fifth discipline. The art and practice of the learning organisation. Century Business, London.

Shaw, E, Levitt, C and Kaczorowski, J (2006) Systematic review of the literature on postpartum care: effectiveness of postpartum support to improve maternal parenting, mental health, quality of life, and physical health. *Birth* **33**(3): 210–20.

Sisson, R (1990) Effects of auditory stimuli on comatose patients with head injury. *Heart and Lung* **4**: 373–8.

Sloan, G and Watson, H (2001) John Heron's six-category intervention analysis: towards understanding interpersonal relations and progressing the delivery of clinical supervision for mental health nursing in the United Kingdom. *Journal of Advanced Nursing* **36**(2): 206–14.

Smith, G (2000) Friendship within clinical supervision: a model for the NHS? http://www.clinical-supervision.com.

Smith, M and Liehr, P (1999) Attentively embracing story: a middle range theory with practie and research implications. *Scholarly Inquiry for Nursing Practice* **13**(3): 3–27.

Smuts, JC (1927) Holism and evolution. Macmillan, London.

Smyth, J (1998) A rationale for teachers' critical pedagogy. Deakin University Press, Melbourne.

Smyth, J, Stone, A, Hurewitz, A and Kaell, A (1999) Effects of writing about stressful experiences on symptom reduction in patients with asthma or rheumatoid arthritis. *Journal of the American Medical Association* 281: 1304–9.

Smyth, WJ (1987) A rationale for teachers' critical pedagogy. Deakin University Press, Melbourne.

Spry, T (2001) Performing autoethnography: an embodied methodological praxis. *Qualitative Inquiry* 7: 706–32.

Squire, S (2001) Clinical governance in action. Pt 11: Encouraging a sense of ownership. *Professional Nurse* 16(9): 1332–3.

Stein, L (1978) The doctor–nurse game. In: R Dingwall and J McIntosh (eds) Readings in the sociology of nursing. Churchill Livingstone, Edinburgh, pp108–17.

Stewart, I and Joines, V (1987) TA today: a new introduction to transactional analysis. Russell Press, Nottingham.

Stockwell, F (1972) The unpopular patient. RCN, London.

Street, A (1992) Inside nursing: a critical ethnography of clinical nursing. State University of New York Press, Albany.

Street, A (1995) Nursing replay. Churchill Livingstone, Melbourne.

Summer, J (2001) Caring in nursing: a different interpretation. *Journal of Advanced Nursing* 35(60): 926–32.

Suzuki, S (1999) Zen mind, beginner's mind, revised edition. Weatherhill, New York.

Sutherland, L (1994) Caring as mutual epowerment: working with the BNDU model at Burford. In: C Johns (ed) The Burford NDU model: caring in practice. Blackwell Science, Oxford.

Talton, C (1995) Complementary therapies: touch-of-all-kinds is therapeutic. *RN* 58(2): 61–4.

Taylor, B (1992) From helper to human: a reconceptualisation of the nurse as a person. *Journal of Advanced Nursing* 17: 1042–9.

Taylor, D and Singer, E (1983) New organisation from old. IPM Management Publications, London.

Thomas, K and Kilmann, R (1974) Thomas Kilmann conflict mode instrument. Xicom, Toledo.

Timpson, J (1996) Towards an understanding of the human resource in the context of change in the NHS: economic sense versus cultural sensibilities? *Journal of Nursing Management* 4: 315–24.

Torbert, WR (1978) Educating toward shared purpose, self direction and quality work. The theory and practice of liberating structure. *Journal of Higher Education* 49(2): 109–35.

Tosch, P (1988) Patients' recollections of their post-traumatic coma. *Journal of Neuroscience Nursing* 20(4): 223–8.

Trihn, M (1991) When the moon waxes red: representation, gender and cultural politics. Routledge, New York.

Trnobanski, P (1994) Nurse–patient dialogue: assumption or reality? *Journal of Advanced Nursing* 19: 733–7.

Tschudin, V (1993) Ethics in nursing, 2nd edn. Butterworth Heinemann, Oxford.

Tuffnell, M and Crickmay, C (2004) A widening field. Dance Books, Alton.

Turton, P (1989) Touch me, feel me, heal me. *Nursing Times* 85(19): 42–4.

Tversky, A and Kahneman, D (1974) Judgement under uncertainty: heuristics and biases. *Science* 185: 1124–31.

Tyler, J (1998) Nonverbal communication and the use of art in the care of the dying. *Palliative Medicine* 12: 123–6.

Tzu, Lao (1999) Tao Te Ching (trans. S Mitchell). Frances Lincoln, London.

UKCC (1987) Advisory paper: confidentiality – an elaboration of clause 9. UKCC, London.

Vachon, M (1988) Battle fatigue in hospice/palliative care. In: A Gilmore and S Gilmore (eds) A safer death. Plenum Publishing, New York.

Vaught-Alexander, K (1994) The personal journal for nurses: writing for delivery and healing. In: D Gaut and Boykin A (eds) Caring as healing: renewal through hope. National League for Nursing, New York.

Van Manen, M (1990) Researching lived experience. State University of New York Press, New York.

Visinstainer, M (1986) The nature of knowledge and theory in nursing. *Image: The Journal of Nursing Scholarship* 18: 32–8.

Wade, S (1999) Promoting quality of care for older people: developing positive attitudes to working with older people. *Journal of Nursing Management* 7: 339–47.

Wagner, L (1999) Within the circle of death: transpersonal poetic reflections on nurses' stories about the quality of the dying process. *International Journal for Human Caring* 3(2): 21–30.

Wainwright, P (2000) Towards an aesthetics of nursing. *Journal of Advanced Nursing* 32(3): 750–5.

Wall, TD, Bolden, RI and Borril, CS (1997) Minor psychiatric disturbance in NHS trust staff. *British Journal of Psychiatry* 171: 519–23.

Walsh, D (2006) The ontology of childbirth. *British Journal of Midwifery* 14(11): 662.

Ward, K (1988) Not just the patient in bed three. *Nursing Times* 84(78): 39–50.

Waterworth, D (1995) Exploring the value of clinical nursing practice: the practitioner's perspective. *Journal of Advanced Nursing* 22: 13–17.

Waterworth, S and Luker, K (1990) Reluctant collaborators: do patients want to be involved in decisions involving care? *Journal of Advanced Nursing* 15: 971–6.

Watson, J (1988) Nursing: human science and human care. A theory of nursing. National League for Nursing, New York.

Watson, J (1990) The moral failure of the hierarchy. *Nursing Outlook* 38(2): 62–6.

Wheatley, MJ (1999) Leadership and the new science. Discovering order in a chaotic world. Berrett-Koehler, San Frascisco

Wheatley, M and Kellner-Rogers, M (1999) A simpler way. Berrett-Koehler, San Francisco.

White, A (1993) The nursing process: a constraint on expert practice. *Journal of Nursing Management* 1: 245–52.

White, J (1995) Patterns of knowing: review, critique and update. *Advanced Nursing Science* 17(4): 73–86.

Whittemore, R (1999) Natural science and nursing science: where do the horizons fuse? *Journal of Advanced Nursing* 30(5): 1027–33.

Wilber, K (1998) The eye of spirit: an integral vision for a world gone slightly mad. Shambhala, Boston.

Wilkinson, J (1988) Moral distress in nursing practice: experience and effect. *Nursing Forum* 23(1): 16–29.

Winterson, J (2001) The powerbook. Vintage, London.

Woodward, V and Webb, C (2001) Women's anxieties surrounding breast disorders: a systematic review of the literature. *Journal of Advanced Nursing* 33(1): 29–41.

Woolf, V (1945) A room of one's own. Penguin Books, London.

Worwood, V (1999) The fragrant heavens. Doubleday, London.

Wray, J (2006) Postnatal care: is it based on ritual or a purpose? A reflective account. *British Journal of Midwifery* 14(9): 520–6.

Wuest, J (1997) Illuminating environmental influences on women's caring. *Journal of Advanced Nursing* 26(1): 49–58.

Young, M and Cullen, L (1996) A good death. Routledge, London.

Younger, J (1995) The alienation of the sufferer. *Advances in Nursing Science* 17(4): 53–72.

Index

Page numbers in **bold** represent tables, those in *italics* represent figures.